Leadership, management, and role delineation

ISSUES FOR THE DENTAL TEAM

Leadership, management, and role delineation
ISSUES FOR THE DENTAL TEAM

Irene R. Woodall, R.D.H., M.A.

Assistant Professor and Chairperson, Department of Dental
Hygiene, Assistant Professor, Department of Dental Care Systems,
School of Dental Medicine, University of Pennsylvania,
Philadelphia, Pennsylvania

with 41 illustrations

The C. V. Mosby Company

Saint Louis   1977

Printed in the United States of America

Distributed in Great Britain by Henry Kimpton, London

The C. V. Mosby Company
11830 Westline Industrial Drive, St. Louis, Missouri 63141

Library of Congress Cataloging in Publication Data

Woodall, Irene R   1946-
    Leadership, management, and role delineation.

    Bibliography: p.
    Includes index.
    1. Dentistry—Practice.   2.   Dental auxiliary
personnel.   3.   Dental care—United States.   4.   Dental
laws and legislation—United States.   5.   Dental ethics.
I.   Title.   [DNLN: 1.   Dental care.   2.   Patient care
team.   3.   Practice management, Dental.   WU77 W881L]
RK58.W67   617.6′023   77-8533
ISBN 0-8016-5621-4

GW/CB/CB   9 8 7 6 5 4 3 2 1

To
Conrad Woodall and our children,
Charlotte Claire and **Amanda Marie,**
for the light in their eyes,
the love in their hearts,
and the joy and peace they bring me

FOREWORD

In this volume, Irene Woodall has defined subjects that are cogent to the oral health care provider of today, whether dentist or auxiliary. While these topics unfortunately are often overlooked in the curriculum of many centers of dental education, they may have greater impact on the future of our profession than the development of technology and may result in improved skills for dental care delivery. The need for this text is a reflection of the deficiencies in the average, present-day dental curriculum, since the behavior of most providers is directly correlated to their educational experience.

Ms. Woodall has demonstrated her expertise as an educator and planner in assembling the information in this volume. Her style of communication is direct and lucid. It is hoped that the many members of the oral health professions will review this material carefully and objectively. If dental educators and health planners utilize the subjects in this book, they should have an important basis for discussion within the profession, as well as between those responsible for the oral health of the population.

I would like to compliment the author on her ability to compile and synthesize material from the literature and to present it in a manner that is easy for the reader to comprehend.

D. Walter Cohen, D.D.S.

Dean,
Professor of Periodontics,
School of Dental Medicine,
University of Pennsylvania,
Philadelphia, Pennsylvania

PREFACE

This book was written for students and for practitioners who wish to become involved in the changes that are confronting the health care professions. While it focuses primarily on the problems unique to the delivery of dental care, it contains many elements that are common to all providers of care, regardless of their field of practice.

The book can serve as a resource for learning facts and in sharing opinions that have been voiced regarding the changes that confront the professions. But more than that, it provides a forum for discussion. The chapters provide an opportunity to assimilate the primary issues so that students, study club members, organizational leaders, and informal groups of health care providers have a basis for informed debate. The group activities are suggested as a means for guiding the "forum" of individuals who wish to better formulate their own ideas regarding change and who wish to have a better understanding of the perceptions that others have developed. The primary goal is to stimulate thinking and to facilitate decision making and problem solving so that health professionals may take positive measures to shape the future in the best interests of the public who seek their care.

The way in which this book is used in stimulating thought and interest will, of course, vary with the group using it. One approach that may prove successful is to have the members of the group independently read one or more chapters, assess their knowledge using the study questions at the end of each chapter, and then gather in groups of five to twenty people to implement one or more of the suggested group activities. This procedure may enhance the effectiveness with which the stated objectives for each chapter may be learned. The first chapter provides a group activity for the first group session, setting the stage for the issues of the remainder of the text and introducing the group participants to the style of group activity that is best suited to the development of awareness of complex issues and multifaceted solutions.

Irene R. Woodall

Acknowledgements

A special acknowledgement and thank you are due to my husband, Conrad, and to Lotte and Mandy, for their continuing support during the preparation of the manuscript. I wish to acknowledge Conrad's editorial assistance and his indexing skills in the manuscript preparation.

I gratefully acknowledge the editorial assistance of, and content review by, Dr. Charles Jerge and Dr. Patricia P. Cormier, Department of Dental Care Systems; Dr. Arnold Rosoff, Leonard Davis Institute for Health Economics; and Ms. Sally Verity, Visiting Professor, Department of Dental Hygiene, University of Pennsylvania.

A special thank you is extended to Dr. Patricia Cormier of Dental Auxiliary Programs, Ms. Emily Mintz, administrative assistant, and the entire dental hygiene faculty who made it possible for me to complete the manuscript despite the demands of my new position and my continuing teaching responsibilities: Debbie Arnett, Bonnie Dafoe, Karen Flickinger, Debbie Frazier, Jane Griffin, Carol Holland, Susan Joyner, Joyce Levy, Pamela Morgan, Penny Miller, Marsha Morrow, Nancy Stutsman, Roberta Throne, Rosemarie Valentine, and Leslie Weed. A special acknowledgement is due, also, to the students who were patient with my limited visibility and who trusted my desire to serve them well as an administrator, a teacher, and a mentor.

I also wish to acknowledge the photographic assistance of Dr. Daniel Boston, Joyce Levy, and Donnis Newman and the graphics preparation provided by Elizabeth Hiser.

CONTENTS

PART I

ROLE DELINEATION FOR DENTAL HEALTH CARE PROVIDERS

Dental auxiliary means different things to different people. A definition should be preceded by a careful analysis of the issues and trends that have brought about the development and utilization of the "auxiliaries" in dental care delivery. In addition, current trends require consideration.

This text identifies those issues and trends and explains how dental health care providers have influenced and been influenced by each. It offers suggestions for seeking employment and developing a practice mode most compatible with the "real world" of the provision of care and with the "high ideals" of a patient-centered health care delivery system. As a result, the reader should be in a position to define for him/herself the concept of dental auxiliary in terms of its origin, its development, and its direction for the future.

However, for many persons who qualify as auxiliaries, the very term is unacceptable. Those persons believe that its connotation of "extra help" is inappropriate for educated and credentialed persons who provide direct patient care. Some believe that each kind of dental care provider should be referred to by the more specific occupational title of dental hygienist, dental assistant, or expanded function (duty) dental auxiliary (EFDA or EDDA). A small contingent believe such health care providers should be called allied health professionals in dentistry, paralleling the terminology of medicine where terms such as auxiliary and ancillary personnel were discarded many years ago.

Many persons who support the specific titling of each kind of dental care provider hope that, with the titles, roles will remain distinct and well defined. Generally, those who support the collective titles, "auxiliaries" or "allied health professions," view a merger of resources and roles as desirable, particularly when defining how health care delivery settings should be staffed. For them, the skills, knowledge, and experience each person possesses should define the role each person has in patterns of delivering care. The traditional role delineation is theoretically based on clearly defined parameters of practice. The collective titles reflect recent blurring of those parameters. Overlap is increasing and it complicates the process of credentialing the various dental health care providers and of assigning functional practice roles in health care delivery.

The fact is that the "auxiliaries" are changing before their definitions. They are defining themselves as they adopt new patterns of practice and as the educational programs and legal constraints on practice change.

1

In order to address the challenges that face those persons who are actively defining themselves, some common term needs to be adopted, one that avoids the stigmas of the traditional roles and one that points toward responsibility and self-concept development. For this reason, the term *dental health care provider* is used often in this text. Where there is a specific need to differentiate dentists from non-dentists, the term auxiliary or one of the more specific occupational titles is used.

Regardless of the terms used to describe those persons who provide direct care, it is important to develop an awareness of the patterns of change. The first portion of the text provides the reader with the basic information and appropriate group activities to accomplish this.

Building on this initial portion, the text will provide the reader with the tools to enter the continuing debate in the professional forum and to develop a keener appreciation of the forces in the movement toward a more workable health care delivery system in this country.

CHAPTER 1

Values clarification for the dental health care provider

OBJECTIVES: The reader will be able to:

1. List personal experiences that have helped shape his/her perceptions of dental health care providers while viewing the profession.
   a. As a patient.
   b. As a beginning student.
   c. As a clinician (either in school or in practice).
2. Discuss how technological change and rapidly changing life styles may impact the "security" of a well-defined occupational role in the years ahead.
3. Participate in a values clarification process by:
   a. Identifying at least six descriptive statements regarding dental health care providers with which he/she agrees.
   b. Forming a partnership (dyad) with another person whose six descriptive statements are compatible.
   c. Forming a group of four with another dyad, whose collective descriptive statements are compatible with the partnership's.
   d. Describing why each statement is agreed upon and ranking the group of statements according to their "importance."
   e. Sharing the choices and ranking with other groups.
4. Participate in active listening.
5. Identify how others' perceptions of dental health care providers differ from his/her own and explain why the others have chosen different points of view or beliefs.
6. Begin to debate the issues related to the role delineation and function of dental health care providers.

Most persons enter a career as a result of the perceptions they have acquired regarding its attractiveness. Men and women entering health professions may base their decision on how they perceived the profession while seeking care as patients. Or they may have been influenced by family members who are in the profession. The attractiveness may be defined in terms of self-esteem, financial reward, service to people, job security, independence, scope of responsibility, or pleasantness of the working environment.

Those perceptions are altered or reaffirmed as the persons enters educational preparation for the role and once again after having entered practice.

Depending on what an individual's total experiences are in relationship to the health career, the person develops a perception of the career. People's perceptions therefore differ as greatly as their personal experiences. For a person in a health profession to acquire a better understanding of what the career "really" is, there must be a sharing of perceptions among its members and with persons who stand outside the profession.

This may occur by accident as a health

care provider overhears a conversation in which his/her career is being discussed. He/she may hear a rather inaccurate description of the activities or responsibilities that such a provider of care is supposed to perform or hear him/herself being cast into a stereotype. The humorous, albeit less than complimentary, ways in which the dental profession is often portrayed in films and on television programs are a hint of what the consumer may think about dental health care providers. An awakening may come from a conversation with another dental health care provider who has quite a different perception of the role of the profession. Each new experience as a patient, as a student, and as a practitioner will either alter or reaffirm certain aspects of a professional's view of his/her career.

For purposes of focusing on the variations in people's perceptions, a planned group activity, referred to as values clarification, can point out clearly where the differences lie as well as provide insight into why certain people hold the views they identify as their own. Different solo or group methods can be used in values clarification. One method involves simply noting various incidents or encounters that prompted the participant to develop his/her perceptions of the profession. Incidents in early childhood, during primary and high school years, and during professional preparation should be written down and then shared with a group of three people who are also participating in the exercise. The perceptions and their reasons should be clearly stated for the group. Each member of the group then feeds back one facet of what he/she heard each speaker saying, in order to facilitate active listening. As each person in the group has a turn in describing personal perceptions of the profession and then hears them reflected by the other group members, the person's values and beliefs should become clearer and more available for discussion and analysis. As the same person hears others' perceptions and others' feedback regarding those perceptions and then hears him/her-

self reflect some facet of the description and the reasoning, the participant becomes more aware of the unity of belief on some issues and the disparity between certain views with regard to others.

A second, more structured, approach to values clarification involves a sorting of values statements that are prepared for the participants in advance and that reflect the broad spectrum of beliefs and values about the profession.* Each participant is given six cards on which values statements are written (one statement per 3 × 5 card). Participants move around the room, trading cards with other participants until each person is satisfied with the six cards he/she holds. "Satisfaction" is described as holding cards that are acceptable as an expression of that person's beliefs or values. In other words, the person generally agrees with the statements on the six cards. There are no "right" or "wrong" cards. No one should have prejudged the appropriateness or "truth" of any of the cards. Each card should be considered neutral in terms of any external evaluation. The cards should be evaluated only in terms of the person's own particular beliefs.

When each person has six cards with which he/she feels reasonably comfortable, each participant should begin to form a partnership with one other person whose cards also seem to be reasonable reflections of his/her own values. The dyad (twosome) may discard two or three cards upon which they do not agree in order to form the partnership. The dyad should have between nine and twelve cards upon which they both agree.

The dyad then sets out to form a foursome. A total of four more cards may be discarded if the formation of the foursome is blocked by them. A settled foursome should therefore have at least twenty cards and a maximum of twenty-four cards. Forming a group of four people may not be possible for

---

*This exercise was first described by the National Training Laboratory. It has been adapted for use in this context by the author.

all participants, in which case dyads may wish to remain unattached.

Once the foursomes are settled, each group should identify the four most important and four least important statements included in their values cards. The group should rank the four least important and then rank the four most important.

Depending on the size of the entire group of participants, the foursomes may need to write out their choices on sheets of newsprint with a felt-tip marker. This may assist the sharing process that follows, when each foursome or dyad explains its top and bottom four choices and the reasons why they were ranked as they were. Each person in the foursome should explain two of the eight choices.

During the discussion, noticeable similarities and disparities among the various groups will appear. On some points there may be general agreement in the entire group of participants, while on other points polar opposites may be apparent between two or more groups.

What is important to achieve is a thorough discussion of why people believe or value certain points. At the close of the session, each participant should be able to state the basis for six of his/her own personal convictions regarding dental health care providers and be able to state and explain the basis for six beliefs others have, with which the person does not necessarily agree.

It is helpful to include faculty members and dental care providers currently in practice as long as these persons do not dominate the group discussions or become too influential in the decisions the students make about the values. If this exercise is conducted in a professional association as a beginning session of a study club, it may be helpful to invite several student members or consumers to participate. The shades of valuing should expand with the variety of persons involved in the process.

The entire process should take approximately 1½ hours, with 20 minutes allocated for initial trading of cards, 15 minutes for forming dyads, and 20 minutes for forming foursomes and ranking statements. Thirty minutes or more should be allowed for discussion.

The discussion can easily grow into a debate. In most instances it may be wise for the group facilitator to help participants focus on the open expression and sharing of beliefs, values, and the reasons people hold them rather than allowing the group to begin condemning some and supporting others. This exercise should prepare people to be more interested in the differences and in the sources of their own beliefs, so that subsequent group activities can be opportunities for a more in-depth analysis of the issues that arose.

GROUP ACTIVITY

1. Conduct a values clarification session in which foursomes identify the sources of their perceptions of their profession and explain the beliefs they hold and why. Other members in the foursome feed back what they heard the person say. Each person participates in both the sharing and the reflective feedback exercise.

2. Conduct a values clarification session using card sorting as described in the text. Below are listed samples of "values statements" that may be transferred to 3 × 5 cards for distribution and the sorting process. Multiplying the number of participants by six will provide the correct number of cards that must be prepared. The group facilitator may add more if necessary, or duplicates of especially controversial ones may be prepared for circulation if the total number needed exceeds 240.

Dental hygiene is an ideal profession for a person who plans a lifetime career.

Auxiliaries should unionize in order to improve working conditions and benefits.

There are too many dental hygienists in certain parts of the country.

Dental hygiene and dental assisting are best suited to females.

Unionization would deprofessionalize auxiliary practice.

Dentists have no reason to unionize.

Assistants stay in practice longer than hygienists.

Despite all the controversy about expanded functions, dental hygienists spend most of their time performing prophylaxes.

Hygienists who receive a commission tend to be more dollar-oriented.

Hygienists should work under the direct supervision of a dentist.

Dental hygienists in community programs should be free to provide clinical services without a dentist physically present.

Dental hygienists should be free to practice independently if they wish, making appropriate referrals to dentists.

A dental hygienist needs a chairside assistant to function most efficiently and economically.

An expanded function dental auxiliary is another term for a traditional hygienist with added skills and knowledge.

Hygienists should always remember that their primary role is to prevent disease.

The white uniform is an important symbol of dental auxiliaries that should be retained.

A dental auxiliary must have and maintain good oral health.

The most important aspects of a dental hygienist's expertise are clinical (instrumentation) skills.

The most important aspects of a dental hygienist's expertise are problem solving and decision making skills

The most important aspect of a dental auxiliary's expertise is the ability to communicate effectively with patients.

A dental auxiliary is a decision maker.

A dental auxiliary implements the dentist's decisions.

A dental hygienist should wear a white uniform and cap.

A dental auxiliary should participate in continuing education.

Dental auxiliary practice should be regulated by dentists.

Dental hygiene should be regulated by dental hygienists.

Many hygienists do not stay in practice very long because they are unchallenged.

Hygienists remain in practice a long time because of their commitment to oral health.

Auxiliaries remain in practice a long time because of their excellent working conditions.

Auxiliaries have excellent opportunity for personal growth and career advancement.

Auxiliaries leave practice because of the lack of opportunity for personal growth and career advancement.

Dental hygienists are a basically happy, fulfilled group.

Dental hygienists seem rigid in their ways.

Dental hygienists are as eager to change themselves as their patients.

Dental hygienists like things carefully defined and uniform.

Dental hygienists are suspicious of change that affects them.

Hygienists should be willing to change their name and their self-image in order to meet a changed need in dental health care delivery.

Dental hygiene is a therapeutically oriented profession.

Dental hygiene has a strong tradition that should be maintained.

A good dental hygienist will work him/herself out of a "job."

Decision-making and working for a dentist are incompatible roles for a dental auxiliary.

A dental hygienist has the skill to diagnose caries.

A dental hygienist performing gingival recontouring cannot be expected to do as well as a dentist.

A dentist and a dental auxiliary, who have been given equivalent education to perform a given skill, should be able to do equally well.

Patients see the dental hygienist as the "person who cleans my teeth."

Dental hygienists soon drop patient education from their scope of practice after graduation.

Dental auxiliary programs emphasize total patient care more than mastering individual skills.

Dental auxiliary programs emphasize clinical expertise that is not needed in practice.

Dental hygienists are full members of the dental team.

Dental assistants are full members of the dental team.

A dental practice that does not have a hygienist is missing an important team member.

A dental hygienist can and should be able to supervise other auxiliaries in a practice setting.

The best feature about dental assisting is its prestige.

The best feature about dental assisting is its flexibility.

The best feature about dental assisting is the pay.

The best feature about dental hygiene is the pay.

A dental hygienist is not really a full member of the dental team.

Current dental practice does not permit a dental hygienist to perform all the services learned in school.

Dental hygiene is a relatively static profession.

The dental hygiene organization (ADHA) provides little leadership for the profession to change.

The dental hygiene organization (ADHA) is a primary source of leadership for changes in the profession.

Dental hygiene should expand its scope of responsibility in practice.

Dental hygiene should stay as it is.

Dental auxiliaries tend to be introverts.

Dental auxiliaries tend to be extroverts.

Dental hygienists should be women.

Dentists tend to be introverts.

Dentists tend to be extroverts.

When I think "dentist," I think "man."

When I think "dental auxiliary," I think "woman."

When I think "dental auxiliary," I think "girl."

Male dental auxiliaries cannot provide the same caring service that women can.

Male dental auxiliaries can be just as competent as their female counterparts.

Dentists view auxiliaries as subservient.

The idea of a dental hygienist practicing without a dentist on the premises is frightening or at least makes me uncomfortable.

An auxiliary usually is hired largely on the basis of appearance.

Dental hygienists should be the group to examine candidates for dental hygiene licensure.

Dental hygiene is a widely recognized health profession.

Dental hygiene is more of a vocation than a profession.

Hygienists should maintain their status above dental assisting.

The oral prophylaxis is the most important function of the dental hygienist.

Patient education is the most important function of the dental auxiliary.

Patients fully appreciate the knowledge and skill of dental auxiliaries.

Patients prefer to receive care from dentists rather than from auxiliaries.

Auxiliaries are legally responsible for the quality of care they provide.

Hygienists are fully capable of assuming responsibility for the quality of care they provide.

Dental auxiliaries are not fully appreciated by most dentists.

Dentists are not fully appreciated by most dental auxiliaries.

Auxiliaries are receptive to suggestions for change and improvement.

Hygienists are prima donnas.

The best aspect of dental hygiene is its economic stability.

The best part of clinical practice of dental hygiene is the sense of completion when a prophylaxis is finished.

Hygienists really are more technically oriented than people-oriented, despite their protests to the contrary.

It is easy to get into a rut when practicing dental hygiene.

The clinical skills of a dental hygienist are not very sophisticated.

Dental assisting is a high status profession.

Men will not become dental assistants because *they* need more money to support a family. Women do not need as much money as men.

A dental auxiliary needs a full complement of basic sciences in order to be competent clinically.

Dental hygiene is an excellent profession for a women until she gets married but is quite unrewarding as a lifetime career.

Dental hygiene and assisting change slowly because practitioners are so isolated in various practice settings.

Dental hygiene and assisting change slowly because practitioners are reluctant to change traditions.

Dental hygiene and assisting change slowly because they are regulated by dentists.

Dental hygienists and dental assistants should ally themselves if the dental team is to function more effectively.

Dental hygienists and other auxiliaries should remain relatively independent of each other if they are to maintain their role in the dental team.

There will always be a dental auxiliary known as the "dental hygienist."

If dental hygiene or assisting loses its prestige, I will leave it.

If dental auxiliaries become more unified, I will leave dental hygiene.

If dental auxiliaries become more assertive, dentistry will crush them.

If the preventive orientation of dental hygiene is lessened, the profession will be lost.

Future research discoveries in the control of dental disease will put hygienists out of business.

Dentistry will always be a viable profession.

Dental hygiene will always be a viable profession.

Dental assisting will always be a viable profession if it changes with the health needs of the public.

Pantsuit uniforms are unprofessional attire for female auxiliaries.

Colored uniforms are unprofessional attire for auxiliaries.

Dental auxiliaries learn cooperation skills rather than competitiveness in dental auxiliary programs.

Dental auxiliaries learn competiveness rather than cooperation skills in school.

Auxiliaries need to have most intraoral procedures evaluated by a dentist.

Assistants for the most part are pleased with the relationships they have with their employers.

Most dental hygienists function to the maximum in terms of their ability to accept responsibility and perform complete clinical services.

Dental hygiene functions could fairly easily be expanded to be important components of most dental specialties.

A dental auxiliary is limited to general practice settings because of limited education and skill.

Most hygienists could not function adequately in a periodontics practice without additional training by a periodontist.

An orthodontics practice could find little use for a dental hygienist.

I would be reluctant to learn new clinical procedures through continuing education.

I would like to stay in one employment situation for as long as I can—even for a lifetime.

The adventure of change would make me want to change employment situations at least every 5 years.

A raise in salary is the primary reason I would want to change employment situations.

Hygienists are not able to assess the level of quality of dental care provided by a dentist.

There are areas of responsibility where the dental team leader should be the dental auxiliary.

The leader of the dental team is the dentist.

As long as there are many people with dental diseases, dental hygienists are needed.

There are not too many hygienists in some parts of the country; there are only too few mechanisms for people to receive the care hygienists could provide.

I would feel most comfortable practicing in an upper middle class dental practice.

Dental auxiliaries should not be expected to learn to provide emergency care requiring administration of drugs.

The dental auxiliary's main goal is to provide service to dentistry.

The auxiliary's main goal is to provide service to patients.

The traditionally subservient role of women has accounted for many of dental auxiliaries' problems in relationship to dentistry.

If dental auxiliaries want more responsibility, they should go back to dental school and learn to be dentists.

The practice of dental hygienists is in most instances intellectually and emotionally rewarding.

The practice of dental assisting is in most instances intellectually and emotionally rewarding.

The dental patient is a member of the dental team.

The dental patient in most instances does not care to be very much involved in treatment planning.

The only reason most hygienists didn't become dentists is because they didn't want the additional responsibility.

Male dental hygienists are more assertive than female hygienists.

Auxiliaries need the security of a daily routine.

Auxiliaries are not paid well enough for what they do.

Direct patient care auxiliaries should be free to work on salary or commision.

Working on commission does not necessarily lead to lower clinical standards.

A hygienist's attire really is unrelated to his/her professionalism.

Dental hygienists need to change their image to be more closely associated with the concept of total patient care.

Dental hygiene should remain primarily interested in education of patients in preventing dental disease.

Dental auxiliaries have always been oriented toward both therapy and prevention.

Some dental auxiliaries should be legally able to practice with no direct dental supervision.

Dental hygienists should be able to practice in school settings, providing a full range of preventive and therapeutic services.

Dental hygienists should be able to practice in hospital and nursing home settings, providing a full range of preventive and therapeutic services.

Dental hygienists should be able to practice in county and state health department programs providing a full range of preventive and therapeutic services.

Dental hygiene's variety lies in the wide range of skills its members can provide for patients.

Dental hygiene's variety lies in the wide range of practice settings from which its members may select.

Dental hygiene's variety lies in the number of patients for whom one of its members provides regular care.

Dental assistants are generally overworked.

Dental hygienists earn unreasonably large amounts of money compared to what their level of expertise is.

Dental assistants generally earn reasonable salaries in return for their expertise and effort.

Dental auxiliaries generally have low salaries.

Auxiliaries should have a complete understanding of the costs of operating a health care delivery setting.

Dentists are overpaid for what they do.

Dental assistants are underpaid for what they can do.

Auxiliaries receive salary increases regularly in most private practice settings.

Fringe benefits for dental auxiliaries are excellent.

Auxiliaries generally have a "ceiling" on their salaries that rarely is raised despite length of service or quality of performance.

Most dental auxiliaries are content with their financial rewards.

Dental hygienists' skills can be learned through on-the-job training.

Dental hygienists' skills require formal education.

Dental auxiliaries should be licensed by the state in order to practice.

Dental auxiliaries should be certified by their professional association in order to practice.

Dental auxiliaries need no legal regulation (licensure or certification) in order to practice.

Dental hygienists should be required to have continuing education each year in order to retain licensure for practice.

Dental hygienists do not need mandatory continuing education in order to retain licensure, since voluntary systems work as well.

Dental auxiliaries in most cases are members of their professional organization.

Dental auxiliaries should be members of their professional organization.

There is little reason why dental auxiliaries should join their professional organization.

Junior membership while in dental hygiene school usually results in the person joining ADHA after graduation.

Junior membership meetings and projects are good preparation for local membership responsibilities in ADHA.

Junior membership meetings and projects are poor preparation for ultimate professional membership responsibilities.

Dental assisting skills can be learned through on-the-job training.

Dental assisting skills require formal education.

Local component activities of professional associations should be mostly social.

Local component activities of professional associations should be mostly scientific/educational sessions.

Local component activities of professional associations should be mostly political/business sessions concerned with the role of the profession.

Local component activities are worth attending.

Local component activities are not worth attending.

A large percentage of dental hygienists are inadequate clinicians.

People change their prevention routines for the better as a result of the efforts of dental hygienists.

Dental auxiliary practice should attract persons of all age groups into its ranks.

Dental auxiliary practice should primarily attract people into its rank in the age range of 18 to 22 years.

Graduates of 2-year auxiliary programs have only a skeleton education for clinical practice.

Graduates of 2-year programs are not prepared to practice in sites other than private practice.

Graduates of 2-year programs are not as clinically competent as graduates of 4-year programs.

Graduates of 4-year dental hygiene programs in most instances are better able to make decisions regarding patient care.

Graduates of 4-year dental hygiene programs in most instances have higher status in the eyes of employers.

Graduates of 2-year programs are clinically competent for most community clinical practice settings as well as for private practice in dental hygiene

For most dental hygiene functions, 2-year graduates are as well prepared as 4-year graduates.

The source of professional leadership lies mostly with 4-year and master's degree graduates.

The source of professional leadership lies with 2-year and 4-year graduates.

The main source of leadership for the dental assisting profession lies in dentistry.

Dental assisting should rely on dentistry for its leadership.

Dental auxiliaries should ally themselves with other health professions for strength.

Dental auxiliares should ally themselves with other health professions in order to capitalize on scientific/educational events and sessions of mutual interest.

Dental auxiliaries should ally themselves with other health professions in order to create a health care delivery team that extends beyond dentistry.

Dental hygiene has much in common with nursing.

Dental hygiene is a unique health profession with little in common with other health providers.

Dental hygiene and traditional dental assisting have little in common.

Dental hygiene and traditional dental assisting have much in common.

Dental hygienists and expanded function dental assistants have little in common.

Expanded function assistants and dental hygienists have a great deal in common.

Expanded function dental auxiliaries should not perform the oral prophylaxis.

Expanded function dental auxiliaries should not perform patient education procedures.

Expanded function dental auxiliaries are not dental hygienists.

Dental hygienists are not expanded function dental auxiliaries.

Dental assistants can easily learn clinical skills currently delegated only to dental hygienists.

Dentistry has tried to unify dental auxiliaries.

Dentistry has responded favorably to auxiliaries' efforts to modify their own future roles.

The fact that auxiliaries are almost exclusively women and dentists are almost exclusively men has little effect upon the roles each have in decision-making for the dental team.

Expanded function dental auxiliaries should have formal education.

Expanded function dental auxiliaries should be licensed.

Dentists are not interested in hiring auxiliaries over 40 years of age.

Age is of little importance to most dentists when hiring auxiliaries.

Dentists would probably prefer to hire women as employees.

The best feature of dentistry is its prestige.

The best feature of dentistry is its flexibility.

The best feature of dentistry is its pay.

The best feature of dentistry is its independence.

The dental assisting organization (ADAA) provides little leadership for the profession to change.

The dental assisting organization (ADAA) provides a primary source of leadership for changes in the profession.

Dentistry is a rewarding lifetime career.

Dental assisting is a rewarding lifetime career.

The term *auxiliary* is an appropriate title for an assistant or hygienist who provides direct patient care.

Allied health professionals in dentistry is a better term than *auxiliary* in describing dental care providers who are not dentists.

The rewards of a lifetime career in auxiliary practice are mostly related to service to people.

Dentists choose their career primarily because it affords them independence.

CHAPTER 2

Origins of direct patient care auxiliaries

OBJECTIVES: The reader will be able to:

1. Briefly summarize the development of the profession of dental hygiene
   (as the first direct patient care dental auxiliary), including
   a. The founder of the profession.
   b. The first dental hygienist of record.
   c. The date the practice of dental hygiene was first defined.
   d. The first continuing dental hygiene education program.
   e. The function the educated dental hygienist was intended to serve in the
      provision of dental services.
2. Compare the purpose and function of the dental hygienist in the United States
   with the other operating dental auxiliaries that have been established as health
   care providers in other countries, including
   a. Dental hygienists other than in the United States.
   b. The New Zealand School Dental Nurse.
   c. The New Cross Dental Auxiliary.
   d. The Canadian dental nurse.
3. Contrast the effects of the care delivered by the traditional dental hygienist
   with those of the care delivered by operating auxiliaries whose scope of practice
   includes restorative functions.
4. List three probable reasons for the disparity between the overall population levels
   of dental health attained in New Zealand and in the United States.
5. Summarize briefly the move to extend additional functions to dental auxiliaries
   (United States), including
   a. Identification of the major experiments and demonstration projects that focused
      on expanded function dental assistants.
   b. An explanation of dentistry's focus on dental assistants rather than on dental
      hygienists as auxiliaries to whom additional duties should be delegated.
   c. Primary experiments in the expansion of functions for dental hygienists.
   d. Overall results of the studies of the delegation of expanded functions to dental
      assistants and dental hygienists.
6. Describe the evolving role of the second direct patient care dental auxiliary in the
   United States.
7. Compare the current scope of practice of the dental hygienist with that of the
   dental hygienist as defined by Fones and Newman.

DEVELOPMENT OF THE DENTAL HYGIENE PROFESSION

The first direct patient care dental auxiliary in the United States that is acknowledged historically and that has continued to exist since the time of that profession's establishment is the dental hygienist. Dr. Alfred Civilion Fones, in 1906, established the profession by preparing Irene Newman to be a provider of care for his patients.[8] There were earlier instances of women serving roles as preventive assistants as the concept of oral hygiene was periodically discussed as a proper role for nondentists.[15] Fones was the person responsible for gaining widespread acceptance of the concept and for developing a lasting program of instruction for those persons. It was his expressed belief that there ought to be an auxiliary whose primary function was the prevention of dental disease and that the auxiliary called the dental hygienist should be educated to remove calcareous deposits from teeth and to instruct patients in the care and maintenance of their teeth and supporting structures.[15] The first educational program was long thought to be the Fones School of Dental Hygiene at the University of Bridgeport in Connecticut. However, recent findings indicate that the first program actually was at the Ohio College of Dental Surgery, from 1910 to 1911; it was closed down because of the opposition of area dentists.[15] Most activity in the development of the profession of dental hygiene occurred in the East, where dental hygienists were employed by school systems to provide dental health education and oral prophylaxis for children. The role was distinctly preventive and did not include restorative treatment.[15]

In the profession's infancy, its members were not licensed. The first legal definition of dental hygiene was the Connecticut Dental Practice Act in 1915.[15] Licensure would be a trend the profession would both enjoy as strong support and later bemoan from time to time as a roadblock to its own evolution in the second 50 years of existence.

In many ways licensure has preserved the profession since health agencies and dentists legally may not hire unlicensed persons to provide hygiene care. To do so is to break the state law.[11b,14] However, licensure has not always worked to the advantage of the profession. The individual licensing jurisdictions often have no reciprocal agreements with other jurisdictions. They may require complete reexamination before granting a hygienist entering the state or district a license

to practice, reducing the ability of dental hygiene practitioners to move from state to state without suffering long waiting periods of unemployment and the complexities of restudying for written examinations and preparing for clinical proficiency examinations.[22]

In addition, the various individual laws define dental hygiene with few common denominators among them.[11b,22] The scope of practice varies greatly from state to state. Laws that define dental hygiene in narrow terms of allowable functions and broad terms of disallowable functions often are the primary barrier to a broadened scope of practice. It takes virtually years to change the dental law so that it can reflect changes in the scope of practice.[14] The legislative process must consider many points of view regarding the best approach to changing the law. The lack of consensus among members of the professions makes legislators' decision making a complex process, and the ultimate changes in the law may be less than ideal from many points of view.

THE DIRECT PATIENT CARE AUXILIARY

Dental assistants are less consistently regulated by the state. For purposes of many licensing jurisdictions, dental assistants are support personnel who do not provide direct patient care. That is, they do not perform intraoral procedures defined as the practice of dentistry or dental hygiene. As a result, dentists are legally free to hire whomever they wish to be their "dental assistants."[11b]

There are, of course, educational programs to prepare trained dental assistants. The American Dental Assistants' Association (ADAA) has a certification program to identify those persons who have demonstrated skill and knowledge in dental assisting through formal education, an examination program, and required continuing education. Despite the educational programs and the certification credential, there is no mandate to hire these qualified persons. Only a few states, responding to an ADAA survey, reported requiring such certification of persons performing expanded functions delegated to dental assistants.[3a] As a result, ADAA has had unique problems both in establishing its credibility as the voice of dental assisting and in establishing economic security for its members who continually compete with the on-the-job trained work force that staffs the vast majority of dental offices.[3a]

However, what dental hygiene has in economic security in licensure, dental assisting has in flexibility of practice. Until recently dental assistants were not defined in the law and therefore not specifically restricted in practice, and they have always been available in large numbers (albeit not all educated or certified). These factors attracted many persons to begin experimentation in more productive patterns for the delivery of care with the focus on the dental assistant as the provider of the newly delegated services.[18]

The first experimentation was conducted in 1959 by the United States Navy at Great Lakes Naval Training Station in Illinois. Setting the pattern for numerous experimental projects to follow, the U.S. Navy discovered that dental technicians with some didactic background could learn to place quality restorations in prepared teeth. Productivity was increased by up to 80% to 100% for the dental officers responsible for the care.[13b] The results in this study were reported to the American Dental Association in 1965.[3]

The University of Alabama initiated a program in 1963, which eventually demonstrated that auxiliaries could successfully place rubber dams, matrices, temporary restorations, and amalgam and silicate restorations[3,11a] The Indian Health Service in 1963 demonstrated that appropriately trained auxiliaries could perform restorative procedures including placing and carving amalgam and silicate restorations.[1,3]

A landmark productivity study was conducted at Louisville, Kentucky, at the Division of Dental Health, U.S. Public Health Service.[3,13a] It demonstrated that assistants could perform the services as well as dentists and that with one dentist and four expanded function restorative assistants, productivity could be improved by up to 140%. Patient acceptance of auxiliaries performing such services was documented in this study, also. The University of the Pacific[17a] and the University of North Carolina[7] conducted studies also, both utilizing specially trained dental assistants to perform restorative functions.

This trend toward delegating additional functions, particularly restorative functions, to assistants created a new breed of auxiliary, the expanded function (duty) dental auxiliary. This person was to be the second direct patient care dental auxiliary in the United States. The scope of responsibility of this auxiliary varies with each experimental program and demonstration project that has been conducted and with each state's legal definition.[3a] This is a concept that varies with the developers' perceptions of the relative importance of formal education, appropriate certification mechanisms, the autonomy of the employer-dentist, and the usefulness and availability of other dental auxiliaries.

This direct patient care auxiliary may be a completely new entity with some of the skills of the traditional chairside dental assistant and a full array of intraoral skills. Or he/she may be a dental hygienist with additional periodontal and restorative functions.[3a] Regardless of the expanded function dental auxiliary's ambiguous definition, it seems apparent that a third operating auxiliary is emerging in the United States. It may take decades for the specific role of this provider of care to be delineated, agreed upon, and then functionally integrated into the delivery of care in this country.

DENTAL AUXILIARIES IN OTHER COUNTRIES

Other countries have introduced various kinds of dental auxiliaries as direct providers of care, with many patterned after the scope of practice and the educational programs of those of the United States. Nigeria, Argentina, Brazil, Canada, Columbia, Mexico, Uruguay, Iran, Egypt, the Netherlands, Norway, Sweden, the United Kingdom, India, Thailand, Australia, Fiji, Japan, and Korea each have one or more educational programs to prepare dental hygienists.[16] The first country to follow suit in developing the profession of dental hygiene was the United Kingdom, which introduced this auxiliary in 1944. In 1948, Japan introduced the dental hygienist and now has at least 63 programs to prepare persons for practice.[16] Italy, Germany, and Israel are considering establishing dental hygiene programs to meet their specific needs.

The United States may have established the model for dental hygiene, but it cannot claim the development of the dental nurse. New Zealand, in 1921, introduced the dental nurse concept.[9,10] Dental nurses in New Zealand provide direct patient care to children in schools, but in addition to providing oral examinations, prophylaxes, fluoride applications, and patient education they are trained to prepare (cut) and restore deciduous and permanent teeth, to polish amalgam restorations, to perform pulp capping, to extract deciduous teeth, and to refer patients to private dentists for more complex services, including extraction of permanent teeth, restoration of fractured permanent incisors, and orthodontic care. They perform diagnosis and treatment planning. While the dental hygienist was developing in the United States in a preventive mode, the dental nurse was developing in New Zealand, providing both preventive and therapeutic services for children.[9,10,11,19]

Just as a number of countries adopted the dental hygiene model in developing dental auxiliaries, many of the same countries and other countries opted for auxiliaries similar to the dental nurse model, permitting such direct patient care auxiliaries to provide, in varying ways, many basic restorative and therapeutic as well as preventive services to patients. Ghana, Senegal, Uganda, Canada, Columbia, Cuba, Jamaica, Paraguay, Sudan, the United Kingdom, Sri Lanka, Indonesia, Thailand, Australia, Hong Kong, Malaysia, Papua, New Guinea, and Singapore have all introduced such auxiliaries at various points in time during the five decades of the New Zealand scheme.[16] The papers developed for the International Symposia on Dental Hygiene during the 1970s provide a great deal of interesting information about the specific patterns of development and utilization that characterize many of the dental hygiene and other operating auxiliary concepts adopted by various countries.

In some countries there are distinctly separate role delineations for the dental hygienist and the restorative dental nurse. The United Kingdom provides a case in point. There are educational programs to prepare dental hygienists who perform the traditional functions related to prevention. And there is one educational program to prepare New Cross Dental Auxiliaries who provide restorative and other "expanded" functions that are not in the realm of the dental hygienist. These two auxiliaries are not educated together, nor do they usually function in the same practice setting after their education is completed. Dental hygienists mostly work in the private sector for individual practitioners, but the New Cross Dental Auxiliary is required to work within the dental hospital facilities or school health clinics.[14a]

Dental nurses have been functional in the northwest territories of Canada and in Saskatchewan for some years.[5,19] Countries with large underdeveloped areas such as Canada have found the dental nurse to be a primary means of extending care where dentists are not available. In at least one country, the dental hygienist has been in a position to accept expanded functions in addition to the more traditional preventive role. Canada has done this to a large extent, beginning with efforts in the mid-1960s to add prosthetic skills to the expertise of the licensed hygienist and later abandoning that thrust and turning to operative functions, delegating prosthetic functions to dental technicians. The dental hygienist in the United States has experienced some of this trend, largely through experimental programs that have shown that restorative and periodontal functions can be delegated to dental hygienists.

UTILIZING DENTAL HYGIENISTS IN EXPANDED FUNCTIONS

The four primary experiments and training programs utilizing dental hygienists in restorative expanded functions were conducted at the University of Iowa,[20] Howard University,[17] the University of Kentucky,[21] and Forsyth Dental Center.[12,13] Experimentation included dental hygienists cutting tooth structure to prepare the tooth for a restoration as well as placing and carving the restoration, functions dental nurses have had but which had been carefully avoided by United States dentists in experimenting with dental assistants in restorative functions in the 1960s. The studies were conclusive in proving that cutting hard tooth structure and replacing it with amalgam or tooth colored restorative materials could be delegated to specially educated dental hygienists without loss of quality. It was also demonstrated that dental hygienists could administer local anesthetic agents.[3a] The University of Iowa also assessed hygienists' abilities to accept expanded functions (cutting soft tissue) in periodontics. A similar study was conducted at the University of Pennsylvania.[2a] Both demonstrated again that expanded functions could be delegated to dental hygienists without loss of quality and with patient acceptance.

On the basis of quality of care, patient acceptance, relative cost of educating auxiliaries rather than dentists, and the effect such personnel utilization could have on productivity in delivering dental care, the studies pointed directly toward delegating those functions to dental hygienists.[12,13,17,21]

Supporters of that move cited the dental hygienist's substantial background in behavioral and clinical sciences as a solid basis on which to build expanded functions.[1a,6,12,13] The fact that hygienists have an established, national educational system and licensure mechanism was offered as further reason to consider the hygienist as a primary person to accept expanded functions in cutting hard and soft tissue and in administering local anesthesia.[3a] For persons concerned about a systematic program for preparing expanded functions personnel and then regulating their practice, these arguments were convincing.

There have been almost no opportunities, however, for implementation of these concepts in the health care system since few dental practice acts have been sufficiently altered to permit the delegation of restorative or advanced periodontal functions to licensed dental hygienists, regardless of their advanced educational preparation.[3a] Except for a few licensing jurisdictions, the dental hygienist is still primarily described legally and in practice as the "prevention oriented" person who may legally perform only the oral prophylaxis, preliminary oral examinations, fluoride applications, and patient education.[11b]

As the debate continues regarding which functions should be delegated and which auxiliary (if any) should perform expanded functions under the supervision of a dentist, dental hygienists find their role delineation basically unchanged in the law. But they have gravitated away from the public health sector and toward the private sector of health care (usually solo practitioner dental offices); they have often found it difficult to continue to focus on prevention particularly when confronted with the challenge to make prevention "pay," and they have watched a number of their primary functions be delegated to other auxiliaries (both legally and illegally) while their own scope of responsibility has had only tenuous, sporadic growth.[3a]

EFFECTIVENESS OF TRADITIONAL DENTAL HEALTH CARE

Perhaps one of the most startling, sobering realizations is an honest assessment of how effective the professions' efforts have been in the irradication of dental disease, particularly when compared with the effectiveness of the concurrent dental nurse program in New Zealand. What have the professions of dental hygiene and dentistry accomplished, particularly in comparison with the efforts of dental nurses? Certainly the individual dental hygienist can identify those particular patients whom he/she has affected, whose oral health is significantly improved. Perhaps there are hundreds of patients for each practicing dental hygienist who have established oral health routines that keep them virtually plaque-free and in a state of near-ideal dental health.

However, dentistry cannot claim that dental hygienists in the United States have decreased tooth mortality rates from 88.2 to 12.6 extractions per 100 children over a 36 year period. The New Zealand dental nurse can. Seventy-two percent of the carious teeth in New Zealand children under 13 have been restored.[9,10] Also, the program in New Zealand seems to have directly modified the behavior of patients to continue to seek dental care long past the time they cease to be eligible for the school programs. Sixty-seven percent of men and 77% of women continued to seek dental care (at their expense and effort) after attaining adulthood.[9,10] In the United States 15% to 20% of adults seek regular dental care,[4] and only 23% of children's carious lesions are restored.[4]

To place any "blame" on the profession of dental hygiene for not matching the achievements of the dental nurses is unfair. For years there were hardly sufficient numbers of dental hygienists to begin to tackle the problems of children and adults. Even with the current burgeoning numbers of dental hygienists, the functional role of dental hygienists still depends almost entirely on the judgment of the employing solo dentist,[2] with the scope of practice still defined narrowly in most states. Dental hygienists are often not able to extend their efforts to the people who need preventive care most. Practice acts often require that a dental hygienist have a dentist physically present when he/she is providing dental care of any sort, hampering dental hygienists from provididng intraoral care in community programs. Dental hygienists are not legally able to establish a preventive practice of their own, regardless of the dire need of the identified population group and the scarcity of dentists to open such practices legally.[11b]

And, of course, functions that are legally restricted to primary prevention do not greatly assist patients who have access to a dental hygienist but no access to a dentist and who need one. Could dental hygienists have accomplished as much as their dental nurse counterpart if they had been able to provide immediate restorative and pain relieving care to children in need of such services rather than merely to hope that the parent could locate a dentist, schedule an appointment, and pay for the services? If dental hygiene had been defined differently from the beginning, there is some chance that the dental health problems of the country today would be greatly reduced. If there had been a planned, national program (with the scope of practice *still* defined as preventive) to prepare adequate numbers of dental hygienists and to ensure that children had ready access to continuous assessment, prevention, and referral for treatment, there is reason to believe the current dental health levels of the public could have been significantly higher.

However, this did not happen. Individual states licensed hygienists according to their individual needs. The first 30 years of the profession saw only minimal growth, and as a result, minimal impact on the health of the public. Despite the fact that Dr. Fones envisioned the hygienist as improving health levels, the nation did not see the need for comprehensive planning and did not develop dental hygienists to their full potential.

The dental hygienist continues to be a primary deliverer of dental care. And for many, the hygienist is the logical answer to many of the dental health care problems of this country and others. However, there are a great many others who have ceased acknowledging the existence of that provider and who look to other, new auxiliaries to fulfill a role that blends restorative and preventive functions and that is not encumbered by state-by-state licensure and stereotypes associated with a profession that has never had the full opportunity to impact dental health in a measurable, significant manner.

Review questions

1. The founder of the profession of dental hygiene was _____ .
2. The first dental hygienist was _____ .
3. The original role delineation of the dental hygienist can be briefly described as:
4. The functions of the New Zealand dental nurse differ from those of the dental hygienist in the United States because of the inclusion of:
5. What have the relative impacts of the dental hygienist in the United States and the New Zealand dental nurse been on the dental health of their respective populations?
6. What basic expanded functions have most often been included in experimentation with:
   a. Dental assistants
   b. Dental hygienists
7. List three probable reasons for the disparity between the overall population levels of dental health attained in New Zealand and in the United States.
   a.
   b.
   c.

ANSWERS

1. Alfred C. Fones
2. Irene Newman
3. A preventive role in which the profession removed calcareous deposits (oral prophylaxis), performed oral examinations, and provided patient education. The role developed primarily in public school systems in the East.
4. The preparation and placement of restorations, extraction of deciduous teeth, pulp capping, diagnosis, treatment planning.
5. New Zealand population has 72% of its children's carious lesions restored. Tooth mortality has reduced from 88.2 to 12.6 extractions over a 36-year period and 67 to 77% of adult patients continue to seek routine dental care. Twenty-three percent of United States' children's carious lesions are restored, and 15% to 20% of adults continue to receive care regularly.
6. a. Placement of amalgam and tooth colored restorations
   b. Preparation of teeth and placement of restorations, local anesthesia, periodontal functions including surgery on soft tissues.
7. a. There were insufficient numbers of hygienists to impact the public.
   b. The laws have restricted the hygienist from providing needed care.
   c. The laws have restricted hygienists to limited practice settings.

GROUP ACTIVITIES

1. Locate the original publications of data of the various experimental programs in extending restorative and periodontal functions to auxiliaries. Discuss the implications and findings of each study in terms of the dental health needs of the population of the United States.
2. Locate articles describing the various operating dental auxiliaries in other countries. Compare and contrast their function and their effectiveness with that of dental auxiliaries in the United States.
3. Conduct an inquiry regarding the feasibility of introducing the dental nurse program to the school system in your community. Role play the parts of the local dental society, the dental hygiene society, the consumers interested in improving the oral health of the children in the community, the school board, the representative of the state board of dental examiners, and consultants from New Zealand who have agreed to begin the educational program. Research each of those roles and conduct the mock hearing or inquiry with various group members assuming and acting out one of the identified parts. Each person should conform his/her behavior to that which would be predictable for the role assigned.

REFERENCES

1. Abramowitz, J. and Berg, L. E.: A four-year study of the utilization of dental assistants with expanded functions, J. Am. Dent. Assoc., **87**:623.
1a. Barish, Anna M. and Barish, Nathanial H.: Will dental hygiene become obsolete? J. Am. Dent. Hyg. Assoc., **45**:47.
2. Born, David Omar: Research in expanded duties auxiliary utilization: The past and the future. In Lucaccini, Luigi F. and Handley, Jack, editors: Research in the use of expanded function auxiliaries, Bethesda, 1974, U.S. Dept. of Health, Education and Welfare, PHS-HRA, Bureau of Health Resources Development, Division of Dentistry.
2a. Cohen, D. Walter: University of Pennsylvania: Personal communication.
3. Council on Dental Education Annual Report, Chicago, 1970, American Dental Association.
3a. Council on Dental Education Annual Report, Chicago, 1976, American Dental Association.
4. Current estimates from the Health Interview Survey, United States—1973, Data from the National Health Survey, Series 10, Number 95, Rockville, Maryland, 1974, U.S. Dept. of Health, Education and Welfare, National Center for Health Statistics, Health Resources Administration.
5. Curry, T. M. and others: Saskatchewan studies with the British dental auxiliary model. In Lucaccini, Luigi F. and Handley, Jack, editors: Research in the use of expanded function auxiliaries, Bethesda, 1974, U.S. Dept. of Health, Education and Welfare, PHS-HRA, Bureau of Health Resources Development, Division of Dentistry.
6. Diefenbach, Viron: The 1970's—a new era for dental auxiliaries, J. Am. Dent. Hyg. Assoc., **45**:50.
7. Douglass, Chester W.: Utilization of expanded duty dental assistants in a solo private practice. In Lucaccini, Luigi F. and Handley, Jack, editors: Research in the use of expanded function auxiliaries. Bethesda, 1974, U.S. Dept. of Health, Education and Welfare, PHS-HRA, Bureau of Health Resources Development, Division of Dentistry.
8. Fones, A.C.: The origin and history of the dental hygienist movement. In Fones, A. C., editor: Mouth hygiene, Philadelphia, 1927, Lea & Febiger.
9. Friedman, Jay W.: The New Zealand School Dental Service: Lesson in radical conservatism. Presented at the Conference of Dental Examiners and Dental Educators, February 11-12, 1972, Chicago, Ill.
10. Gladstone, Rhoda Nash: International dental nurse programs, Dent. Hyg., **49**:169.
11. Goldhaber, Paul: Improving the dental health status in the United States—putting your money where your mouth is, J. Dent. Educ., **41**:50.
11a. Hammons, P. E., Jamieson, H. C., and Wilson, L. L.: Quality of service provided by dental therapists in an experimental program at the University of Alabama, J. Am. Dent. Assoc., **82**:1060.
11b. Johnson, Donald W. and Holz, Frank M.: Legal provisions on expanded functions for dental hygienists and assistants, Bethesda, Md., 1974, U.S. Department of Health, Education, and Welfare, PHS-HRA, Bureau of Health Resources Development, Division of Dentistry.
12. Lobene, Ralph R.: The Forsyth study of new duties for dental hygienists. In Lucaccini, Luigi F. and Handley, Jack, editors: Research in the use of expanded function auxiliaries, Bethesda, 1974, U.S. Dept. of Health, Education and Welfare, PHS-HRA, Bureau of Health Resources Development, Division of Dentistry.
13. Lobene, Ralph R., and others: The Forsyth experiment in training of advanced skill hygienists, J. Dent. Educ., **38**:369.
13a. Latzkar, S. J., Johnson, D. W., and Thompson, M. B.: Experimental program in expanded functions for dental assistants: Phase III experiment with dental teams, J. Am. Dent. Assoc., **82**:1067.
13b. Ludwig, William E. and others: Report of clinical tests, Greater utilization of dental technicians, Dental Research Facility, U.S. Navy Training Center, Great Lakes, Ill., May 1964.
14. Manual for consultants to state boards of dentistry.

Chicago, 1976, American Dental Hygienists Association.

14a. Milward, E.: Dental auxiliaries—four years on, Dental Health (Brit.) 6:15.

15. Motley, Wilma: Ethics, jurisprudence and history for the dental hygienist, ed. 2, Philadelphia, 1976, Lea & Febiger.

16. Myers, Sharon E.: Operating dental auxiliaries, WHO Chron., 26:511.

17. Powell, William O., and others: Comparison of clinical performance of dental therapist trainees and dental students, J. Dent. Educ., 38:268.

17a. Redig, Dale and others: Expanded duty dental auxiliaries in four private dental offices: the first year's experience, J. Am. Dent. Assoc., 88:969.

18. Report of the Inter-agency Committee on Dental Auxiliaries, J. Am. Dent. Assoc., 84:1027.

19. Roemer, Ruth: Credentialing dental auxiliary personnel in the United States and selected other countries. In Proceedings of the Workshop on changing roles of dental auxiliaries, Bethesda, 1975, U.S. Dept. of Health, Education and Welfare, PHS-HRA, Bureau of Health Manpower, Division of Dentistry.

20. Sisty, Nancy L.: Expanded-function dental hygiene student performance evaluations, Dent. Hyg., 49:401.

21. Spohn, Eric: Background and transition of the expanded duty program. In agenda material for the meeting of the Educational Advisory Committee for the University of Kentucky expanded duty dental hygiene research program, June 1975.

22. Woodall, Irene: Changes in state licensing acts allowing for expanded use of dental auxiliaries. In Mescher, Kay, ed.: Proceedings of a workshop on adaptation of dental hygiene practice to changing concepts in delivery of oral health services, Little Amana, Iowa, 1972, American Dental Hygienists Association.

PART II

HEALTH CARE DELIVERY AND THE PRESENT AND FUTURE ROLES OF DIRECT PATIENT CARE DENTAL AUXILIARIES

The origin of dental auxiliaries and their role in dental care delivery are integrally related to the way in which the health care delivery system has developed and the ways in which delivery of dental care is related to the overall health system. Auxiliaries are the result of the expressed needs of the dental profession in attempting to provide better care for patients and in attempting to improve the productivity and the ease with which care can be delivered.

Unlike medical care, dental care has seen the establishment of few new categories of care providers. While there are presently literally hundreds of categories of health workers in the field of medicine, each with its own educational and credentialing process, dentistry has identified only three primary auxiliaries (dental assisting, dental hygiene, and dental laboratory technology) as providing services to augment the practice of dentistry. As seen in previous chapters, other auxiliaries that might fulfill some expanded role in dentistry have received considerable attention, but they remain as yet basically undefined as a distinct group of persons with specified education qualifications.

Whether the current three traditional auxiliaries, plus a fourth, expanded functions dental auxiliary, will comprise the field of providers who are supporting dentistry will be dependent on how the system for delivery of care evolves in the coming years.

That evolution will be shaped in part by the influence of consumers and by the profession's efforts to resolve the issues of cost, access, quality of care, and the utilization of manpower.

CHAPTER 3

Health care delivery settings and systems and the concept of team health care delivery

OBJECTIVES: The reader will be able to:

1. Describe briefly the current system of delivery of dental health care services, including:
    a. Practice settings
    b. Payment mechanisms
    c. Patient access to care
    d. Utilization of health care providers in the system
    e. Its uniqueness in contrast to delivery systems for medical care
2. Identify, chronologically, the basic components of the movement toward dental care systems that utilize auxiliaries and that are described as "team" health care.
3. Identify the sources of influence that have shaped the dental health care delivery system, describing the "vested interest" each source of influence has in the outcome of the system.

PRESENT SYSTEM OF DENTAL HEALTH CARE SERVICES

Dentistry for the most part has been and continues to be perceived as a cottage industry. Delivery of dental care occurs in isolated practice settings where individual providers of care (dentists) provide dental services to which the patient agrees. The dentist typically makes him/herself available for appointments during given hours in an office or clinic setting and attempts to meet the needs of the patients as they appear. There is no concerted, organized program to attract patients to dental care, and for the most part dental care is quite separate from any of the other health care experiences a patient may have.[32] The efficiency, pleasantness of care, and settings of the dental profession have been modified to a certain degree over the past 100 years as dental equipment became more functional, attractive, and more in keeping with minimal patient and operator discomfort. Practice settings have moved from Spartan environments to comfortable bungalow offices and medical arts buildings, but essentially the system for delivering care has changed very little. The patient presents him/herself for care often only when disease is apparent. The goal for dentistry, in shifting away from the role of repairing disease and treating emergencies, was to have patients appear regularly for check-ups.[41] For some, oral prophylaxis was added as a routine procedure, particularly if the individual dentist wished to employ and could locate a dental hygienist to perform the prophylaxis at each recall visit.

The American Dental Association (ADA) has gone on record over the last 30 years as stating that the membership desires to be viewed as a prevention-oriented profession rather than as a pain alleviator. Many dentists expressed priorities for prevention and

25

carried on full-scale preventive practices well before the renewed prevention thrust of the late 1960s. However, an important fact about dentistry is that people do not view dental disease as a life or death matter. Dental problems may cause a person great discomfort, but they rarely involve the life threatening impact of many medical problems. As a result, the public often views dentistry as a luxury rather than a necessity, especially when financial resources are minimal.[28a]

Dental care, particularly regular, preventive dental care, has therefore been more common among the middle and upper classes of the United States. This was partly a result of the community's view of the relative unimportance of dental care in overall health, but it was also caused by an economic factor.[28a] Dentistry, until the mid-1960s was almost exclusively a fee-for-service enterprise.[32] Patients paid for services from their private financial resources. There were almost no mechanisms for prepaid dentistry that would ensure that an individual would be able to pay for care when it was needed. Dental services, therefore, tended to be available only to those persons who were financially secure. Now, with the advent of health maintenance organizations (HMOs) and comprehensive group practices, persons can subscribe to health care on an annual basis and be assured that needed care will be paid for. The large labor unions have been able to negotiate for and obtain dental care benefits so that workers and their families are able to have dental care reimbursed through the company's insurance plan when it is needed or prepaid through a capitation plan. In addition, public funds are more readily available to pay for care for special beneficiary groups, such as the aged and children.[32]

However, improved access to health care implies more than providing the financial resources to pay for the care. Despite the fact that the patient may be able to have dental care paid for in its entirety, people still are not always able to receive the care

they need.[15b] Several reasons for this include the fact that the health care facility may be open on weekdays from 9 A.M. to 5 P.M., but the patient may not be able to come at those times because of conflicts with a work schedule. Perhaps transportation is not available to the site; the number of forms that need to be completed for each visit and the complexity of making an appointment may be more than the patient is able or willing to endure in obtaining health care. The more complex reasons include the possibility that patients covered by an insurance plan cannot locate a care facility willing to accept the plan. Or the plan itself may not provide realistic levels of payments for services provided, causing reimbursement to be insufficient for the requirements of various procedures, unless the patients supplement the plan's allotted amount with their own funds.

A broader issue related to access to health care is the problem of geographic distribution of health care providers.[29] Certain segments of the population may not have access to care because the providers are not available in certain areas. This is often the case in rural areas and sometimes in the inner city. Very often the treatment facilities are clustered together in areas where care is already plentiful and accessible.[13,24,33]

The issues of access to and cost of care are problems common to both medicine and dentistry, but they may be compounded in dentistry since the providers are operating largely independently of any larger system of health care planning to assess where care is most needed and how plans can be made to provide it.

Ensuring the quality of care is an issue related to past and current health care delivery systems. In hospital environments or clinics where a number of providers have frequent opportunities to review each other's performance in diagnosis and treatment, the elements of at least a rudimentary peer review mechanism have existed. And in instances where third party payors such as insurance carriers and public agencies are paying for the cost of care, there may be more formal review mechanisms for individual providers and individual patient cases. For these reasons, medicine has been involved on a more continuing basis with the issue of assessing the quality of care delivered. In dentistry, especially in solo practices where it is unlikely that another dentist may regularly see the work of the dentist and where third-party payors have been less common, the external constraints and reviews are less frequent. Only recently has dentistry begun to formalize a review mechanism to assess the quality of care being rendered.

The federal government recently enacted legislation to establish Professional Standards Review Organizations (PSROs) to monitor certain providers of medical care.[45] This may be extended to dentistry and perhaps to other levels of health care providers such as nurses and allied health personnel once a reasonable mechanism is developed and the public extends its concern for quality care to all segments of the health care workforce.[47a]

Another characteristic of the dental care delivery system is the proportionately fewer numbers of auxiliary personnel or lower level providers who are fully utilized in the provision of care. The dental hygienist, as noted earlier, is the only long standing direct patient care auxiliary in dentistry. Dental assistants have been utilized as support personnel for many years, but to full advantage since only 1961, when attention was turned to the most efficient ways to provide care in dentistry. Recent literature indicates that many practitioners still use few if any auxiliaries and perhaps do not utilize the auxiliaries they do employ to their fullest potential.[24,31,34] The advent of the expanded function dental auxiliary who may provide restorative services or who may be involved in advanced periodontal skills certainly indicates a trend toward the development of a new auxiliary, but the extent to which this source of manpower will be fully utilized in dental practice is not easily predicted.

The dental laboratory technician is viewed by organized dentistry as an auxiliary, along with the dental hygienist and the dental assistant. The dental laboratory technician fabricates appliances and prostheses according to the specifications of the dentist. The dental laboratory technician is not viewed by dentistry as a direct patient care auxiliary since he/she supports dental services in the laboratory rather than the operatory. Dental laboratory technicians, however, often choose to disavow themselves of the auxiliary concept and prefer to be acknowledged as free-enterprise business persons who contractually provide dentists with services they need performed by constructing intraoral appliances and prostheses. Those technicians who work directly with the dentist at the delivery site are more amenable to accepting the role or label of an auxiliary to the dentist. The American Dental Association concurred with this role distinction in its 1976 House of Delegates transactions.[9]

There has been a continuing controversy between dental laboratory technicians and organized dentistry among those elements who cannot agree upon the appropriate role of the technician in providing care. Various elements in laboratory technology wish to have authority to provide direct care to patients. This movement has been labeled "denturism." The basic argument is whether a technician ought to be legally allowed to prepare dentures from start to finish for edentulous patients. Some technicians argue that their expertise ought to permit them to see patients directly. In their testimony before various state legislatures in an attempt to modify the law to permit denturism, they cite the high cost of dentures prepared by dentists compared to the actual construction cost of the devices. Their primary argument is that they can provide dentures to patients at a lower cost than dentistry can—and that care may be more readily available if technicians are allowed to provide these services for patients.[19a]

Dentistry's response has been definite and powerful in arguing against denturism. The dental literature is replete with articles concerning the denturist movement, particularly since its startling growth in Canada in the middle and late 1970s.[19a,21b] Dentistry views the denturist movement as a threat to the health care of patients whose special needs cannot be identified or met by the limited skill and knowledge of the technician.[1a] Dentistry's other basic objection to the denturist movement is that it would allow an "auxiliary" to provide care without the direct supervision of a dentist, a trend dentistry has identified as undesirable.[2,3,5,9,16]

In summary, dental care delivery systems tend to be separated from other health care providers. Individual practitioners provide care as people present themselves for treatment, usually on a fee-for-service basis. Access to care breaks down geographically and financially. Practice sites may cluster in some areas and be totally inaccessible to others. There has been no formal widespread system of formalized peer review in dentistry, and auxiliary personnel remain underutilized and continue to function under the direct supervision of the dentist.

Dentistry is in contrast to medicine, where much of the provision of care occurs in hospitals and other health center facilities and where the delivery of services involves teams of personnel. The fee payment mechanism consists largely of third-party payment systems such as prepaid programs, insurance, and public assistance programs. Although medical care is not totally subjected to preplanning for accessibility to target populations in need of care, area health planning agencies have a more direct involvement in the establishment of health care facilities. The medical profession is currently involved in formalizing peer review mechanisms associated with PSROs and with third-party payors who review diagnoses and treatment prior to authorizing payment for services. Medicine relies heavily on the services of a myriad of health care providers. Hundreds of categories of allied health personnel, with specialized skills to support medical treatment, are available and utilized in the provision of care. Many function quite apart from the direct supervision of the physician.[21,30]

The literature indicates that medicine has been confronted by each health care system issue (cost, access, quality assurance, utilization of auxiliary manpower) before dentistry's confrontation with such issues. The third-party payment system, the responsibility for ensuring or at least planning for improved access to care, peer review, and all the battles of "which person should perform which support service" for medicine are all issues that medicine has confronted and responded to, for better or for worse. Many writers suggest that the wise organization of health care providers who have not yet faced these issues might learn from medicine's successes and mistakes. This suggestion was particularly frequent in the literature when Medicare was enacted in 1965 by the federal government despite the opposition of the American Medical Association (AMA). Predictions were that dentistry would soon be embroiled in a very similar debate over the way in which dental care should be funded by state and federal agencies, particularly as the Congress heightened the discussion of enacting national health insurance. According to some of the proposals such a law would provide all citizens with prepaid medical and dental care. Dentistry did follow the advice to some extent, and ADA drafted its position on national health care programs in 1971.[26] It attempted to establish a very positive statement with regard to imminent changes in the manner in which people were going to have at least financial access to care. Several of its more recent position statements appear to reflect a reconsideration of those guidelines, particularly in the area of manpower utilization.

A comparison of dental care delivery in the United States with that of other countries may be essential in order to begin to understand the shift in policy of organized dentistry in the late 1970s. The literature of the early 1960s includes proposals for improving the United States health care delivery system; these proposals often included the "team" approach to dentistry with the primary objective being greater productivity. Little attention was given to assessing the quality of care. The stimulus for change was to offer more care for more people, in anticipation of the projected enormous population growth that was to occur during the 1970s and 1980s.[17,33] Essentially, the concern was with continuing the level of care for the population and coping with large numbers of people who would overburden the dental manpower force.

In New Zealand and Great Britain the primary objective stated for altering the dental care system was to improve the dental health of the public.[15,23,24,43] Statistics were examined regarding the dental health of children and adults, and programs were initiated in which dental manpower (including auxiliaries) would be available to extend care to those whose current level of health was poor. As described in the previous chapter, New Zealand designed a system of dental nurses to provide preventive and restorative treatment to children at school based clinics. The data reveal that this was a most successful approach since the levels of health of the population have risen considerably as a direct result. In Great Britain the traditional dental hygienist and a restorative therapist (known as the New Cross Dental Auxiliary) were introduced to provide preventive and therapeutic treatment to persons through the National Health Service, which was intended to ensure its citizens of funded comprehensive medical care and many basic dental services.

MOVEMENT TOWARD TEAM HEALTH CARE

The focus of effort in the United States was to improve the efficiency with which specific intraoral services were performed.[17,33,38] The 1960s saw the era of time and motion studies, when the procedures performed by dentists were analyzed for the stress and strain they placed on the operator and for the amount of time they consumed. Systems analysts and efficiency experts analyzed the traditional stand-up dentistry approach that used few if any support personnel. They assessed the design of equipment and the manner in which storage was located in the dental operatory. The age of four-handed, sit-down dentistry resulted from these first efforts and established the "chairside dental assistant." This assistant became an active participant in the intraoral procedures provided by the dentist. The assistant passed instruments, aspirated fluids from the oral cavity, prepared materials at chairside for intraoral use, and generally facilitated the efficiency with which each given procedure was performed. The chapter on the management of time and motion describes these services in greater detail.

In 1961 the federal government funded Dental Auxiliary Utilization (DAU) programs at dental schools and supported the preparation of instructional materials and courses to bring to the practicing dentist a new approach to practice.[33] Dental meetings almost always included lectures and seminars on how to implement four-handed dentistry. A good deal of effort was spent on designing dental equipment that would be compatible with these approaches to the delivery of care. The dental units of the 1940s and 1950s were immovable objects with little flexibility for accommodating dental assisting procedures. It was during this period of time that the ADA expressed its first significant interest in experimentation with the delegation of additional functions to auxiliaries. The success of four-handed dentistry in reducing chair time and in improving the ease with which various procedures could be performed prompted others to speculate how components of various clinical procedures could be delegated to auxiliaries. Increased efficiency could be achieved to an even greater extent by freeing the dentist to spend more time with the more demanding aspects of dental practice.

The first real focus on the low levels of health in the United States rather than on low productivity came with the Carnegie Commission Report of 1970, and a series of national health surveys that cited the shortage of dentists and physicians to provide reasonable levels of health care and drew attention to the differences between the need and demand for health care.[12,14,48]

The reports projected that there would be a critical manpower shortage in the years to come unless more physicians and dentists were educated and unless additional functions could be delegated to allied health personnel and that there was a current unmet need in the population based on health statistics.

The reports stimulated Congress to appropriate large amounts of money to assist dental and medical schools to improve their educational programs and to increase the numbers of students they were preparing. Congress also funded a new grants program in 1971 called TEAM (Training in Expanded Auxiliary Management),[33] which would extend beyond the four-handed dentistry concept and support the learning of methods of delegating intraoral functions to dental auxiliaries. Federal legislation also supported the development of allied health education programs that would prepare personnel for assuming supportive roles in the provision of medical and dental services. Dental hygiene and dental assisting were defined as a part of allied health for purposes of funding. With federal support available, numerous community colleges and technical institutes started dental assisting and dental hygiene programs along with the myriad of other eligible allied health programs. The biggest growth period in dental hygiene programs in their entire 60-year history occurred when the numbers of programs increased from 56 in 1965 to 183 in 1975. The emphasis was to increase the number of persons available to provide services and to extend various delegatable services to auxiliaries.

As described in the previous chapter, dentistry turned first to dental assisting in designing experimental programs for delegating expanded functions. The reasons most frequently cited were: (1) dental assistants were not governed by restrictive licensing laws that would inhibit the possibility of expanding their scope of function; (2) there were far more dental assistants (albeit many on-the-job trained) than there were dental hygienists[25,38]; (3) dental hygienists are ren-

dering an important service, the oral prophylaxis, and would find it difficult to add expanded functions to their responsibilities[50]; (4) it would be difficult to logistically involve a dental hygienist in the provision of restorative care in a dental practice, whereas it would be relatively easy to involve the dental assistant; and (5) dental hygienists demand a higher salary than do dental assistants and therefore are an economic detriment to containing the cost of dental services. Another reason occasionally referred to in the literature is the dental hygienists' collective reticence with regard to expanding their scope of function.[10,24]

A significant number of dental hygiene leaders, however, began to reexamine the role of the dental hygienist and to suggest ways in which new functions could be delegated to hygienists. The broad educational base of the dental hygienist, the already existing curricula, the growing number of dental hygiene programs, and the fact that many dental hygienists felt that they were underutilized in terms of their education[15,22,28,47] prompted a new perception on the part of the profession. Hygienists, with the support of interested dentists, began to pursue experimental programs within their own ranks.[18,39] The Forsyth, Iowa, Kentucky, Howard, and Pennsylvania programs all went beyond the scope of study of the expanded duty dental assistant, since the experiments with dental hygienists involved the administration of local anesthesia, the cutting of preparations for the placement of restorations, and in two studies, gingival recontouring.[15a,36,40,44,46]

An interesting historical note is that an experimental program to assess how well dental hygienists could learn to prepare children's teeth for the placement of restorations was proposed and funded in 1949 for the Forsyth Dental Center.[35] Opposition from within both dentistry and dental hygiene[29a,37] caused the program to close, with the House of Representatives of Massachusetts passing legislation to end the program in 1950.

RESISTANCE TO CHANGE

In October, 1975, after hearing testimony and reviewing the data available from the experimental programs, the ADA adopted a number of position statements that indicated their decision to pursue such experimental interests no further.[4] A policy adopted in the early 1960s that supported experimentation with auxiliaries and that recommended extending every possible delegatable function to auxiliaries was reversed. The House of Delegates of the ADA adopted a position statement that expressed its opposition to auxiliaries placing restorations in teeth that had been prepared by the dentist, thus disclaiming the numerous experimental studies performed with dental assistants as well as the more controversial studies utilizing dental hygienists. The Association has continued to state its opposition to permitting auxiliaries to diagnose and prescribe, to administer anesthetics, or to cut hard and soft tissues.[8] Some critics cite these policy statements as denial of the evidence of experimental programs that demonstrate that hygienists and assistants, when properly trained, can perform many of the functions previously reserved for the hands of the dentist. Organized dentistry contends that much of the research has been conducted in settings not reflective of the economic and logistical realities of most practice settings. They say that further research would be needed to determine the efficacy of how such procedures could be delegated. The discussions within the ADA, as described in reports of its continuing workshops regarding appropriate delegation of functions and as voiced in its reference committee hearings at its annual meetings, indicate that the dentists acknowledge that those functions *can* be delegated, but they are not convinced that they *should* be delegated.

The ADA's position in the early 1960s was that state dental practice acts would have to change in order to provide for the delegation of functions to auxiliaries. At least 44 licensing jurisdictions since that time have amended their laws to permit broader scopes of practice for at least the dental assistant, and often for the dental hygienist.[19]

Programs preparing dentists to utilize dental auxiliaries in expanded function practice and programs preparing dental auxiliaries have revised their curricula to provide the educational base for team practice involving expanded duties. These programs are now faced with coming to grips with the trichotomy among federal recommendations, the policy of organized dentistry, and what is known from research about delegating functions.

The federal government continues to fund educational programs to prepare persons to perform expanded functions and to utilize expanded function dental auxiliaries.[27] The consumer continues to question the high cost of dental health care. Demand and need are becoming more equal, and the profession now finds itself in a dilemma in terms of defining utilization of personnel in practice and in stabilizing the rising costs of dental health care.

The forces of state boards of dentistry, education, federal funding, and the consumer do not seem to be compatible with the force of the ADA. Both the ADAA and ADHA continue their support of the delegation of expanded functions to dental auxiliaries, with their only conditions being that the person be educated to perform the service and that a single minimum standard of quality of care be utilized to assess the services provided, regardless of who is providing the care (dentist, hygienist, assistant, or EFDA).

The state boards of dentistry have a legal mandate to enforce legislation passed by the individual state legislatures. The legislative changes have defined dentistry and auxiliary practice in response to input from organized dentistry and consumers, and often from auxiliary associations as well. They have adopted the legislation in order to extend appropriate opportunity for care to the people of the state. As an agency of the state, the board is required to enforce the dental law and to interpret it according to the way it is written. Laws that clearly identify the allowed duties for auxiliaries in the wording of the statute cannot be ignored. However, the ADA position statements may have an impact on the way in which rules and regulations are written by the state boards of dentistry. Many of the dental law changes provide a brief explanation of the practice of the defined auxiliaries, listing some of their functions, but more than likely only those functions that they may *not* perform. These laws often contain a phrase that empowers the state board of dentistry to specify which functions the auxiliaries may legally perform.[19] There are some states where the law has changed but where rules and regulations have not been prepared by the state board and where board rulings have been reversed. The "open" practice act that gives this power to the board may provide an avenue for state boards to conform to ADA policy.

The educational programs have already expressed, by means of a position statement from the American Association of Dental Schools (AADS), that they will not endorse pre-1960s utilization patterns in preparing their students for practice. This strong stand has caused an unfortunate separation in philosophical approach to education and practice between dental educators and organized dental practitioners in some segments of the profession.[31] Much of the controversy is being waged in the arena of academic freedom, where individual programs claim the right to teach whichever functions they choose in their educational institutions, regardless of the particular dental law of the state in which the school is located.[20,42] ADA does not support schools teaching functions that cannot be legally performed in practice in that state. AADS policy states that they ought to be free to do so, since they have an obligation to prepare students to obtain licensure and practice in any licensing jurisdiction without requiring extensive additional education beyond traditional, basic preparation.[1] The legal entanglements have upheld the state's right to enjoin those educational programs from teaching beyond that allowed in the letter of the law,[42] thus limiting the opportunity for continued experimentation and precluding the preparation of large numbers of personnel for other states where the laws are less constraining and where health workers are needed.[21a]

The nuances of each state's law are causing "basic dental hygiene education" to offer a less generally understood, predictable curriculum. The basic courses may include one or more or none of the various expanded functions depending upon the state in which the program is located. Although there is one title for all the persons graduating from those programs, the graduates are in actuality often drastically different from each other in terms of levels of knowledge and in terms of the services they are able to perform and the competency levels at which they are able to perform them. This is a problem not only in the practice of the profession but in the identification of qualified teachers for educational programs.

The federal government and the consumer movement continue to respond in their programs to the need for additional manpower with a broad range of expanded functions. However, the EFDA guidelines for funding dental auxiliary programs do require that the state law permit the teaching of those functions in that educational institution before funding can be awarded.[27] Private foundations that have funded expanded function experimental programs are influenced by the position statements since they too are now assessing the relative likelihood that such persons will be employable and whether the state in which the educational program is located allows the performance of those functions in practice or allows them to be taught regardless of the legality of their being put into practice.[46]

For many auxiliaries it is difficult to understand why, despite the quality of care they have learned to provide, dentistry chooses to oppose its being delegated to them. The hygienist who has learned to provide periodontal therapy may view the policy reversal as an unreasonable narrowing of his/her scope of function and as a step backward into a less challenging role in providing care. Dental assistants may see their opportunity for a long-overdue proper recognition of certification slipping away, along with the potential for a reasonable income level. And the expanded function dental auxiliary, trained specifically for restorative functions may feel, and be, totally obsolete.

The reversal is easily understood, despite its relative impact on the forces that be. It is frequently described as a reaction to a very real threat that dentists feel when they see the functions they have routinely performed—and which for some individual dentists actually comprise the operating definition of dentistry—being delegated to auxiliaries with 2 or less years of education. Dentists have described the phenomenon as a gradual eating away of their role in delivering dental services.[49]

Despite the theoretician's descriptions of the important, evolving role of the "oral physician" who engages in complex diagnosis, treatment planning, sophisticated therapy, and team management,[12] the dentist who has been comfortable in a more simplified role may not become terribly excited about the changes.[49] The concept of "team" dentistry involving multiple personnel performing multifaceted services is not necessarily the goal of the contented solo practitioner. It may be that the results of the experimental programs and the accompanying legal and educational changes have pointed too clearly toward radical change that would begin to have a strong impact on

the grass roots dentist. Some dentists prefer to support changes that are good for the practitioner, saying that what is good for dentistry will provide the best outcome for the population.[11] The dentists of the early 1960s may have enjoyed speculating about radical change and they may have enjoyed tinkering with management of time and motion, but they may now be shocked to discover how closely the speculations have come to being transformed into reality. The ADA has called for dentists to be utilized to fullest capacity before auxiliaries receive expanded functions.[6,7] Dentistry is, quite understandably, interested in utilizing the available manpower in dentistry before developing roles for dental auxiliaries.

The only certainty for the future is that of change. The movement to develop a system of team dentistry that provides comprehensive dental care to every patient as a right rather than as a luxury is reliant on the resolution of the issue of which functions may be performed by whom and under what degree of supervision. The resolution will come from organized dentistry, the individual states, education, the federal government, auxiliaries, and the consumer. It will need to be generated among them, cooperating, all working toward a common goal. The issue yet to be addressed is whether the team concept described will indeed have impact on the oral health of the nation's people. That objective and yet-to-be-measured outcome must emerge at the top of the priority list. The question remains: Is the goal to provide more health services or to improve health?

Review questions

1. Describe briefly the current system of delivery of dental health care services:
2. The primary stimulus for attempts to modify the delivery of dental care in the early 1960s was:
3. The two early 1970s reports that shifted the reason for modifying dental care delivery are:
   a.
   b.
4. List three reasons why dentists turned to dental assistants in conducting experimentation in expanded functions:
   a.
   b.
   c.
5. Describe briefly the ADA's response to results of experiments that demonstrate the degree to which auxiliaries can perform services traditionally defined as the practice of dentistry.
6. List the sources of influence that have shaped the dental care system and that are affected by proposed changes.
   a.
   b.
   c.
   d.
   e.
   f.

ANSWERS

1. It is a cottage industry comprised mainly of solo dentist practitioners who have little contact with other health care providers. It operates primarily on a fee-for-service basis, although this is rapidly changing. It is not often involved in comprehensive area health planning and often is characterized by geographic maldistribution of providers. There is no formal widespread system of peer review. Dentists use few categories of health care providers for auxiliary support, and they exercise considerable control over the care such auxiliaries provide.

2. The threat of a population explosion in the 1960s and 1970s.

3. a. Carnegie Commission Report of 1970.
   b. National Health Surveys

4. a. There were more of them.
   b. They are not restricted by licensing laws.
   c. They seemed to be more readily integrated logistically into the provision of restorative services.

5. The ADA has acknowledged that services *can* be delegated to auxiliaries, but they question whether they *should* be. Position statements of the late 1970s indicate that dentistry has adopted a more conservative view of auxiliary utilization, essentially reversing its position of the 1960s and early 1970s.

6. a. ADA
   b. State licensing laws and boards of dentistry
   c. Educational programs
   d. Federal government
   e. Consumers
   f. ADAA and ADHA (auxiliaries in general)

GROUP ACTIVITIES

1. Trace the ADA's position with regard to expanded functions for dental auxiliaries by reviewing their policy statements from 1960 to the present.
2. Trace ADAA's and the ADHA's positions with regard to expanded functions from 1960 to the present.
3. Review the literature for descriptions of the debate surrounding the 1950 and the 1975 closings of the Forsyth experimental projects. Identify similarities as well as differences in the debate.

REFERENCES

1. American Association of Dental Schools, 17-76-H, Amendment of 27-73-H.
1a. American Dental Association, 217-1972-H.
2. American Dental Association, 77-1972-H.
3. American Dental Association, 78-1972-H.
4. American Dental Association, 50-1973-H.
5. American Dental Association, 87-1973-H.
6. American Dental Association, 8-1976-H.
7. American Dental Association, 33-1976-H.
8. American Dental Association, 24-1976-H.
9. American Dental Association, 127-1976-H.
10. Barish, Anna M. and Barish, Nathan H.: Will dental hygiene become obsolete? J. Am. Dent. Hyg. Assoc., **45**:47.
11. Bhaskar, S. N.: Expanded-duty auxiliaries: opinions and perspectives, Dent. Surv., **52**:17.
12. Bohannon, Harry M., and others: A concept of the flexible dental curriculum. Presented at the Conference of Dental Examiners and Dental Educators, American Dental Association, February 12, 1971, Chicago.
13. Born, David Omar: Factors affecting the distribution of dental auxiliaries. In Proceedings of the workshop on changing roles of dental auxiliaries, Bethesda, Md., 1975, U.S. Dept. of Health, Education and Welfare, PHS-HRA, Bureau of Health Manpower, Division of Dentistry.
14. Carnegie Commission on Higher Education. Higher education and the nation's health: policies of medical and dental education. Special report and recommendation, New York, 1970, McGraw-Hill Book Co.
15. Cavicchio, Patricia Monahan: An overview of dental hygiene expanded duties projects and consideration of relevant changes in state dental practice acts. In Hayden, Hermine, editor: Training workshop on expanded functions for dental hygienists, Honolulu, 1971, District XI, American Dental Hygienists Association.
15a. Cohen, D. Walter: University of Pennsylvania, personal communication.
15b. Colchamiro, Stephen: The challenge of dentistry in neighborhood health centers, J. Public Health Dent., **36**:254.
16. Council on Dental Education–Commission on Accreditation of Dental and Dental Auxiliary Educational Programs 1975 Annual Report (Excerpt). In Proceedings of the workshop on changing roles of dental auxiliaries, Bethesda, Md., 1975, U.S. Dept. of Health, Education and Welfare, PHS-HRA, Bureau of Health Manpower, Division of Dentistry.
17. Cooper, Thomas M: Four-handed dentistry in the team practice of dentistry, Dent. Clin. North Am., **18**:739.
18. Cramer, John R.: Development of a local anesthesia course, Presented at American Association of Dental Schools, Dental Hygiene Section, 1973.
19. Dental practice act provisions for delegating expanded functions to dental hygienists and dental assistants, Chicago, 1976, American Dental Association, Division of Educational Measurements, Council on Dental Education.
19a. Denturism in Ontario—a case study, Insights, February 15, 1977.
20. DiBiaggio, J. A.: Academic freedom—a test case, Dent. Student News, **5**:1.
21. DuGas, Beverly Witter: Nursing's expanded role in Canada, Nurs. Clin. North Am., **9**:523.
21a. Eglit, Howard C. and Hauber, Carl H.: The constitutionality of state restrictions imposed upon the dental hygiene education system, Educational Directions, **1**:15.
21b. Fight against denturism in the U.S.A., Insights, March 15, 1977.
22. Gilman, C. W.: Comments on the inter-agency committee on dental auxiliaries, J. Am. Dent. Assoc., **45**:32.
23. Gladstone, Rhoda Nash: International dental nurse programs, Dent. Hyg., **49**:169.
24. Goldhaber, Paul: Improving the dental health status in the United States—putting your money where your mouth is, J. Dent. Educ., **41**:50.
25. Greene, John C.: Dental auxiliaries and national health insurance, J. Am. Dent. Hyg. Assoc., **46**:97.
26. Guidelines for dentistry's position in a national health program, J. Am. Dent. Assoc., **83**:1226.
27. Guidelines for the expanded function dental auxiliary (EFDA) training program, Bethesda, Md., 1975, U.S. Dept. of Health, Education and Welfare, PHS-HRA, Bureau of Health Manpower, Division of Dentistry.
28. Hayden, Hermine, editor: Introduction, Training workshop on expanded functions for dental hygienists, Honolulu, 1971, District XI, American Dental Hygienists Association.
28a. Helfman, Murry: The dentist-to-patient ratio: what should it be? JADA, **93**:525.
29. Hobbs, Evelyn R., Morgan, Joann S., and Irby, David M.: Factors influencing the need for dental auxiliary curriculum changes: Washington state—

1974. A report prepared for Curriculum Task Force, Washington State Coordinating Committee for Dental Auxiliary Education.

29a. Hygienists in Massachusetts to receive training in dentistry for children, JADA, **40**:77.

30. Invitational conferences on certification in allied health professions, reference materials, College Park, Md., 1971, American Society of Allied Health Professions.

31. Jacobs, Richard M.: Reflections on the controversy over expanded function dental auxiliaries, J. Dent. Educ., **40**:332.

32. Jerge, Charles R., and others, editors: Group practice and the future of dental care, Philadelphia, 1974, Lea and Febiger.

33. Jones, Patricia Faust: The changing role of the dental hygienist. In Boundy, Suzanne Styers and Reynolds, Nancy J., editors: Current concepts in dental hygiene, St. Louis, 1977, The C. V. Mosby Co.

34. Kerr, I. Lawrence: Changing roles of dental auxiliaries, keynote address. In Proceedings of the workshop on changing roles of dental auxiliaries, Bethesda, Md., 1975, U.S. Dept. of Health, Education and Welfare, PHS-HRA, Bureau of Health Manpower, Division of Dentistry.

35. Legislation: Massachusetts, JADA, **40**:115.

36. Lobene, Ralph R., and others: The Forsyth experiment in training of advanced skills hygienists, J. Dent. Educ., **38**:369.

37. Maas, Evelyn: President's corner, J. Am. Dent. Hyg. Assoc. **24**:37.

38. McGovern, Frederick J.: Expansion of duties of dental assistants and dental hygienists. In Hayden, Hermine, editor: Training workshop on expanded functions for dental hygienists, Honolulu, 1971, District XI, American Dental Hygienists Association.

39. Murdock, Gerald I.: Implementation of expanded duties in two-year dental hygiene programs, Unpublished paper, 1973.

40. Powell, William O., and others: Comparison of clinical performance of dental therapist trainees and dental students, J. Dent. Educ., **38**:268.

40a. Quality Assurance System Field Test, Letter from C. Gordon Watson to Maynard K. Hine, American Dental Association, June 14, 1977.

41. Redig, Dale F.: The team program and its implications for expanded duties for dental hygienists. In Hayden, Hermine, editor: Training workshop on expanded functions for dental hygienists, Honolulu, 1971, District XI, American Dental Hygienists Association.

42. Robinson, Hamilton B. G.: Academic freedom and the issue of expanded-duty auxiliaries, Dent. Surv., **52**:12.

43. Roemer, Ruth: Credentialing dental auxiliary personnel in the United States and selected other countries. In Proceedings of the workshop on changing roles of dental auxiliaries, Bethesda, Md., 1975, U.S. Dept. of Health, Education and Welfare, PHS-HRA, Bureau of Health Manpower, Division of Dentistry.

44. Sisty, Nancy L.: Experimental program for dental hygienists at the University of Iowa, In Mescher, Kay, editor: Training workshop on adaptation of dental hygiene practice to changing concepts in delivery of oral health services, Little Amana, Iowa, 1972, Iowa Dental Hygienists Association.

45. Social Security Amendments of 1972 (P.L. 92-603).

46. Spohn, Eric: Background and transition of the expanded duty program. In agenda material of the meeting of the Educational Advisory Committee for the University of Kentucky expanded duty dental hygiene research program, June 1975.

47. Mescher, Kay, editor: Summary of workshop discussions in Training workshop on adaptation of dental hygiene practice to changing concepts in delivery of oral health services, Little Amana, Iowa, 1972, Iowa Dental Hygienists Association.

47a. Trends for the future—quality assurance in ambulatory health care, Insights, April 15, 1977.

48. U.S. Public Health Service, Dept. of Health, Education and Welfare, National Health Surveys, 1969 to 1972.

49. Waldman, H. Barry: Is dentistry's future threatened? Dent. Surv., **51**:50.

50. Williams, Carlton H.: Are dental hygiene concepts changing? J. Am. Dent. Hyg. Assoc., **45**:30.

CHAPTER 4

Educational requirements and credentialing procedures and standards for health care providers

OBJECTIVES: The reader will be able to:

1. Briefly explain the purpose and role of educational standards and credentialing in the regulation of health care providers.
2. Define *accreditation*.
3. Identify three problems created by the fragmented system of accreditation of allied health education programs.
4. Given descriptions of credentialing processes for health care providers, identify whether the process is an example of:
   a. *Licensure*
   b. *Certification*
   c. *Registration*
   d. *Institutional licensure*
5. Explain the legal and economic constraints placed upon employers that enforce the utilization of persons credentialed by licensure or certification.
6. Describe the advantages and disadvantages of licensure and certification.
7. Describe briefly the allied health movement.
8. Explain briefly the cause of the great variety of methods of credentialing allied health personnel.
9. Describe the trend toward national certification of health personnel and explain the rationale for this trend.
10. Identify two similarities and two differences between:
    a. Nursing and dental hygiene
    b. Dental assisting and dental hygiene

The primary reason for standards of education and credentialing for health care providers is to ensure that the public receives quality care. Accreditation and credentialing, by themselves, cannot guarantee appropriate care, but they can influence programs to offer curricula that will adequately prepare persons for practice and they can establish whether the candidate for practice possesses the knowledge and skill to deliver adequate care. Both accreditation and credentialing are focal points of control over the delivery of care and the maturation of the professional group of providers.

ACCREDITATION

Accreditation has been defined as a form of "regulation or control which is exercised over educational institutions and/or programs by external organizations or agencies."[11] It is a "process whereby an association or agency grants public recognition to a school, institute, college, university, or specialized program of study having met certain established qualifications or standards as determined through initial and periodic evaluations."[11] Institutions typically seek accreditation from a regional accrediting agency that evaluates the institution as a whole and from the individual specialty accreditation agencies for the specific programs offered that require accreditation for recognition.

In addition to serving as a determinant of an educational program's quality, accreditation has served as a means for establishing control over a specialty area of education by a special interest group.[12] The accrediting body has great power in determining the future of a professional group or subspecialty by specifying which educational components and which educational structures are appropriate for that group. For instance, the profession of nursing has control of its own accreditation process.[7] The individual state boards of nursing accredit the programs established within their jurisdiction. The authority to accredit is granted to the boards of nursing and the National League for Nursing. The fact that nursing controls accreditation gives it far greater control over the growth and direction of its profession than dental hygiene and dental assisting, for instance, have in the control of their respective professions. Both dental hygiene and assisting programs are accredited by the American Dental Association (ADA) Commission on Accreditation of Dental and Dental Auxiliary Educational Programs.[11] In this case, dentistry has control over the "growth and direction" possible in educational programs. The two auxiliaries rely on the input of their representation on the Commission and on the wisdom of the dentists in control.

FRAGMENTATION OF ACCREDITING SYSTEMS

With the tremendous growth in the number of allied health professions during the 1960s, mechanisms for accrediting educational programs to prepare those professionals proliferated as well. This caused several difficulties to develop for (1) institutions offering allied health programs, (2) the federal government, and (3) potential employers,[11,12] especially in terms of role definition.

With the proliferation of accrediting agencies and mechanisms, educational institutions could expect a separate interest-group accreditation visit for every health program offered, in addition to that of the regional accrediting agency. For an institution offering fifteen allied health programs, an inordinate amount of time could be expected to be spent preparing for numerous individual accreditation site visits and preparing reports—each with a different format.

The United States Office of Education of the Department of Health, Education and Welfare has identified the proliferation of accrediting agencies as a serious problem.[12] That Office, as well as the health education divisions of the Public Health Service, has consistently deferred to accreditation as the "primary criterion base for federal funding." The federal government, through the Office of Education and the Public Health Service, has directed large amounts of federal funds to support special projects and improvements, as well as program development, in educational institutions. Reviewers of grant applications have used "accreditation" as a primary way of establishing whether the institution is able to carry out what it proposes to do if awarded funds. The government has expressed its discomfort with blanketly accepting accreditation status when so little has been known about the process that has been so fragmented.

Employers, particularly in large health care facilities, who have had no central source of information regarding the accreditation requirements enforced for various allied health professions, have had difficulty determining appropriate role definitions and staffing patterns.[8,9]

At the 1970 Annual Meeting of the Association of Schools of Allied Health Professions, Dr. William K. Selden described a study of accreditation that would address the complexity and fragmentation of accreditation. The seven specific areas that were to be considered in the study were listed as: (1) accountability, (2) structure, (3) expansion, (4) financing, (5) research, (6) the relationship between accreditation and licensure, and (7) the relationship between accreditation and certification.[19]

The study was completed by the National Commission on Accrediting and a report filed in 1972, recommending that an independent Joint Council for the Accreditation of Allied Health Education be established. The Council was to be national (but not federal), thereby minimizing redundancy in evaluation but remaining free of government control.[18]

CREDENTIALING PROCESSES FOR HEALTH CARE PROVIDERS

Credentialing of the individual health care provider is different from accreditation of an educational institution.[11] It addresses itself to the capabilities of the person who has completed a formal education and wishes to enter the workforce to provide care. It is similar to accreditation in that it is often administered by the same group who controls the accreditation process and because it is a force that shapes the nature of the profession for which the person is being credentialed. Both accreditation and individual credentialing involve standards for approval and utilize measurement processes to determine whether the standards are met.

Licensure and certification

Licensure and *certification* are utilized for credentialing allied health personnel. "Licensure is the credentialing mechanism or process by which an agency of the government (usually the state) grants permission to persons meeting predetermined qualifications to engage in a given occupation and/or use a particular title, or grants permission to institutions (such as hospitals, nursing homes) to perform specified functions."[19] Dental hygiene, dentistry, optometry, nursing, osteopathy, medicine, and pharmacy are examples of health professions that are licensed in all states and the District of Columbia. Legislation enacted by the state grants that licensing power to an agency, such as a state board, in order to protect the public from unqualified persons. The individual state dental practice acts are examples of such legislation. They empower the state boards of dentistry to regulate dentistry and dental hygiene by examining candidates for licensure and by ensuring that licensees remain within the law while providing care.[10,19]

Certification refers to the "process by which a non-government agency or association grants recognition to an individual who has met certain predetermined qualifications specified by that agency or association. Such qualifications may include: (1) graduation from an accredited or approved program of study, (2) acceptable performance on a qualifying examination or series of examinations, and/or (3) completion of a stated amount of work experience." The primary distinction between licensure and certification is that the former is granted by the state whereas the latter is granted by a nongovernmental agency, usually the professional association.[19]

Both licensure and certification imply a "restraint of trade."[15] The credentialing process does prohibit unqualified persons from entering the workforce to perform services reserved for the licensed or certified person. In the case of licensure, the law specifies that an employer may not hire an unlicensed person to provide those services. The law also warns charlatans that to perform restricted services is a criminal offense. In the case of certification, the enforcement is economic rather than legal. In order for a health care facility, such as a hospital, to receive third-party reimbursement for services delivered at the facility, the facility must be accredited by the Joint Commission on Accreditation of Hospitals.[6] In order to be accredited, the facility must employ only those persons who are qualified to provide care. The Joint Commission recognizes professional associations' certification of their members as an appropriate credential to designate persons as "qualified."[6] Therefore, in order to collect third-party payments, only certified persons must be employed in the key positions specified by the Joint Commission.

In order to enforce licensure restrictions, the state must send out investigators to scrutinize the credentials of persons providing care, an insurmountable task in a cottage industry such as dentistry. The enforcement of accreditation requirements to employ only certified persons occurs every few years for every hospital.[6]

The dental hygienist and dental assistant provide excellent examples of two allied health personnel who provide patient care but who are regulated under different mechanisms. The dental hygienist is licensed by the state according to the criteria stated in the law, after a minimum 2-year educational program.* The dental assistant is certified by the American Dental Assistants Association (ADAA) after graduating from an approved (accredited) dental assisting program of at least 1 academic year and successfully completing an examination. It is also necessary that continuing education be demonstrated each year.

Licensure has worked to the advantage of the hygienist more than certification has worked to the advantage of the dental assistant because of the nature of the health system in which dental care is delivered. It should be remembered that dentistry has been a fee-for-service enterprise, rarely located in a hospital facility. With no accreditation visits provided by the Joint Commission in individual dental offices and (until recently) little reason to be overly concerned about preferential status in the eyes of third-party payors, dentistry had no economic reason to employ only certified dental assistants. There was, however, a legal mandate to employ only licensed hygienists to perform dental hygiene care.

There is some possibility that certification will be meaningful in dentistry, just as it is in the delivery of medical care. Dentists in group practice saw the need to establish a mechanism by which group practices could be "accredited" for purposes of being "excepted" from the scrupulous scrutiny of third-party payors. In November 1976 the American Academy of Group Practice Dentists agreed to an accreditation mechanism and standards of practice.[1] If the employment of only certified personnel is added to the standards, dental assisting may, for economic reasons, enjoy the same security dental hygiene has enjoyed for legal reasons.

Registration

The term *registration* is often used interchangeably with licensure and certification. Actually it is synonymous with neither. Registration is the process by which an individual is listed on an official roster maintained by the state or the nongovernmental agency offering certification. The registration process is used to describe the rostering process rather than the credentialing process.

Institutional licensure

Another distinct form of credentialing that has been discussed in medical fields is *institutional licensure*.[5] Institutional licensure would grant to an institution such as a hospital or health maintenance organization the authority to define the role and responsibility of personnel on the basis of manpower need in the facility and on the basis of the individual skills of the personnel employed. The institution would in effect control credentialing internally and be free to create staffing patterns based on its assessments. Few health care providers have voiced support for this alternative, despite the flexibility it would provide. It removes credentialing control from the professions and places it in the hands of administrators of health care facilities.

The primary reason for suggesting the alternative is the need to sort out the vast array of certification requirements that the myriad of categories of allied health personnel have developed. Each category of worker has distinct criteria and a unique registration process, which again causes many headaches for employers attempting to create reasonable staffing patterns that meet accreditation standards.[9]

---

*Alabama is the only state that licenses persons as dental hygienists without requiring formal education.

DEVELOPMENT OF PROFESSIONAL REGULATION

Historically, health professions began to adopt standards of professional competence prior to 1800 when the medical profession was concerned about the training and conduct of practitioners and had appealed to the individual states to establish and enforce controls. The most notable move toward the development of professional regulation occurred in the midnineteenth century when professional associations were founded and licensure became more prevalent. The associations began to exert control over the educational institutions in order to improve and standardize educational programs. The American Medical Association was formed in 1847, the American Pharmaceutical Association in 1852, and the American Dental Association in 1859.[11]

Those professions that were established to support medical and dental services were organized and regulated toward the late nineteenth and early twentieth centuries. The American Nurses Association was established in 1896, and the American Dental Hygienists Association (ADHA) in 1923. Licensure was the primary mechanism for regulation during that period since there was no source for an economic mandate for employers to hire only those persons who held appropriate credentials. The legal constraint was the only mandate available.

The period for the development and delineation of health care providers as supporters of dentistry and (primarily) medicine occurred after World War II, with greatest growth during the late 1960s. The allied health movement began when the necessities of war proved that persons could be prepared to perform various medical procedures without being physicians. Schools of allied medical professions were established and new categories of health workers developed to extend care to civilians in the postwar era. They were known, at first, as paraprofessionals or paramedical personnel. The terms auxiliary and ancillary were also used in the early years of development, but those terms were dropped as being nonreflective of the scope of responsibility the providers had in the delivery of health care.

The terms allied health professional, physician extender, and mid-level practitioner were used to describe the rapidly growing group of health workers who were established as the complexities of comprehensive health care demanded greater specialization among providers, particularly those who carry out the orders of the physician with specialized equipment and therapy. New advances in renal care, cardiology, medical technology, respiratory therapy, and nuclear medicine dictated that highly skilled technicians would be needed to operate the sophisticated equipment and to carry out the prescribed orders of the physician. With the health manpower scare of the early 1960s and the Allied Health Manpower Training Act of 1966 that funded new programs for such personnel and that supported enrollment increases, new categories of health workers burgeoned. There was a specialist for every type of medical equipment and often an assistant for that person, each with a specified curriculum and specific standards to be met for association certification. No comprehensive plan was developed or followed.

THE ALLIED HEALTH MOVEMENT

Certification was almost always the credentialing mechanism of choice for the new categories of health personnel.[8] Licensure had proved to be effective in mandating that only qualified personnel perform the stated health services, but it had also proved to be a cumbersome mechanism with which to work when the scope of practice of the licensed person needed to be altered to meet the changing demands of health care delivery and to be in conformance with the changes in the educational programs of the profession.[7a] Licensure changes required legislative change.[15] Certification usually required only a change in association policy and procedure.

Therefore as a matter of expediency in

credentialing the new categories of workers and as a means of ensuring professional control over health workers the professional associations assumed the responsibility of credentialing those persons. The variety of criteria and processes to which the new categories of health care providers were subjected caused, as noted earlier, considerable difficulty for those employers and agencies concerned with determining whether an individual health care worker was indeed properly credentialed.[9] In 1971 the Department of Health, Education and Welfare funded a contract with the American Society of Allied Health Professions to convene an invitational conference at the University of Maryland. The purpose of the conference was to identify the problems and commonalities of the various allied health organizations with regard to credentialing procedures. The major recommendation that evolved from that conference was the need for a study of the possibility of formalizing a national voluntary system for certification that would serve allied health professionals in establishing competency to practice and that would award appropriate certification. The Institute of Public Administration conducted a 2-year study. In 1975 another conference was convened to review the results of the study. The recommendation from that conference was that the workability and possible creation of such a commission be explored.[14] The American Society of Allied Health Professions worked with fifteen health organizations to define such a structure and to describe its purpose and the mechanisms for funding such a commission. Both the ADAA and the ADHA were involved, as was the ADA. At its final certification conference the Steering Committee for the development of a National Commission for Health Credentialing Agencies (as it was called) presented eight recommendations that were modified and agreed upon by the conference participants. The recommendations called for the creation of a national, voluntary commission of health certification, with the primary purpose being to estab-lish standards for recognizing certifying bodies and to monitor their adherence to those standards, thereby promoting public accountability. Membership in the commission was described as including certifying agencies that attest to the competency of health practitioners, professional associations of those certified occupations, professional health societies, groups of lay public representatives, and governmental agencies.[17]

COMPETENCY ASSURANCE

This type of regulatory agency, which is directed to establish criteria for assessing the effectiveness of certifying agencies, is an attempt to standardize the way in which people are assessed for their competence to practice. It is *not* a federal or governmental bureau. Its intention is not to create one mechanism for all health care providers, but rather to direct credentialing processes into predictable patterns. The direction is *competency assurance*, a move away from norm-referenced evaluation of practitioners and toward criterion-referenced evaluation.[2]

The move toward competency assurance has followed a decade or more of delineation of practice roles in terms of *task analyses*, where professional functions were described in increments of activities and in behavioral terms.[20] Educational programs used these task analyses to identify and justify the components of learning necessary for their students to master the defined tasks. Professional organizations have used them to identify levels of competence for practice by developing measures for entry and for continued assessment of practitioners with continuing education packages prepared to bolster those areas of each person's expertise in need of improvement. No longer is the provider measured against what the average provider knows or does. Rather, the provider is measured against *standards of competence* that are agreed upon by educational programs, agencies responsible for credentialing health care providers, and those organizations measuring continued competence and providing continuing education.[2,3,20]

The shift from measurement against peers to measurement against standards has been a slow process, partly because of the necessity that standards be defined in reasonable, explicit, measurable behavioral terms. This required a great deal of skill on the part of those preparing the standards—skill that developed as educators and professionals continued to draft and refine the objectives in an effort to specify exactly what it is they look for in evaluating a student or practitioner.[13,20] Judgments about attitudes needed to be specified in observable behaviors, with the question, "What do I see that leads me to conclude that?" asked repeatedly.

It had usually been the practice to gather a number of test items or practical exercises for a group to be evaluated and then to determine the number who passed or failed on the basis of how the *group* performed. Those who performed better than the group scored well. There was usually a larger portion who did about average. A certain percentage who did worse than the rest of the group failed. No specific, minimum, predetermined performance level was required in most instances. As a result, even if a person were to have correctly performed only 60% of the tasks in the evaluation, if most of the group achieved 50%, the person would pass with a high percentile ranking. Likewise, if a person were to score 80% when the group scored 90%, there would be a possibility that he/she would fail the examination, or at least be in a low percentile. Students may recognize this process as "curving" grades. The "curve" refers to the ignominious bell curve that educators used for years as a measure of teaching success. The curve relates to a line drawn on the *x* and *y* axes showing a few very low grades, a few very high grades, and a large number of average or mediocre grades.

In an age of accountability, when the student and the consumer expect appropriate performance, "norming" is becoming less acceptable. What is growing in acceptance is criterion-referenced or competency based measurement that specifies the performance, measures the performance, and provides a diagnosis of skill deficiencies and mastered competencies.[2,3]

The *Curriculum Essentials* document of the ADHA details the competencies of the dental hygienist. It is the result of a decade of task analysis, course content specification in behavioral objectives, and educational technology in mastery teaching and learning.[22] It is a benchmark for developing a system of education, competency assessment, and continuing education in terms of predetermined statements of that competence.

Other allied health professions are in various stages of role delineation and in developing criterion-referenced proficiency tests. The American Occupational Therapy Association, the American Association for Respiratory Therapy, and the American Medical Records Association are three such groups. Proficiency examinations have been prepared for diagnostic radiologic technology, clinical laboratory technology, respiratory therapy, and occupational therapy. The American Society of Radiologic Technologists has developed a self-assessment continuing education program for all medical diagnostic x-ray machine operators. The allied health professions are moving ahead in competency assurance, partly in response to consumer expectations and partly in response to the newly acquired skills of the professions' leaders in defining those expectations.[2,3]

In the areas of accreditation, development of educational programs, and credentialing of personnel, the dental auxiliary professions have found a great deal in common with other allied health professions. The dental assistant, a certified health care provider, has been able to identify appropriate liaison activities with the many other certified professions. Dental hygiene has been able to establish a liaison in assessing its educational and credentialing systems and to call upon other group's experiences in measuring levels of competence.

There is no total agreement that increased affiliation with other allied health professions is a wise step for dental auxiliaries; however, it has served to identify the commonalities among providers of health care and has resulted in a sharing of resources and interests as the dental auxiliary professional organizations have attempted to achieve greater self-direction and to look for sources of leadership and guidance beyond the dental profession.

NURSING AND DENTAL HEALTH CARE PROFESSIONS

Many leaders in dental hygiene have identified nursing as the profession to which ADHA should turn for direction. This follows mostly from the fact that nursing is a well-established, *licensed* profession, which has successfully extricated itself from the dominance of the medical profession. Having started out as the handmaiden to the physician, nursing has established itself as a distinct profession. It has its own nursing practice acts and therefore its own state boards of nursing, accredits its own educational programs, and licenses its own members.[16] It is not controlled by the medical practice acts, nor is it subject to the American Medical Association. Nurses often practice quite independently of the physician's supervision. They dispense and administer prescribed medications, provide direct patient care, and are able to provide care that a decade ago was restricted to licensed physicians.[7] In Washington State, nurses are able to diagnose, prescribe medications, and perform minor surgery, predicated on appropriate educational preparation for these functions.[21]

Nursing is in some ways giant steps ahead of dental hygiene. Long before the development of the various allied health professions, nursing had gained control of its destiny. Its primary uphill fight in recent years has been to achieve consensus among its ranks regarding what its destiny should be.[7] Role delineation became a major concern

as the licensed practical nurse (LPN), a 1-year graduate, encroached on many of the functions of the traditional nurse. Hospital-based 3-year diploma programs have been phased out as 2-year associate degree programs based in junior and community colleges developed. In addition, 4-year colleges and universities offer baccalaureate programs in nursing. Masters programs prepare nurses for clinical specialties and teaching. There are even doctoral programs for nurses. The task has been to sort out the functions of "a nurse" who has graduated from any of the various levels of educational preparation in terms of appropriate job descriptions in health care delivery settings, while maintaining a system of state-by-state licensure regulation.

With the delegation of many traditional nursing services to the various allied health personnel (particularly the physician's assistant) and with services previously *not* legally delegated to nurses being delegated to other providers of care, nursing found itself in the midst of shifting occupational boundaries. It was during this period that nursing intensified its efforts to have greater responsibility in the delivery of care—particularly in communities or geographic regions where physicians are rarely available for care. Midwifery, for example, was revived as an appropriate clinical specialty for masters degree nurses specially educated for such a role. The pediatric nurse practitioner was developed as a direct patient care provider substituting in large part for the physician. This shifting of roles has created a credentialing problem for nursing, just as it has for allied health personnel.[7,16]

With various levels of nursing defined, there must be a provision for a series of competency measures. Despite the fact that nursing does not view itself as an allied health profession,[17] it shares problems and concerns with those newer groups of health care providers. It is struggling with the issues of proficiency testing, mandatory versus continuing education, foreign trained nurses, and standardized curricula.[7]

Dental hygiene leaders smile at the way in which the term *dental hygiene* can be read in place of *nursing* in the various articles written by and for nurses. The developmental struggles of a century of nursing now confront dental hygiene, and many of nursing's current struggles are concomitantly dental hygiene's.

DENTAL ASSISTING AND DENTAL HYGIENE

Another source of unity and strength exists between dental assisting and hygiene. ADAA and ADHA leaders attempted to formalize this unity in the early 1970s with "Project Alliance,"[4] a plan to consolidate the two associations' resources and to avoid duplication of effort in reaching members. The plan itself was never approved, but the two groups have moved closer to one another by means of the "Partners in Progress" annual meetings, where ADHA and ADAA present educational and scientific programs of interest to both auxiliaries. The two associations publish *Educational Directions*, a journal for dental auxiliary educators. The direction generally has been toward more frequent and more meaningful communication between the two groups. The late 1970s appears to be a time when the similarities outweigh the differences.

The issues for the future with regard to alliances with allied health, nursing, and dental hygiene and assisting are primarily related to what direction the dental health care providers will take in defining practice roles and degrees of supervision. Dentistry currently is in strong opposition to greater independence of auxiliaries and has blocked the few moves that have been made in that direction. It is likely that any major effort to assume responsibility for credentialing of dental hygiene practitioners and accreditation of educational programs for dental assisting or hygiene would be met with the disfavor of the ADA and the state boards of dentistry. Regardless of the direction for change and the outcome of efforts to guide dental auxiliaries toward a more responsible role, there is no question that liaison with other health care provider groups has helped dental assisting and hygiene acquire the skills for competent self-regulation and knowledge of the most progressive modes of assessment of students and practitioners.

Review questions

1. Why are accreditation and credentialing important components of the health care delivery system?
2. What are three problems created by the fragmented system of accreditation in the health care delivery system?
   a.
   b.
   c.
3. A state agency governed by a state practice act is empowered to (license/certify) a health care provider.
4. A professional association sets up criteria for assessing candidates for (licensure/certification) as health care providers.
5. Certification is not currently a strong mandate in dentistry for the employment of dental assistants because:
6. Why is there such great variety in the methods of credentialing allied health personnel?
7. Two similarities between nursing and dental hygiene are:
   a.
   b.
8. Two differences between nursing and dental hygiene are:
   a.
   b.
9. Two similarities between dental assisting and dental hygiene are:
   a.
   b.
10. Two differences between dental assisting and dental hygiene are:
    a.
    b.

ANSWERS

1. Together accreditation and credentialing provide methods for ensuring the quality of care delivered to the public. They also serve as a control over the growth and direction of the professions.
2. a. Multiple site visits by multiple interest groups to educational institutions
   b. The government relies on accreditation as a measure of an institution's ability to carry out grant projects and contracts.
   c. Employers are frustrated in attempting to define roles and responsibilities with such a scattered accreditation process.
3. License
4. Certification
5. Dentistry does not yet rely on third-party payment reimbursement and has had little reason to be "excepted" by such payors. Therefore, they have not been active, until recently, in accreditation of practices by any group that might specify *certified* personnel.
6. With the rapidly growing allied health movement of the 1960s, numerous categories of workers were created, each with its own certifying process. No comprehensive plan was followed.
7. a. Both are licensed.
   b. Both are long-standing, well established professions.
8. a. Nursing has its own practice act; dental hygiene is within the dental practice act.
   b. Nursing accredits its own educational programs; dental hygiene programs are accredited by the American Dental Association Commission on Accreditation.
9. a. Both auxiliaries' educational programs are accredited by the American Dental Association Commission on Accreditation.
   b. Both must work under the supervision of a dentist when providing intra-oral services.
10. a. Dental hygienists are licensed; assistants are certified.
    b. Dental hygienists have a minimum 2-year education; assistants have a 1-year minimum.

GROUP ACTIVITIES

1. Compare the specific credentialing requirements for:
   a. Respiratory therapists
   b. Dietitians
   c. Medical technologists
   d. Nurses
   e. Other health personnel of choice.
2. Review the requirements for accreditation of the Joint Commission on the Accreditation of Hospitals and those of the American Academy of Group Practice Dentists.

REFERENCES

1. American Academy of Dental Group Practice: Accreditation program for dental group practice: program description and requirements for accreditation, Madison, Wisc., 1976, The Academy.
2. Competency Assurance: Invitational Workshop materials, Bethesda, Md., 1976, U.S. Dept. of Health, Education and Welfare, PHS-HRA, Bureau of Health Manpower, Manpower Utilization Branch, Division of Associated Health Professions.
3. Conant, Robert M. and Hatch, Thomas D.: Policies for the development of credentialing mechanisms for health personnel, Am. J. Occup. Ther., **28:** 288.
4. Gandy, Kay: Project Alliance—The implications for the future of our association and cooperative working relationships with other allied oral health organizations. In Hayden, Hermine, editor: Training workshop on expanded functions for dental hygienists, Honolulu, 1971, District XI, American Dental Hygienists Association.
5. Guy, Joan S.: Institutional licensure: a dilemma for nurses, Nurs. Clin. North Am., **9:**497.
6. Joint Commission on the Accreditation of Hospitals, Accreditation manual for hospitals, Chicago, 1976, The Commission.
7. Kelly, Lucy Young: Nursing practice acts, Am. J. Nurs., **74:**1310.
7a. Kolar, Mary Jane: Viewpoint from a licensed profession, Dental Assistant, **45:**17 (Sept.).
8. Light, Israel: Development and growth of new allied health fields, J. Am. Med. Assoc., **210:**114.
9. Mansfield, Edgar O.: How the health care administrator looks at certification of allied health personnel in a changing health care system. An abstract in conference materials for an Invitational Conference on Certification in Allied Health Professions, College Park, Md., 1971, American Society of Allied Health Professions.
10. Manual for consultants to state boards of dentistry, Chicago, 1973, American Dental Hygienists Association.
11. Pennell, Maryland Y., Proffitt, John R., and Hatch, Thomas D.: Accreditation and certification in relation to allied health manpower, Bethesda, Md., 1972, U.S. Dept. of Health, Education and Welfare, PHS-NIH, Bureau of Health Manpower Education, p. 3.
12. Proffitt, John R.: Accreditation as a stabilizing force in allied health professions, J. Am. Med. Assoc., **213:**604.
13. Popham, W. James: Measurement advances for educational evaluators. Presented at the symposium on The Expanding Technology of Educational Evaluation, Annual Meeting of the American Educational Research Association, Chicago, April 15-19, 1974.
14. Report of the meeting to discuss the feasibility of a national system of certification for allied health personnel, Bethesda, Md., January 1975, U.S. Dept. of Health, Education and Welfare, PHS-HRA, Bureau of Health Manpower Education, Division of Associated Health Professions.
15. Restrictive licensing of dental paraprofessionals, Yale Law Journal, **83:**806.
16. Stahl, Adele G.: State boards of nursing: legal aspects, Nurs. Clin. North Am., **9:**505.
17. Steering Committee for the Development of a National Commission for Health Credentialing Agencies, Proceedings, Certification Conference, Kansas City, August 1976.
18. Study of accreditation of selected health educational programs, Commission Report, Washington, D.C., 1972, National Commission on Accrediting.
19. Study of accreditation of selected health educational programs. In conference materials for an Invitational Conference on Certification in Allied Health Professions, College Park, Md., 1971, American Society of Allied Health Professions.
20. Terry, David R. and Evans, Rupert N.: Determining behavioral task content of the curriculum in occupational and professional educational programs: The dental auxiliaries, Final report of Grant No. MB 0014 supported by Office of Special Programs, Bureau of Health Manpower, PHS-HRA, U.S. Dept. of Health, Education and Welfare, May 1975.
21. Where R.N.s can diagnose and prescribe, RN, **36:** 31.
22. Woodall, Irene R., editor: Curriculum essentials, ed. 4, Chicago, 1977, American Dental Hygienists Association.

CHAPTER 5

The quality of care: the consumer interest, peer review, and continuing competence

OBJECTIVES: The reader will be able to:

1. State the three issues upon which consumers have focused primary concerns and complaints with regard to the delivery of health care services.
2. Explain three ways in which consumers have gained influence with regard to the way in which the health care system functions.
3. Identify the ways in which health care is monitored for its quality.
4. Differentiate *audit* and *peer review* as two mechanisms for assessment.
5. Describe a mechanism for auditing patient records that can be instituted in a health care practice or local professional organization.
6. Explain two ways in which peer review mechanisms can function to assess the quality of health care in a health care practice or professional organization.
7. Describe a mechanism that can relate assessment of quality of care to programs for continuing education (continued competence).
8. Outline a functional program for continuing education that could satisfy the need to establish a relationship between continuing education and improved quality of care.

THE CONSUMER MOVEMENT

The late 1960s marked a period when consumer awareness was awakened. Ralph Nader, in his book *Unsafe at Any Speed*, described how a major auto manufacturer had designed and was selling a product that was proved to be unsafe and a contributor to a number of accidents.[11] While many at first may have found such a book to be laughable in terms of its having any influence on big business, the auto described in that book was taken off the market a few years later. If the auto manufacturer did not respond immediately to the need to improve the auto's design to improve its safety, it did eventually respond to the fact that people were no longer purchasing that product in sufficient numbers to warrant its continued production. The consumer had triumphed, in a landmark confrontation, in causing business to improve or retract its faulty merchandise.

Ralph Nader has since continued his mission, investigating a number of industries, including the dental profession. He took the dental profession to task for what he believed was the unscrupulous use of x-radiation.[12] The article resulted in practicing dental personnel needing to explain again and again to patients the rationale for the radiographs that needed to be exposed. There is no question that the article had a dramatic effect upon the public's awareness of their right to question the services they receive, including health care services.

Mr. Nader has reviewed the United States Congress, as well, publishing fact sheets about the attendance records, voting records, responsiveness, and productivity of each of the constituency's representatives. The extent to which this investigative program has affected industry and government is not limited to what that one man could perform. With the advent of the Nader reports came a

52

number of other consumer advocates who formed consumer organizations in order to inform buyers of unscrupulous business and professional persons and to provide advice to those seeking restitution when a product or service they purchased was shown to be inadequate or dangerous.

Dry cereals, long the staple of the American breakfast table, were examined for the nutrition they provided, resulting, in part, in legislation requiring food processors to include nutritive value amounts on their packages. Toy manufacturers were scrutinized for the quality and safety of the products they produce; consumer awareness announcements were carried on national television prior to the December holidays to inform shoppers of the dangers of some toys. Journalism turned increasingly to ferreting out those aspects of private enterprise that were suspect in their handling of the public, with newspaper columns devoted to assisting exasperated customers in achieving satisfaction and with television programming featuring several "in-depth analyses" of corruption in nursing homes, camps for children, hospitals, and any other endeavors, public or private, that squandered people's money or provided less than a fair return for the investment made.

CONSUMERS AND THE HEALTH CARE SYSTEM

As noted previously, health care was not immune to this growing interest in what consumers were receiving in return for their money. Consumers organized to form a strong lobbying force in the state and federal governments.[7a] Numerous pieces of legislation have been influenced by this interest group. As consumers they represent the American public as a whole, which is a force that is difficult to ignore in the legislature. Elected officials are eager to be seen in the light of consumer protectors and as responsive to the needs of the individual.

One of the forms of legislation consumer groups have been active in shaping is the continuing stream of proposals for national

health insurance.[1,7a] The public has been vocal in its displeasure with the health care system in this country. The high cost of care, the frequent inaccessibility of care, and the quality of care received are matters of concern.[1,7a] Congressional hearings include numerous pieces of testimony regarding the inadequacies of the system. The consumers have asked the legislature to enact laws to initiate a program that will improve the situation. With the election of Jimmy Carter to the Presidency in 1976 and the appointment of Joseph Califano as Secretary of Health, Education and Welfare, there is reason to believe that national health insurance will be enacted. Secretary Califano was involved in the "Great Society" era of Lyndon Johnson in the 1960s, during which time Medicare was enacted. He indicated shortly after his appointment that one of his primary objectives as Secretary was to reconstruct the Medicare claims system so that the fraud that has been associated with the operation of that program can be greatly reduced and hopefully eliminated. If this objective is met, the Congress may look more favorably upon establishing a larger scale national insurance program to ensure the health of the public.

While political lobbying has certainly been a strong force in the consumer movement to improve health care, consumers have made other inroads in affecting the health care system. Consumers objected to the way in which state boards controlling the practice of health care providers did not include consumer representation, or "public members." Their goal is to ensure that the state boards are indeed protecting the public as they are mandated in the law and that they are not serving as a guild to control the numbers of practitioners or using questionable procedures in regulating the practice of dental personnel already licensed.[10] The American Dental Association has had limited support for the inclusion of public members on review boards or state boards of dentistry or in any of the other decision-making components of the profession.

Consumers have been involved at least in

the development of systems of peer review. Indirectly, they have affected private and public sector reviews of the quality of care through private insurance carriers and public assistance programs that cover dental care. These third-party payors conduct reviews of work to be performed and often evaluate the quality of the finished product before paying the health care provider.[4,5,16]

In addition to the more overt involvement of consumers in the legislative process and on state and private regulatory agencies, the consumer awareness era has spawned a plethora of articles describing how good dental work can be found and how it can be evaluated by laypersons. These articles are written by inquiring consumers who have made it their business to investigate the health care industry[14] and by providers of care who feel a sense of responsibility for the well-being of the public (and who, perhaps, recognize the ready market for such a publication).[9,15]

The landmark consumer awareness text for dentistry is *Dentistry and Its Victims*, written by "Paul Revere," D.D.S.[15] The book describes what to watch for in dental care and is less than complimentary in its evaluation of the kind of dentistry most patients receive. It stirred considerable wrath in the dental community since it marked a defection on the part of a dentist from the self-protective society of dentists. It had long been an unwritten "ethical rule" of associations to refrain from discrediting the profession.

The most significant impacts consumer awareness may have on the individual provider are: patients' increased confidence in challenging treatment plans, in deciding to change providers when displeased, and in initiating litigation against dental care providers.

Whether the move toward assessment of quality of performance in health care is a direct result of the consumer movement is questioned by some. There have been long-standing "ethics" committees of the state and local dental associations as evidence of den-

tistry's continuing interest in monitoring the quality of care its members provide the public. State boards of dentistry have had the power to revoke the license of any provider who did not meet the "ethical" standards of the state practice act.

These review committees have existed for many years, but their impact in identifying and resolving weaknesses has been minimal because of the limited financial resources and the limited contingency controls they, in actuality, have over practicing dentists. The majority of complaints brought to them by patients may be resolved, but they have limited means to seek out or monitor the quality of care delivered by the individual practicing dentists to whom no disfavorable attention has been drawn. The committees usually do not have provisions for remediating providers whose level of care is unacceptable. License revocation (by the state) is rarely based on lack of quality of care since it is difficult, in the absence of agreed upon criteria, to establish that a person is indeed practicing unacceptably. The state boards of dentistry may review complaints and take official legal action, but there has been no claim that they have had a significant impact on improving the overall quality of care delivered by providers. They ensure that the very minimum of ethical and legal requirements are enforced, but again only within the limited resources they are provided.

ASSESSING THE QUALITY OF CARE
The audit process

Perhaps the most effective available mechanism for reviewing dental care is the private insurance investigator or the claims reviewers for public assistance programs that fund health care. Dental care, as noted in earlier chapters, is not financed by third parties to the same extent as medical care. However, the trend toward prepaid dentistry will continue to grow as more employees receive dental care coverage as a fringe benefit and particularly if national health insurance does include dental benefits. As external audit mechanisms related to financing care apply to more and more dentists, review of dental care provided will be more prevalent. The audit has great potential for monitoring the quality of care since it carries an economic contingency.

In the *audit* process used by insurance carriers, professionals and perhaps specially trained laypersons review a sample of patient records, radiographic surveys, data regarding appointment visits, sequence of treatment and fees, and study models.[4-7] The basic goal is to assess the relevance of planned procedures to the needs of the patient, the emphasis on preserving teeth, and the appropriateness of the fees and filed claims. The economic contingency is that if the service is unnecessary or an obvious case of substandard care, or if the fees are unreasonable, the claim will not be paid.

This audit system of review can be implemented in a group practice environment as an internal check on quality. It can be carried out by the providers or by a person employed to perform those procedures.[7] An audit system could be developed for local professional society review of care.

Peer review

A more sophisticated method of assessing quality of care is *peer review* in which a group of colleague-providers either audit records and evaluate the outcome of care or actually assess the process used in the provision of care.[4-6,16] The results of the group peer review can be measured against specific, predetermined criteria so that recommendations for improvement can be based on an objective, agreed upon definition of quality practice. With the refined behavioral descriptions of diagnostic, treatment planning, preventive and therapeutic services that are available for nearly all phases of dental care, measuring provider performances is a logical step forward in measuring the quality of care. Again, these performance descriptions can be assessed in terms of data available in the patient record, radiographs, and models. This is the simpler approach. However, it does not allow for assessment of the *process*

of care. Records cannot speak to the gentleness and accuracy with which an injection is given. They cannot reflect the trauma induced during an oral prophylaxis or during the application of a rubber dam. The record does not readily reflect the quality of interpersonal communications with the patient.

If the consumer or the provider of care determines that these other "process' components of health care are important enough to evaluate, it may be necessary to include on-site evaluations of patient care or to design a system for videotaping certain components of care for later measurement against predetermined criteria.

Self-assessment

The technology exists to tape components of care with minimal disruption. Unobtrusive portable equipment can be set up to record several appointments. The tapes could be utilized to assess time and motion management as well as the quality of the actual procedures in process. The most important benefit of such an approach may be that the provider of care would be able to step back from him/herself and assess skills, rapport, and ease of operation.

Although the technology exists for this style of peer review and self-assessment, there is some question whether the profession is adequately prepared in group process to participate in such a system without resorting to competitive tactics and without creating a mutual admiration society that is reluctant to identify areas of needed growth or to feel comfortable with the notion of a group review.[17] The peer group will need to identify and agree upon the standards and the criteria and then adopt a pattern of review that focuses on objective observation of behavior that relates to each of the standards. The group will have to develop a support system for members needing assistance, and they will have to share the responsibility of participation and evaluation equally.

The likelihood that such a system could readily be adopted in any component society of organized dentistry or of auxiliaries may be hampered by the "loner" tendency of solo practitioners and because of the way in which many health care providers were evaluated while in school. Evaluation may have been a highly judgmental, arbitrary process, reflective more of authority than of achievement of stated goals and objectives. If evaluation was a negative experience, there is little reason to expect that practitioners would view it any more positively after leaving the school environment.

CONTINUING COMPETENCE

If a system of self-assessment and peer review *is* attempted and does result in both positive feedback and identification of areas needing improvement, it is essential that it be keyed to a source of continuing education that can help the provider of care bolster his/her skills.[2] It will not be sufficient to simply identify weaknesses. If the component has a number of peer review groups (of five or six providers each), it may be possible to develop a support mechanism among the reviewers that will generate study club activities to focus on areas of expertise that providers need to develop.

The national organization may provide a library of continuing education packages tied to the stated performance standards. Continuing education, to be effective in remediating various components of care, must be performance based also. Learning cannot be measured (and therefore neither can improvement) simply in terms of attendance at lectures and seminars. For this reason, systems of continuing education, particularly in allied health fields, are moving toward accreditation of continuing education programs based not only on content, format, and time but on learning outcomes as well.

The American Dental Hygienists' Association has been accrediting continuing education in terms of objectives and outcomes since 1973.[2,3] They are now moving toward a certification program for continuing education faculty based on their specific competencies as content experts and as managers of learning.[2]

The peer review process does have great potential for implementing a cycle of learning, practice, assessment, and prescriptive learning for the provider of care. It could provide a valuable mechanism for measurably bolstering the quality of care and in establishing a new level of credibility with the watchful consumer. It could be integrated into a group practice or be carried out as a local component function. Once again, there could be economic linkages, with participants in such peer review groups being eligible for accreditation by the American Academy of Dental Group Practice and therefore "excepted" by third-party payors from frequent external reviews.

There is a possibility that continuing education will continue to grow as a prerequisite for license renewal, as it is in a few licensing jurisdictions, such as Minnesota[1a] and California. However, unless continuing education is evaluated in terms of learning outcomes and unless the courses most needed by the provider are the ones he/she chooses to complete, there may be only incidental improvement in care.[8,13]

The quality of care delivered and the relationship the provider has with the patient are two critical elements in health care delivery, not only from an economic standpoint but from a legal and ethical point of view as well. Subsequent chapters will discuss those implications in greater detail.

Review questions

1. What three issues have been the focus of consumer complaints regarding health care?
   a.
   b.
   c.
2. Explain briefly three ways in which consumers are gaining influence in the delivery of health care.
   a.
   b.
   c.
3. The (audit/peer review system) involves a monitoring of patient records and other data by a review board or other persons to determine the appropriateness of treatment, outcome, and fees.
4. The (audit/peer review system) involves an evaluation of patient care (perhaps including the process of care) by a group of colleagues to determine the appropriateness and quality of care delivered.
5. Describe how a peer review system could be tied to continuing education.

ANSWERS

1. a. Cost
   b. Access
   c. Quality
2. a. They have successfully influenced state and federal legislators to enact laws to alleviate problems related to cost, access, and quality.
   b. They are more aware as individuals of their right to question treatment; they seek to be involved in decision-making regarding their care.
   c. They have increased litigation against providers who have performed substandard care.
3. Audit
4. Peer review system
5. If peer review is based upon predetermined, behavioral criteria, then deficiencies or areas where skills need improvement could be keyed to continuing education opportunities specific to the weaknesses; the continuing education system, of course, should be tied to those same criteria.

GROUP ACTIVITIES

1. Institute an audit system to review patient records, appointments, and the outcome of care.
2. Institute a peer review system of clinical performance that focuses on end product. Modify it to focus on *process of care*, using available task analyses to define the criteria. Introduce a public member and analyze how he/she affects intragroup competitiveness or reluctance to identify weaknesses.
3. Review articles reflective of consumer awareness of the problems in the health care system.

REFERENCES

1. Angevine, Erma: The consumer's viewpoint of dental hygiene, Dent. Hyg., **47:**380.
1a. Born, David Omar: Dental hygiene participation in a mandatory continuing education system, Dent. Hyg., **49:**215.
2. Continuing education council examining team report. Findings related to the continuing education system of the American Dental Hygienists Association, 1976.
3. Continuing Education Guidelines, Dent. Hyg., **47:**142.
4. Decker, Barry and Bonner, Paul, editors: PSRO: Organization for regional peer review, Cambridge, Mass., 1973, Ballinger Publishing Co.
5. Egdahl, Richard H. and Gertman, Paul M., editors: Quality assurance in health care, Germantown, Md., 1976, Aspen Systems Corporation.
6. Friedman, Jay W.: The potential of group practice for the analysis of the quality of care. In Jerge, Charles R. and others, editors: Group practice and the future of dental care, Philadelphia, 1974, Lea and Febiger.
7. Jerge, Charles R.: Summary of the medical audit procedures utilized at the Promis Clinic, Hampden Highlands, Maine, Unpublished paper.
7a. Jones, Patricia F.: The changing role of the dental hygienist. In Boundy, Suzanne S. and Reynolds, Nancy J., editors: Current concepts in dental hygiene, St. Louis, 1977, The C. V. Mosby Co.
8. Massler, Maury: Continuing education program to meet future needs, J. Dent. Educ., **34:**145.
9. McGuire, Thomas: The tooth trip, New York, 1972, Random House, Inc. and Berkeley, Calif., 1972, The Bookworks.
10. Maurizi, Alex R.: Public policy and the dental care market, Washington, D.C., 1975, American Enterprise Institute for Public Policy Research.
11. Nader, Ralph: Unsafe at any speed: The designed-in dangers of the American automobile, New York, 1965, Grossman Publishers.
12. Nader, Ralph: Wake-Up America—Unsafe X-Rays, Ladies' Home Journal, **85:**126, May 1968.
13. Patterson, William R.: Responsibilities of the practitioner and the dental educator in continuing education, J. Dent. Educ. **28:**311.
14. Quint, Barbara: A closemouthed look at bad dentistry, Money, **3:**11.
15. "Revere, Paul," DDS: Dentistry and its victims, New York, 1970, St. Martin's Press, Inc.
16. Slee, Vergil N.: PSRO and the hospital's quality control, Ann. of Intern. Med., **81:**97.
17. Waldman, H. Barry and Schlissel, Edward: Honor codes and peer review—is peer review really possible? J. Dent. Educ., **41:**126.

PART III

LEGAL CONSIDERATIONS FOR HEALTH CARE PROVIDERS

The way in which a health care provider relates to patients in the efforts to obtain and sustain health has often been regarded as both a matter of common sense and an ethical mandate. To a large extent the "proper" way to relate to a patient can indeed be understood in terms of everyday courtesy and sensitivity to the patient's wants, needs, and expectations. With the addition of the sobering realization that the care to be provided does affect the health and well-being of a person, most health care providers demonstrate an ability to establish a professional, caring relationship with patients.

The law has something to add to the common sense and ethical mandate of relationships between patients and providers. The law has defined, over the years, some specific rights and duties that the patient and health care provider have. Failure to fulfill a duty can mean unhappy days in the courtroom, financial loss, and a tarnished reputation.

This can be avoided by being aware of and following the guidelines that ensure the protection of legal rights in the provider-patient relationship.

CHAPTER 6

Rights and duties in the patient–health care provider relationship

OBJECTIVES: The reader will be able to:

1. Describe the nature of the legal relationship between the health care provider and the patient.
2. Recognize those circumstances under which a health care provider is legally obligated to render care to a patient.
3. Define duty.
4. List the duties legally required of a health care provider.
5. Given a set of circumstances
   a. Indicate if a duty has been breached.
   b. Identify the duty that has been breached.
   c. Specify the possible result of that breach.
6. List the duties that a patient owes a health care provider as a result of the contractual relationship.
7. Define "reasonable care" in terms of the duties the law expects the health care provider to fulfill in a contractual relationship with a patient.
8. Given a set of circumstances in which a patient is claiming that a health care provider did did not exercise "reasonable care," analyze whether the claim is supportable in terms of the duties the patient and the health care provider owe to one another as a result of the contractual relationship.
9. Define
   a. *Negligence*
   b. The legal standard of the *reasonably prudent man*
10. Define *privileged communication*.
11. Recognize that there is an *agency* relationship between dental auxiliary personnel and employers.
12. Provide examples of how the principle of *respondeat superior* affects an employer dentist as well as the accused employee should he/she become liable for a tort committed against the employer's patient.
13. Project the probable impact of expanded functions delegation on the legal definition of standards of skill and care for dental auxiliary personnel.
14. Assess personal rules of conduct in dealing with patients to determine if rights and duties are being respected and alter conduct where necessary.

ESTABLISHING THE LEGAL RELATIONSHIP

When a patient requests that a health care provider perform some service for the assessment, maintenance, or improvement of the patient's health, the health care provider legally has a choice. He/she can agree to provide the service or can refuse. Despite the ethical mandate that health personnel may feel toward providing care where it is needed, the *law* does not require a patient be accepted.[4,9] One exception to the rule is government-funded programs where regulations may stipulate that any and all persons meeting eligibility criteria be accepted as patients by the health care staff.[4] Another is when the patient is enrolled in a prepaid program, such as a health maintenance organization, and the provider has contracted to provide care for enrolled persons.

Once the patient is accepted for care by the provider of care (or once the patient is enrolled in a health maintenance organization), a contract is established.[6] It may be *implied* by the actions of the provider and the patient. Or it may be an *express* contract in which the terms of the agreement are discussed by the two parties or formalized in a written agreement. There are many advantages and disadvantages to be considered in deciding what kind of contract is "best," which will be discussed in the chapter concerning contracts. What is important to consider now is what this *voluntary, contractual* relationship means in terms of basic rights and duties shared by the persons in the contract.[4]

RIGHTS AND DUTIES

A health care provider owes certain duties to the patient, just as the patient owes certain duties to the provider. A *duty* is "that which a persons owes to another. An obligation to do a thing."[2] Corresponding to every duty owed is a *right*.[2] The patient has certain specific rights by virtue of the contractual relationship, and the health care provider is obligated to respect those contractually defined rights. Conversely, the patient has certain duties that correlate to the rights of the health care provider.

The duties of the health care provider include (1) protecting and respecting the personal and property rights of the patient, (2) providing only that care which is necessary and which has been agreed upon with the patient, (3) completing care within a reasonable amount of time, and (4) achieving reasonably satisfactory results if satisfaction was guaranteed.[4,6,9] These four duties are integral to the legal, contractual relationship. Two others, implied by law, are that the provider exercise "reasonable care" in performing

health care services and that the charge for the services provided be a "reasonable fee."[4]

If any of the duties is unmet, the patient has grounds for a civil action against the health care provider. If the patient proves by a preponderance of evidence that a duty was unmet, the patient may be awarded damages (financial restitution) for the wrongdoing.[8]

It should be remembered that the patient has duties to pay the reasonable fee and to cooperate in treatment.[4,9] The patient may very well lose a case against a health professional or even find him/herself the object of a civil suit if either of these duties is unmet.

It should be obvious that the contractual nature of the relationship provides a built-in set of checks and balances established by the law that helps ensure equitable and "reasonable" business as well as professional procedures.[9]

What is most crucial, however, in daily clinical practice is a full understanding of what those duties mean. The description provided here, after all, is really quite vague. What does it mean to protect the personal and property rights of a patient? How should that be interpreted?

Does it mean that the dental hygienist refrains from asking prying questions of the patient's personal life that have no relevance to dental health? Does it mean that the physician ensures that the walkways in the office are free of obstacles that could harm a patient? Does it mean that the dentist must respect the patient's right to ownership of dentures and, in some instances, x-rays? The answer to these questions is yes. And the law offers additional practical interpretations.

The patient has a right to confidentiality regarding the care he is receiving.[6,9] Displays, presentations, and publication of photographs of patients are a breach of the right of privacy of each patient.* Written permission to use patient records, photo-

---

*Radiographic surveys that do not readily identify the person are an exception to this rule.

graphs and the patient's name in any public manner is absolutely necessary.[6] The patient may understandably not want his/her ailments or cures to be known to others, and the health provider has the duty to ensure confidentiality. This includes permitting only personnel contributing to the performance of health care services to be present in the treatment room. Specific permission must be obtained from the patient before nonessential persons may be admitted.[6]

This right to privacy includes not only the particulars of the health care procedures but also any information about the patient acquired in the course of treatment.[6] The law considers such information to be *privileged communication,* and the health care provider is bound by the law not to reveal the information even in a court of law. This right is personal to the patient and can be waived by him/her, for example when the patient asks the provider of care to testify regarding his/her condition. The only exceptions relate to information regarding child abuse and communicable disease. Some states expect such information will be revealed in a court of law.[4,6]

The second duty mentioned in defining the obligations of the health care provider to the patient relates to the requirement that the provider complete the agreed upon care and not abandon the patient.[6,9] The explicit condition of entering a contract is that the agreed upon treatment be completed—and within a reasonable period of time. Long waiting periods to commence or complete treatment violate this duty. If treatment is going to exceed 1 year, it is best to secure the patient's agreement in writing.

It is *not* the provider's right to terminate treatment before it is completed.[4] There are appropriate ways to withdraw from the contract to perform health care services, including a written notice of intent to withdraw, a statement of what care remains to be performed, and suggestions for obtaining the described care. But under no circumstances may the provider purposely extend treatment over an unreasonable amount of time or

simply stop making appointments for a patient. To do the latter is to abandon the patient in the eyes of the law.[4]

In order for a patient to prove abandonment he/she would have to show that the prescribed series of treatments was left incomplete and that it was unreasonable to expect the patient to resume treatment under the care of another provider. In the case of temporary or extended absence on the part of the provider, the patient will need to show harm as a result of not having had access to another provider of care. In any case, the provider does have an obligation to see treatment to its completion and to make some provisions for access to care during periods of absence.

Experimental or nonstandard drugs and procedures should not be used in the care of any patient.[4,9] The patient has the right to expect that commonly accepted, standard care that would be provided by at least a "respectable minority" of practitioners will be provided. Even written permission is little consolation in the courtroom if the innovation fails and harm is caused to the patient.

A closely related duty requires that the provider perform *only* those services to which the patient has agreed.[4] Performing a procedure that the patient has not agreed to constitutes technical assault. It can be a relatively simple legal matter to prove that something was performed that was not in the treatment plan the patient agreed to.

There are, of course, instances where the law assumes implied consent, such as when a patient is unconscious and is in need of oxygen, cardiopulmonary resuscitation, or medication to reverse the medical emergency.

It is the health care provider's duty to ensure the safety and well-being of patients by making certain that there are no hazards present on the premises.[9] All equipment used should be safe, and the patient should have a clear pathway to and from treatment rooms.

Other duties included in the concept of providing "reasonable" care are: keeping the patient informed of the progress of treatment and his or her condition, arranging for care of the patient during periods of temporary absence, referring the patient to a specialist if necessary, and achieving reasonable results.[4]

STANDARDS OF CARE

With the introduction of the word "reasonable" in describing duties, the concept of legal standards or guidelines to ascertain whether a duty has been breached is likewise introduced. What does "reasonable" mean—especially as it relates to the law?

The dictionary definition of "reasonable care" is care that is "just; proper. Ordinary or usual. Fit and appropriate to the end in view."[2] And the measure the law uses in determining whether a provider has exercised reasonable care is known as the standard of what would be exercised by the *reasonably prudent practitioner.*[2,7,9]

This measure of conduct applies to all persons in society in their daily activities with other human beings. When a person does not measure up to the reasonably prudent person and harm results to another, *negligence* may be charged.[8] When the charge specifically relates to a professional person's lack of reasonable care in serving a patient or client, the charge of negligence is referred to as *malpractice.*[9,11]

So, essentially there are three main classifications of charges that a patient may bring against a health care provider as a consequence of the explicit and implicit duties the provider owes the patient as a result of the voluntary, contractual nature of the relationship. The patient may charge *breach of contract* if his/her property and privacy rights have been violated or if the services agreed to are not performed or if they are delayed for an extended period of time. The patient may charge *technical assault* if the provider performs some service that the patient has not agreed to.[4,8] Or the patient may charge *negligence* if the care provided does not satisfy the duty of reasonable prudence *and* causes harm to the patient or if a hazard

is allowed to exist in the office, which harms the patient.

All of the previous charges are covered by civil law since they relate to disagreements between two individuals and do not connote any wrong against society (the basis for criminal law).[9] Only in the case of gross, wanton negligence may criminal proceedings also be appropriate actions against the defendant.[2] Civil law has two branches relevant to this discussion: contracts and torts. Breach of contract is considered under contract law, whereas charges of negligence and technical assault are parts of tort law.[2] Later chapters will discuss the distinctions between these branches of the law.

LEGAL ASPECTS OF EVOLVING ROLES

The implications of the basic issues of contracts and torts have a special meaning for health care providers whose roles in delivery of health services are evolving. The growth of the role of the dental auxiliary in providing care is quite obvious in some states where it is now legal for dental hygienists to administer block and infiltration anesthesia and where other services previously performed only by the dentist are now delegated to the dental hygienist or dental assistant.

Just as every right has a correlative duty, this expansion in role brings an accompanying increase in responsibility. The auxiliary with the legal right to provide direct patient care has the duty to provide that care with the caution, foresight, and quality expected of the "reasonably prudent person."

The contemporary issue that becomes obvious is whether the auxiliary performing a service is properly held to the standard of other auxiliaries or to the standard of the dentist, whose function it also is to perform those services.[7] The law has historically said that the auxiliary will be measured against other auxiliaries and that the dentist will be measured against other dentists.[7] But this may imply a dual standard of quality for the patient.

In 1975 the American Dental Hygienists

Association adopted a position statement that expresses the expectation that dental auxiliaries be regulated on the basis of a "single standard of proficiency for every state regulated intra-oral procedure" in performing direct patient care.[1] ADHA policy supports the development of a single national board examination instrument to be used in assessing dental auxiliary candidates for licensure to practice expanded functions. ADHA expects the construction of the instrument to be based on test items currently used to assess candidates for licensure to practice dentistry.

If the profession is saying that dental auxiliaries should provide the same standard of care as dentists in those functions delegated to them and if learning objectives and mastery levels used in teaching programs for auxiliaries are the same as those used in dental schools, will the law begin to measure the behavior of the auxiliary against the "reasonably prudent provider of dental care"? In other words, will a new standard be created that is the same for dentists and auxiliaries?

In any case, it is apparent that with each step toward greater responsibility in providing health care, the health care provider is held against a greater measure in terms of the law. This fact has been confronted by nursing, which has an ever-expanding definition of practice and which often includes practice without any direct supervision. Irene Murchison describes the situation in nursing this way:

Although there has been no change of legal doctrine, the advances of medical science have been accompanied by radically new developments in nursing practice which require careful legal evaluation. As the nurse assumes increased responsibility for complex acts requiring greater skill, she should be aware that the boundaries of reasonable conduct are shifting. Indeed, were a nurse to harm a patient today, she could well be held to a level of knowledge of medical science and medical practice unknown a generation ago.[7]

The proper caution of the evolving health care provider certainly includes adequate preparation to knowledgeably perform new functions before accepting them as part of the scope of practice.[7] No new function should casually be added to that scope, even as a response to urgent health care needs. Educational preparation and a careful assessment of the legal implications of such an additional function should precede its acceptance.

RISE IN MALPRACTICE ACTIONS

This is particularly true in an age of consumerism when the public is becoming aware of its rights and is learning how to protect those rights.[5] The recent increases in civil actions against physicians and dentists are a sign of that new awareness. Higher premiums for professional liability insurance, the growing difficulty of obtaining such insurance at any price, and the significant increase in the incidence of claims and suits along with larger damage awards should be strong indicators that the public will not tolerate lack of reasonable care and should warn the health professions that reasonable care had better be provided.[6]

In the past this threat of malpractice or breach of contract action was felt primarily by the physician and to a lesser extent by the dentist. Health professionals, such as nurses and dental auxiliaries, whose scope of practice usually finds them employed by physicians and dentists, have suffered from the delusion that all liability for their own negligence would be absorbed by the employer. However, the law relating to the *agency relationship* between the employer-physician and the employee-nurse is clear on the fact that even though the employer may be vicariously liable, the employee *is* personally responsible and liable for his/her actions while furthering the objectives of the practice.[2,3,7,10]

Therefore, it is necessary that the employed health care provider (including the dental hygienist) conduct his/her professional affairs with the same respect for the patient's rights as that of the wise physician or dentist.[10]

It is true that the employer is often named

in a suit in which the employee caused some harm to a patient. And this is legally allowable under the concept of *respondeat superior*, which means literally, "let the master answer" for the wrongful acts of his servants or agents.[2] The attraction of using the master is a practical, economic one.[10] "It is in the interest of every plaintiff to have as many financially responsible persons as defendants as he can legitimately find."[7] However, this does not mean that a dental hygienist, dietician, nurse, respiratory therapist, or other allied health professional does not need personal malpractice insurance. Despite the person's position as an employee, a suit brought solely against him/her for a tort or one brought jointly against him/her and the employer may result in devastating financial losses to the individual if no personal malpractice coverage is in effect.

It should be apparent that the legal ramifications of health care practice can have a profound impact on the individual health care provider. A good reputation, as well as financial assets, requires the application of these basic legal principles in daily practice to ensure that the duties owed the patient are fulfilled.

Review questions

Case 1

A 25-year old male arrives for the first time at a dental office for an oral examination and necessary treatment.
1. Is the dentist legally obligated to provide dental care?
2. Under what conditions is the dentist obligated to provide care?

Case 2

A patient has been accepted for medical treatment. The physician provides a treatment plan and fee schedule to which the patient agrees, in writing. The physician indicates that the patient will be called for his first treatment appointment. Given that the physician has indicated that he will call the patient for the first appointment, what duty must the physician be especially careful in fulfilling?

Case 3

A patient trips over the rheostat in a dental operatory and fractures her arm in the fall. The rheostat had been left directly in the path of the patient.
1. Has a duty been breached?
2. If so, what duty has been breached?
3. What could be the likely legal consequences of the harm the patient suffered?

Case 4

A patient has been highly offensive in his mannerisms and language while receiving care from a dental hygienist. The dental hygienist tells the patient that she will call him for his next appointment. She never does, despite the fact that the treatment plan is incomplete.
1. Has a breach of duty occurred?
2. If so, which one?
In this case, the dental hygienist is employed by a hospital in the outpatient clinic.
3. Legally, the hygienist is an _____ of the hospital.
4. Because of this relationship of the hygienist to the hospital, liability for any breach of duty on the part of the hygienist is charged to _____ .

Case 5

A dental hygienist is doing clinical research in the area of myofunctional therapy. "Before-and-after" study models and photographs are prepared for all patients included in the program. The models and photographs are displayed at a professional meeting as a part of a presentation of the clinical results.

1. What procedures must the clinician follow in order to legally display those articles?
2. What duty, if any, would be breached if the procedure was not followed?
3. What legal action could be taken against the dental hygienist, if any?

In this case, the dental hygienist often invites dental hygiene students to observe therapy sessions. The hygienist always asks the patient's permission to allow these "nonessential" persons into the therapy room.

4. Is this a necessary procedure?
5. Why or why not?

Case 6

A patient has had full-mouth reconstruction completed by his dentist. The verbal contract between the dentist and patient called for three separate, equal payments of $250.00. The last payment was due at the final visit. The first two payments were made on schedule, but at the last visit the patient left without paying, explaining that he had forgotten his checkbook. Six months and a collection agency later, the patient still owed the last payment.

1. Has a duty been breached?
2. If so, which one?
3. What legal action, if any, can be taken as a result?
4. Is there any countercharge the patient could make?

Case 7

A patient is under general anesthesia for the extraction of two impacted molars. The dentist notices that there is a badly decayed tooth next to the first extraction site and decides to remove it, also. When the patient regains consciousness, the dentist tells the patient that three teeth were removed rather than just the two agreed upon.

1. Has a duty been breached?
2. If so, which one?
3. What legal action may result?

Case 8

A dental hygienist is scheduled to perform a root planing and curettage for a reluctant patient. The patient clearly needs the services to be performed, so in his zeal to have the patient consent and cooperate he promises that the patient's mouth will feel much better within a week after treatment. As luck would have it, the patient's teeth become very sensitive even after 2 weeks.

1. Has a breach of duty occurred?
2. If so, which one?
3. Why?
4. What legal action can the patient take against the dental hygienist?
5. Assuming that the patient wins the case, what harm will the dental hygienist suffer?

Case 9

A dentist fractures a root tip during an extraction. He does not tell the patient about it and decides he will retrieve it at a later date. The patient develops severe pain, fever, and malaise and is hospitalized. An oral surgeon removes the root tip in the hospital, and the patient recovers.

1. Did the first dentist breach a duty?
2. Is the fracturing of the root tip *in itself* a breach of duty?
3. If there was a breach of duty in the case, what was it?
4. Could it have been avoided?
5. What charge may the patient bring against the dentist, if any?

Case 10

A patient has developed periodontal disease after 20 years of regular prophylaxis and oral examinations. The patient needs $800 worth of periodontal surgery. Curious about how this could develop "over the last 6 months," the patient visits the local library and learns that it is a slow, developing process that can usually be halted by thorough daily removal of plaque in addition to regular prophylaxis. The patient is appalled that the hygienist casually mentioned brushing and flossing but never emphasized the need for plaque control and the real consequences of incomplete removal of those soft deposits on a daily bais. The patient sues the dental hygienist and the dentist for negligence, claiming that she was given substandard care over a long period of time.

1. Does the patient have a legitimate suit?
2. How will the legal standard of care be applied to this case?

Case 11

A dental assistant who has had no formal training is responsible for instrument sterilization. Because of his lack of knowledge, instruments that are autoclaved are stored in the open air or loose in drawers, allowing air contamination before they are used. A patient proves that an oral infection she developed was directly linked to the contaminated instruments.

1. Has a breach of duty occurred?
2. If so, which one?
3. Whom will the patient probably sue?
4. How will the legal "standard of care" be applied in this case?

ANSWERS
Case 1

1. Not necessarily
2. If the dentist is employed in a federal clinic, he is obligated to provide care to eligible persons; if the provider is in the midst of providing care, he must complete the treatment agreed to; if the patient is enrolled as a subscriber to a prepaid dental plan with which the provider has a contractual arrangement, the dentist must accept the patient for care.

Case 2

The duty to commence treatment within a reasonable time

Case 3

1. Yes
2. Breach of the duty to protect the patient from hazards in the office
3. The patient may sue for negligence charging that the "reasonably prudent man" would clear the patient's pathway of such obstacles; the provider could claim contributory negligence on the part of the patient as a defense.

Case 4

1. Yes
2. Duty to complete treatment that has begun; the patient has been abandoned.
3. Agent
4. The hygienist and the hospital (and perhaps an intermediate dental supervisor)

Case 5

1. Secure written permission from the patients to use the photographs and models; omit patient names from the display unless specifically allowed, in writing, by the patients.
2. Duty to protect the patient's right to privacy
3. Patient could sue for breach of contract or invasion of privacy (if harm resulted to the patient as a result of the display) or sue under quasi contract grounds for reasonable compensation. (The loss in this case assumes a contract exists if a person earns money from the use of one's picture.)
4. Yes
5. The patient has a right to privacy and the dental hygienist has a duty to protect that right.

Case 6

1. Yes
2. Duty to pay a reasonable fee
3. Dentist can sue for breach of this duty to recover payment.

4. The patient may attempt proceedings charging negligence or failure to provide "reasonable" results.

Case 7

1. Yes
2. Duty to perform only those services agreed to
3. Patient may charge technical assault. However, recovery will be minimal unless the patient can show some significant harm.

Case 8

1. Yes
2. Breach of duty to satisfy the patient *if* satisfaction (or a given result) is promised and breach of duty to obtain informed consent regarding the possible outcome of treatment
3. A health professional is not expected to guarantee his results, but if he does promise or guarantee a result, the law holds him to that promise as a matter of contract; the provider is expected to inform the patient of outcome before commencing treatment.
4. The patient can charge breach of contract.
5. The dental hygienist will suffer time and anguish in court, a tarnished reputation and financial loss (especially if he has no personal liability insurance).

Case 9

1. Yes
2. Not necessarily. A reasonably prudent dentist could fracture a root tip. The fracture *in itself* is not proof of negligence.
3. The dentist breached the duty to keep the patient informed.
4. Yes, the dentist could have told the patient about the fracture and suggested they wait to remove it.
5. The patient may bring a breach of contract charge since the duty to keep the patient informed is a contractual matter, or the patient may bring a negligence charge since she suffered so much harm as a result of a breach of professional duty.

Case 10

1. Yes, if she can prove that she was not given "reasonable care" by not having the benefits of plaque control information.
2. The question will be: "Would the reasonably prudent dental hygienist and dentist in that locality have done more in plaque control?" An interesting note is that if the patient can prove that plaque control programs are an integral part of dental hygiene programs and that licensing procedures include examination of skills in plaque control, the patient may be able to use the national standard in proving negligence on the part of the dental hygienist.

Case 11

1. Yes
2. Duty to protect the safety of the patient

3. The patient will probably sue both the dentist (invoking *respondeat superior*) and the dental assistant (since he actually performed the harmful act).
4. The assistant's behavior will be measured against "the reasonably prudent dental assistant" and an educated assistant at that. Whether a person is certified, licensed, or not, if he sets himself up as having the skills to perform his services correctly, he is held to the standards of the qualified person. The dentist is liable because of the agency relationship, but he may also be measured against "the reasonably prudent dentist" for not ensuring that the person responsible for sterilization is performing that service correctly.

GROUP ACTIVITIES

1. Research law review articles to determine the typical size of financial damages awarded to patients winning civil cases against health care providers.
2. Survey local dental hygienists to determine how many carry malpractice insurance, what type, coverage limits, etc.
3. Visit a courtroom during malpractice proceedings. Report to the class on how the legal principles of rights and duties, negligence, breach of contract, standard of care, and *respondeat superior* were applied.
4. Conduct a seminar discussion involving graduating dental hygienists and licensed hygienists at the local society meeting regarding the application of these principles in clinical practice.
5. Recall any incidents in clinical practice that should have been handled differently in order to protect the patient's rights.

REFERENCES

1. American Dental Hygienists Association: Minutes of the Fifty-second Annual Session of the House of Delegates. R-5-Amended-75-H, 1975.
2. Black, M. A.: Black's law dictionary, ed. 4, St. Paul, Minn., 1968, West Publishing Company.
3. Creighton, H.: Law every nurse should know, ed. 2, Philadelphia, 1970, W. B. Saunders Co.
4. Miller, S. L.: Legal aspects of dentistry, New York, 1970, G. P. Putnam's Sons.
5. Morganstern, S.: Legal protection for the consumer, Dobbs Ferry, N.Y., 1973, Oceana Publications, Inc.
6. Morris, R. C. and Moritz, A. R.: Doctor and patient and the law, ed. 5, St. Louis, 1971, The C. V. Mosby Co.
7. Murchison, I. A. and Nichols, T. S.: Legal foundations of nursing practice, New York, 1970, Macmillan, Inc.
8. Prosser, W. L.: Handbook of the law of torts, ed. 4, St. Paul, Minn., 1971, West Publishing Co.
9. Sarner, H.: Dental jurisprudence, Philadelphia, 1963, W. B. Saunders Co.
10. Seavey, W. A.: Handbook of the law of agency, St. Paul, Minn., 1964, West Publishing Co.
11. Willig, S. H.: The nurse's guide to the law, New York, 1970, McGraw-Hill, Inc.

CHAPTER 7

The contract relationship

OBJECTIVES: The reader will be able to:

1. Describe the health care provider-patient relationship as both contractual and consensual.
2. Differentiate express and implied contracts.
3. Given hypothetical situations, identify whether the health care provider may be subject to a breach of contract suit.
4. Given hypothetical situations, identify when the health care provider has taken reasonable precautions to prevent a breach of contract suit.
5. Given hypothetical situations, identify when the contributory action or lack of action on the part of the patient may negate a charge of breach of contract against the health care provider.

As mentioned in the previous chapter, when a person seeks the care of a health professional and the professional agrees to provide a service, a legal contract exists between the person and the professional. The professional has the *legal* right to accept or reject a patient (unless the professional is employed in a federally funded health care program or the patient is enrolled in a prepaid plan, such as a health maintenance organization, with which the provider has a contract). The patient has the right to agree to or reject the proposed care. Therefore, the patient–health care provider relationship is both consensual and contractual. Once both parties *consensually* agree to the service, they have contractual obligations to each other.[1-3]

This contractual relationship may be *express* (stated orally or in writing), or it may be *implied* (agreed to by the actions of the two persons).[1-3] The former is readily identifiable when a treatment plan is presented to the patient, and the patient agrees orally to the plan or actually signs the treatment plan. The latter type is more difficult to identify since it is implied by the actions of the health care provider and the patient.[2,3]

An example of an implied contract to permit an oral examination is: The patient opens his mouth for the dentist, and the dentist looks in. The patient has implied a request for professional assessment of his oral health and the dentist has, by action, agreed to provide that service. Another is: A patient offers his arm for an injection, and the nurse injects a prescribed medication. No words or signed statements may have been exchanged between the patient and the professional. Yet another type of implied contract is the *quasi contract*, which the law recognizes when a provider of care renders necessary emergency treatment to an unconscious person. Implied contracts are viewed as valid in a court of law as long as there is compensation for the service.

In the years that preceded the consumer movement, the vast majority of health care providers relied heavily on the implied contract. It seemed logical that a person behaving in a manner that said, "Provide me with health care," really wanted it, and the implied contract requires no special series of forms nor a lengthy discussion of procedures and alternatives.

However, in the current age of consumer

awareness of rights and privileges, the implied contract is a less tenable approach to health care. If nothing is said or written about what care is to be provided or what cooperation is needed on the part of the patient, the nature of the contract is open to wide interpretation. What *was* the patient agreeing to in his silent submission? What *was* the health care provider expecting of the patient? Simply stated, a charge of breach of contract is difficult to defend when the contract was never specifically stated. Conversely, the charge of breach is difficult to prove, and the plaintiff bears the burden of proof. A written express contract offers greater protection to both parties than does an oral express contract, which relies upon good expressive and listening skills and which fades with the memory.[2] However, a written contract provides firm grounds for proof of breach of contract if it is not fulfilled by one or more parties to the contract.

Breach of this contractual relationship is one of the two most frequently filed charges against health care providers. A breach of contract suit may be initiated whenever a partner in the contract does not perform as agreed. So, in the contractual relationship with a patient, the provider is liable for breach of contract if he/she fails to attend to the needs of the patient agreed upon, until care is completed. For instance, unreasonable delays in providing care may trigger a breach of contract suit. If the health care provider *promised* satisfactory results, and reasonable satisfaction is not obtained, the charge of breach may result. (NOTE: Promising satisfaction is an extremely unwise practice in an inexact field such as health care.[2])

There are several defenses against a charge of breach of contract. A health care provider faced with such a suit may be able to demonstrate that the patient did not cooperate in the contractual relationship. If the patient missed appointments, did not adhere to the prescribed pre- and post-treatment procedures, or refused certain integral phases of the proposed care, the health care provider may be able to prove that there was

no opportunity for the agreed-to procedures to be performed or to be successful. If it can be demonstrated that ample opportunity for successful care was not possible as a result of the patient's lack of cooperation, and that the provider made every effort to perform the agreed upon services, the health care provider will likely be able to turn aside a charge of breach of contract.[2]

The best avoidance of breach of contract is the explicit statement of proposed treatment, in writing, which provides the patient with the following information: (1) a description of the condition the patient has, (2) the treatment proposed, (3) the possibilities that that treatment will or will not be successful, (4) the probable results of not treating the condition, (5) the risks involved, and (6) other possible ways to approach treatment of the condition. Providing the patient with this information will permit the patient to provide an *informed consent*,[2] either orally or in writing.

In addition, estimates of cost and the number and length of appointments should be included in the treatment plan. If payments are expected during the course of treatment, the patient should be informed of this expectation. Otherwise, the patient is not legally obligated to pay until treatment is completed. The patient should have an accurate appraisal of how much time will be necessary to complete all phases of the treatment. If the time is to exceed 1 year, the patient should acknowledge in writing having been informed of that fact.[2,3]

The best precaution is to put *all* this information in writing and to share a copy signed by both parties with the patient. A format or checklist should be obtained from an attorney.

There are times when a health care provider may file a breach of contract suit against a patient—usually when the services have been satisfactorily performed and the patient has not paid. The patient, being on the defensive in this case, may contend that the services either were not completed or that they were unsatisfactory and, therefore, nonpayment is justified. However, the breach of contract suit may stimulate the patient toward even further defensive actions.[2] A patient charged with a breach of contract for nonpayment of fee may choose to countersue, charging negligence or malpractice, particularly if he/she is displeased with the outcome of treatment.

Logically enough, negligence or malpractice suits constitute the other most frequent charge made against health care providers. The unique considerations surrounding the "standard of care" issue related to charges of negligence will be discussed in the next chapter.

Review questions

1. The relationship between a patient and health care provider is both _____ and _____ .
2. What are the two forms of an express contract?
   a.
   b.
3. How is an implied contract different from an express contract?
4. In the following cases indicate whether the health care provider (a) is subject to a breach of contract suit, (b) has taken reasonable precautions to prevent a breach of contract suit, or (c) could bring a breach of contract suit against a patient.

   Case 1. The written and signed treatment plan stipulates that the fee for the planned restorative dental services be paid in three equal installments during the course of treatment. Six months after treatment is completed, only one installment has been paid. _____

   Case 2. A dental hygienist promises her patient that if he brushes and flosses daily, he will not need periodontal surgery. _____

   Case 3. A dentist develops a case presentation form that directs itself to the requirements for *informed* consent. For each patient he completes the form, has the patient sign the agreed upon treatment, and provides the patient with a copy. _____

   Case 4. A dentist leaves on a world tour for 4 months. No provisions for care are made for his patients in treatment. _____

ANSWERS

1. Consensual, contractual
2. Oral, written
3. An implied contract relies upon the "consenting" actions of the patient and health care provider. No oral or written agreement is made.
4. Case 1   c   The patient has breached the contract.
   Case 2   a   Satisfaction "promised" *must* be achieved.
   Case 3   b
   Case 4   a

GROUP ACTIVITIES

1. Using hypothetical treatment plans, prepare case presentations for the patients which include the six necessary components for consent to legally be considered "informed."
2. Consult with an attorney regarding the likelihood of a countersuit, if the health care provider sues the patient for payment of a fee.
3. Identify additional examples of implied consent. Speculate for each what assumptions or expectations could be involved in the contract.

REFERENCES

1. Black, M. A.: Black's law dictionary, ed. 4, St. Paul, Minn., 1968, West Publishing Co.
2. Miller, Sidney L.: Legal aspects of dentistry, New York, 1970, G. P. Putnam's Sons.
3. Sarner, Harvey: Dental jurisprudence, Philadelphia, 1963, W. B. Saunders Co.

CHAPTER 8

The "standard of skill and care" in providing health care

OBJECTIVES: The reader will be able to:

1. Define *negligence* and *malpractice*.
2. Describe the conditions under which a health care provider may be liable for malpractice.
3. Define *proximate cause* and explain how it is a key factor in charges of malpractice.
4. Explain the use of the "prudent-man rule" in litigating charges of negligence.
5. Define *contributory negligence* and explain how it may constitute a defense against malpractice.
6. Explain the importance of informing the patient of any accident or wrong judgment and ensuring that any damage that may have resulted has been rectified.
7. List at least ten errors in dental practice that could be grounds for a malpractice suit.
8. Define "Good Samaritan Law."

In the area of patient–health care provider rights and responsibilities, the most basic considerations are that the patient has the right to expect at least "reasonable" care and the provider has the responsibility to ensure that each patient receives it. When the level of care is not reasonable, the provider may face a tort liability for negligence or malpractice. A *tort* is a civil wrong, such as an injury to another's person, property, or reputation.[1] In discussing levels of quality of care provided by health professionals, *negligence* and *malpractice* are synonymous, referring to the omission of an act that the reasonably prudent health care provider would include in treatment or the commission of an act that the reasonable provider would not perform (or would perform differently).[3,6]

Basically, there are four factors that must be apparent before a person may be liable for negligence. First of all, the provider must have undertaken to care for the patient. Second, the provider must have breached a duty of care owed to the patient. Third, there must be damage or harm to the patient; fourth, this harm must be causally related to the breach of duty. If any of the four factors is missing, the ruling will be in favor of the health care provider and not the patient.[3]

The "reasonably prudent man" rule is applied as the measure of the appropriateness of the action, the basis of the required standard of care. The rule requires only that the practitioner possess and exercise that standard of skill and care that the reasonably prudent practitioner in the same or similar locality would possess and exercise under the same or similar circumstances.[6] An example is: A hygienist agrees to provide an oral inspection and radiographic series for a patient (acceptance of the patient). The patient contracts subacute bacterial endocarditis (harm done) as a result of (causal relationship) the probing for spontaneous gingival hemorrhage points that occurred as an integral part of the oral examination, despite the fact (breach of duty of care) that she has a history of rheumatic fever, as indicated in the patient's medical history.

With all four factors evident, the plaintiff has only to show that reasonably prudent dental hygienists, given the same circumstances, would have the patient premedicated before proceeding with probing for hemorrhage.[3,6] If the plaintiff can show that dental hygienists are expected to exercise this higher level of care according to stated standards, the plaintiff will probably win a judgment against the dental hygienist in question.

The reasonably prudent man is not perfect. And the law does not expect any person to be perfect. But the prudent man "has average courage and average caution,"[5] and he exercises professional foresight and is careful to prevent injury to his fellow human beings. Negligence does not necessarily imply lack of competence "since the competent may be negligent."[1] Negligence implies carelessness, lack of caution or discretion, without the positive intention of harming the person.[1] However, lack of competence may in many instances be the cause of the harm done. The law does expect that a health care practitioner will constantly be seeking to improve his/her level of competence, and a provider is not excused from liability on the grounds of ignorance of proper procedure.

Based on these legal principles, the dental hygienist who probed without premedicating may find him/herself in some difficulty. However, one or two other considerations might spare the dental hygienist from a judgment of malpractice.[3] If the dental hygienist can identify more than one *proximate cause* (the cause directly linked to the harm) of the subacute bacterial endocarditis, the judgment of malpractice will be turned aside. For instance, could the patient have contracted the disease from having brushed her own teeth the day on which the gingiva hemorrhaged? Or what if the patient had seen another dental health care provider that day or one day earlier or later where bleeding occurred and no premedication was provided? If more than on possible cause can be shown and the provider is not the source of

all the identified possible causes, the court may decide that the provider is not liable for the damage. If the court recognizes that the cause, by a preponderance of proof, more than likely *is* attributable to the provider, it may find for the plaintiff.

The second consideration that might spare the dental hygienist from judgment would be proof that the patient contributed to the negligence.[3] For instance, if the patient had a prescription but did not take the medication or if the patient when specifically questioned did not inform the hygienist of the history of rheumatic fever, the patient could be proved to have contributed her own negligence in creating the harm. Failure to follow instructions or disclose pertinent information may be evidence of *contributory negligence* (that is, the patient contributed her own poor judgment to the ultimate harm).

It is quite essential to understand that accidents or instances of poor judgment are not in themselves proof of negligence.[3] The malpractice suit is more likely to focus on how the accident or poor judgment is or is not rectified. Was the patient informed? Did the health care provider take all possible measures to correct the problem? If the provider chooses to hide the error, a judgment against the provider is probable, since not only the duty of reasonable care was breached but so was the provider's duty to inform the patient. Whenever accidental harm occurs to the patient, it is best to calmly inform the patient and then take steps to correct the error.[3,6]

In dental practice, there are several errors that account for the majority of dental malpractice claims. They include errors in judgment, causing harm to a patient by means of slipping with an instrument, extracting too many teeth at one appointment, delivering improperly fitting dentures, using drugs and anesthetics improperly, and allowing a foreign body to be aspirated into the respiratory tract. Failure to refer the patient to a specialist when necessary, failure to keep the patient informed, and failure to sterilize instruments or to prepare adequate x-rays are other frequent errors that may prompt a malpractice suit. If the patient was accepted by the provider and one of these errors can be proved to be the proximate cause of some harm to the patient, the provider of dental care will in all likelihood find him/herself in court. He/she will be compared to the mythical peer, "the reasonably prudent dentist" or "dental hygienist," and if found to have conducted him/herself short of that standard, he/she will probably lose the case.[3]

In many instances, the plaintiff does not need to call upon expert witnesses or create a substantial base of evidence in order to prove negligence. The doctrine of *res ipsa loquitur* (the matter speaks for itself) may be invoked, when injury is obviously directly related to some clear instance of negligence.[1] An example might be harm caused by not recording a medical history or by providing services while intoxicated. Once it is proved that there was no medical history or the provider was indeed intoxicated, the court needs no further proof of fault.

There may be some comfort in the realization that the criteria historically used to determine the appropriate standard of care for health care providers were dependent upon the practice of other health care providers in the profession in the same locale. The plaintiff would then need to call upon professional peers to testify regarding how they would perform under the same circumstances. This is no longer the case, however. The courts now turn to stated professional standards of practice for the criteria rather than to individual peers.[2,5] This trend is in keeping with the "age of accountability," which prompted professions to specify their functions in behavioral, measurable terms and to specify minimum levels of competence. Many educational programs design their curricula with these ultimate competencies in mind. The American Dental Hygienists Association has specified "terminal objectives" that define the scope of practice and the levels of competency necessary for a "reasonably prudent" practicing dental hygienist.[7] Practicing professionals now have greater reason to be aware of the standards the profession has

identified and to participate in continuing education activities designed to raise their levels of competence to that specified by the profession.

During the 1970s malpractice suits have been more frequent.[4] Hygienists are not free from the threat of suit. An awareness of this fact alone may prompt dental hygienists to assume greater responsibility for the quality of care they are delivering.

It is this growth in number of malpractice actions that has caused malpractice insurance premiums to skyrocket. Exorbitant premiums, especially for anesthesiologists, surgeons, and other high risk specialties have driven some insurance companies out of the medical malpractice business and have caused some physicians to consider leaving practice. Annual premiums of $30,000 per practitioner are not uncommon in some specialties. A health care provider who is sued and loses the case will probably never be able to keep insurance coverage, which literally may force him/her from practice. State legislatures and medical societies are attempting to resolve this problem by placing ceilings on malpractice awards and ensuring, by various state measures, that physicians will have coverage available. This situation is particularly critical in those states where no-fault auto insurance was enacted, eliminating a large area of legal practice that was related to proving fault in auto accidents. Observers in those states believe that the increase in malpractice actions is directly related to the decrease in negligence actions resulting from automobile property damage and personal injury.

Ironically, the advent of consumer awareness and the resultant increase in litigation regarding quality of health care resulted in a decrease of certain kinds of care, especially on-the-spot, voluntary emergency care. Physicians may well fear litigation if some harm came to the patient that might be attributed to the inadequacies of first aid efforts.

Most states have felt the need to enact special legislation to protect health personnel from litigation in the event they stop to render emergency care. Such legislative provisions are known as Good Samaritan Laws or clauses.[4] They specifically protect the provider by turning aside litigation charging negligence except when harm is the direct result of wanton or gross negligence. Many Good Samaritan Laws, however, address themselves only to physicians and nurses, making no mention of other persons (such as dentists or dental hygienists) who could provide emergency care. The laws are unclear therefore, in the possible protection they could offer such a provider who "almost" saves a person's life.

The general rule is that the "reasonably prudent man" measure is applied in assessing whether the provider of first aid was negligent. Dentists are "measured" against dentists, physicians against physicians, nurses against nurses, and dental hygienists against dental hygienists.[4] Despite the minimal protection provided by such laws, knowledge of state provisions and just what safeguards they contain is wise for any health care provider.

In the meantime, it is imperative that one develop a constant awareness of the quality of care being provided and the duties owed the patient. Negligence or a violation of a patient's rights can be very costly—in time, money, and reputation.

Review questions

1. Define *negligence*.
2. What is the measure of whether a person is guilty of negligence or not?
3. What four factors must be present for a suit of negligence to be successful against a person?
   a.
   b.
   c.
   d.
4. What is *contributory negligence?*
5. What is *proximate cause?*

True or false:

6. A Good Samaritan Law protects any health care provider against a negligence suit if the provider renders first aid care to an injured person. _____
7. The recently established criteria for determining what is "reasonably prudent" are to determine the average person's quality of activities. _____
8. Hygienists are safe from malpractice suits. _____

ANSWERS

1. Negligence is the commission of an act that the reasonably prudent person would not have performed or the omission of an act that the reasonably prudent person would have performed.
2. Whether or not the reasonably prudent person in that profession and under the same circumstances would have performed similarly, according to defined standards of practice.
3. a. Duty is owed to a person (a contract exists).
   b. There is a breach of that duty.
   c. The person has been injured or harmed.
   d. The breach of the duty is the proximate cause of the harm.
4. The patient "contributed" his own ignorance or action to the situation, "contributing" to the harm.
5. The "proximate cause" is the factor that can be directly and causally related to the harm.
6. False or at least unlikely; check the state law for the exact provision.
7. False; definitive performance criteria are now more commonly used.
8. False; all providers of care *are* responsible for their actions.

GROUP ACTIVITIES

1. Review current literature to identify what suits have been brought against dental auxiliaries, whether the suit was successful, and the amount of damages awarded the plaintiff.
2. Review the literature for the crisis of rising malpractice insurance; review specifically the medical and dental journals and newspapers that are published in states where no-fault auto insurance has been signed into law.
3. Determine whether the state in which you (plan to) practice has a Good Samaritan Law. Analyze it for the actual protection it provides and whom it protects.

REFERENCES

1. Black, M. A.: Black's law dictionary, ed. 4, St. Paul, Minn., 1968, West Publishing Co.
2. Medicolegal Rounds: Shier v. Freedman, J. Am. Med. Assoc., 235:1614.
3. Miller, Sidney L.: Legal aspects of dentistry, New York, 1970, G. P. Putnam's Sons.
4. Morganstern, Stanley: Legal protection for the consumer, Dobbs Ferry, N.Y., 1973, Oceana Publications, Inc.
5. Murchison, I. A. and Nichols, T. S.: Legal foundations of nursing practice, New York, 1970, Macmillan, Inc.
6. Sarner, Harvey: Dental jurisprudence, Philadelphia, 1963, W. B. Saunders Co.
7. Woodall, Irene, R., editor: Curriculum essentials, ed. 3, Chicago, 1975, The American Dental Hygienists Association.

CHAPTER 9

Technical assault

OBJECTIVES: The reader will be able to:

1. Define technical assault.
2. Differentiate between technical assault and breach of contract.
3. Given hypothetical cases, identify instances in which health care professionals commit technical assault or take appropriate precautions to protect themselves from claims of technical assault.
4. Compare express and implied contracts with regard to the protection they provide against charges of technical assault.

It has been shown that when a patient seeks and accepts care from a health care provider, the patient enters a contractual relationship with the health professional and the health care professional is obligated to provide the care agreed to, according to the accepted standard of skill and care. The patient is expected to cooperate in the provision of care and to pay a reasonable fee for the services received.

If the health care provider does not provide the care or if the patient does not pay the fee, one may sue the other for breach of contract. If an appropriate standard of care is not met, resulting in some damage to the patient, the patient may, under tort law, sue for *negligence*. The patient will not be successful in the suit if *contributory negligence* (lack of agreed upon cooperation or other act or omission of the patient significantly contributing to the patient's injury) can be proved.

But what happens if the health care provider performs some service over and above that which is agreed to? Is this some special bonus for the patient? The health care provider may think so. However, if some service other than those specifically agreed to is performed, the patient may sue, charging *technical assault*.[1-5]

Negligence and technical assault are the two components of tort law.[4] The former is applicable when some damage can be proved to be causally related to an act omitted or committed by another person and which is judged to be a dereliction of duty when compared to the action performed by the "reasonably prudent" person. The latter refers to those instances where a "touching" to which the patient has not agreed has occurred.[1,2,4,5] It is different from breach of contract because it generally refers to some procedure *not* included in the contract which *has* been performed rather than to some procedure *not* performed which *is* included in the contract.

The difficulty for health care providers arises when the provider "assumes" that, because the patient has sought his/her care, the patient is agreeable to anything that appears necessary. Many health care providers believe that the trusting patient is providing them with blanket authorization.

Legally, it is not possible for a patient to give up his/her right to be informed by signing any statement that says the provider may do "whatever appears necessary."[2] Nor does a blanket verbal release provide health care personnel with the right to proceed with whatever procedures they choose. Each procedure or combination of procedures must be specifically agreed to by the patient if the provider is to be protected against technical assault. However, the law clearly recognizes an "extension doctrine," which allows the provider to do related things not specifically agreed to, which sound professional judgment requires be done as part of the same procedure and where circumstances preclude consulting the patient.

For example, a child whose parent specifies "oral prophylaxis and fluoride treatment" as the procedures to be provided should not have a radiographic series prepared unless the parent is asked and agrees. A man expecting that one tooth needs to be prepared and restored should not have two teeth receive that treatment unless he is asked and agrees. A woman who agrees to have a biopsy of a lesion should not awaken to realize she has had more extensive surgery, unless prior to the biopsy she has agreed that if surgery is necessary it may be performed.

Persons who participate in express and implied contracts have the legal right to be apprised of intended procedures, and they have the right to agree or to decline.[2,3,5] It should be apparent that the concept of the implied contract leaves the health care professional in a precarious position: the open mouth may legally, contractually imply "You may look in," but it does not provide much protection when the patient claims that it did not imply permission was granted to do what was performed after the provider looked in.

The express contract, where the procedures and conditions are agreed upon either verbally or in writing, provides greater protection,[2] assuming of course that the provider does not deviate from the original written agreement. By discussing the proposed procedures with the patient or by presenting a written treatment plan, the patient has the opportunity to agree or disagree with what is planned. The patient has the opportunity to say "yes," and "proceed," which is all that is necessary, in most instances, to protect the patient from technical assault and to protect the health care provider from the charge that technical assault was committed.[5]

In most instances, the simple request,

"Should we proceed?" following a discussion of the need for and nature of the procedure is adequate. However, a complex treatment or series of treatments would best be agreed to in writing. This may be appropriate especially when a complex treatment plan could result in a less than perfect result because of the difficulty or tenuous nature of the procedures. The patient should be aware of the likelihood of an "imperfect" result prior to agreeing to treatment; a written, signed statement may make it a good deal easier to prove knowledge as well as the agreement.

Often the procedures provided in health care involve more than one "component" of care, depending upon how they are defined.[2] For instance, an oral prophylaxis may include some root planing. Some root planing procedures include soft tissue curettage. It is possible that a patient could successfully sue, charging technical assault, if he were to learn that his roots were planed when all he wanted was to have his teeth "cleaned." The suit would be successful if the definitions of the two procedures were proved to be distinctly different. However, the suit would probably be turned aside if it could be proved that the root planing was an integral part of the oral prophylaxis and necessary for the prophylaxis to be considered complete. Because many treatments are actually composites of more than one distinct procedure, it is probably wise for the health care provider to distinguish components in any treatment when discussing the treatment plan with the patient.

For instance, a routine oral prophylaxis might be identified as scaling and polishing. A complete radiographic survey might be described as a series of fourteen periapical and four bitewing or caries-detection radiographs so that the patient is aware of the scope of the procedure.

Regardless of the scope of the procedure, the best way to avoid technical assault is to explain fully the procedures planned and *ask* for permission to proceed. This relatively simple practice may prove to be invaluable in an era when patients are more aware of their legal rights. Aside from legality, the explanation and permission-seeking may greatly improve patients' cooperation in the delivery of care, since they may have a greater feeling of participation and may more fully understand the nature of procedures.

There is another responsibility owed to patients that is related to performing only those procedures agreed to by the patient. The health care provider may be charged with technical assault if he/she touches the patient in places or in a manner that has no direct relationship to the provision of health care.[2,4,5] Using a patient's chest as a prop for one's arm is one example. Just because the patient agrees to some intraoral procedure does not mean that the patient has agreed to being used as a shelf.

A second easily understood example is the "bear hug" some dental operators give their patients' heads when performing some procedures from behind the patient. If the patient is positioned too high in relation to the operator, it may be convenient for the operator to provide an extra source of support for the patient's head with his/her chest.

The patient has not agreed to this extra contact, and if he/she reacts strongly enough to the touching he/she may sue in tort law, claiming technical assault. The obvious conclusion is that all health care providers ought to be more aware of the liberties they take in touching the patient incidental to providing care.

A second conclusion worthy of some discussion is the possible liability for technical assault a health care provider may have if specific permission is not asked *prior* to commencing palpation examinations. For instance, the oral examination procedure performed for a patient includes extraoral palpation as an integral component. But what if the oral examination the patient thought he agreed to did not include palpation? What reaction may the patient have to having his neck "massaged" when he though he was having his mouth looked at? The patient may immediately react to the palpation procedure as an assault. The patient may sue if his reaction is strong enough. This example may appear to be extreme, but it could occur, and as a practical matter it provides one more reason to describe intended services to patients and to seek their agreement.

A simple precaution is to inform the patient that the oral exam is visual, but that is also includes feeling the face and neck for lumps, texture deviations, and other indicators of normal and abnormal conditions and then to ask for permission to proceed.

Explanation and a request for permission to go ahead with the procedures are the two keys to preventing a charge of technical assault.

Review questions

1. The act of "touching" or performing some procedure for a patient, which was not agreed to is known as _____.
2. Breach of contract occurs when:
3. Breach of contract and technical assault differ because:
4. *Review:* Tort law is comprised of:
   a.
   b.
5. An (implied/express) contract is the better safeguard against technical assault.
6. Identify, for each of the hypothetical cases, whether a charge of technical assault by the patient could be upheld:
   a. A dental hygienist performs a fluoride treatment for a child patient whose mother specified teeth cleaning and x-rays.
   b. A dentist extracts three teeth from a patient while the patient is under general anesthesia. The patient agreed to having only two extracted.
   c. A dental hygienist explains that the oral prophylaxis to be performed will include smoothing roughened roots. He performs an oral prophylaxis and root planes fifteen surfaces.

ANSWERS

1. Technical assault
2. A person in a contract does not perform as agreed to.
3. In technical assault, some procedure *not* agreed to *is* performed, rather than some agreed to procedure not being performed.
4. a. Negligence
   b. Technical assault
5. Express
6. a. Could be upheld
   b. Could be upheld
   c. Not likely to be upheld

GROUP ACTIVITIES

1. Outline a case presentation format that is most likely to prevent technical assault.
2. Consult "consumer awareness" handbooks to determine what guidelines patients should have to protect themselves against technical assault.
3. Record or observe various case presentations to assess whether the express contract is sufficiently comprehensive to prevent technical assault from occurring during the actual provision of treatment.
4. Describe personal experiences as a patient and as a care provider where technical assault occurred.
5. Attend a trial in civil court where technical assault is the charge.

REFERENCES

1. Black, M. A.: Black's law dictionary, ed. 4, St. Paul, Minn., 1968, West Publishing Co.
2. Miller, Sidney L.: Legal aspects of dentistry, New York, 1970, G. P. Putnam's Sons.
3. Morris, R. Crawford and Moritz, Alan R.: Doctor and patient and the law, ed. 5, St. Louis, 1971, The C. V. Mosby Co.
4. Prosser, Wm. L.: Handbook of the law of torts, ed. 4, St. Paul, Minn., 1971, West Publishing Co.
5. Sarner, Harvey: Dental jurisprudence, Philadelphia, 1963, W. B. Saunders Co.

CHAPTER 10

Fees, forms, and good judgment

OBJECTIVES: The reader will be able to:

1. Define *fee* and identify it as an integral part of the contract agreement.
2. Compare the two types of fees with the two types of contracts.
3. Explain how a "reasonable fee" is determined.
4. Explain a patient's likely response to an unexpectedly high fee.
5. Describe the advantages and disadvantages of
   a. Quoting a fee
   b. Estimating a fee
   c. Not discussing fees at all
6. Given a partial payment accompanied by a statement marked "paid in full," identify what consequences may occur if the payment and statement are accepted without comment.
7. Identify the courses of action available to a provider of services whose client or patient does not pay as agreed.
8. Recognize the characteristics of a well-kept patient record.
9. Relate the importance of a well-kept record to its use as evidence in a court of law.
10. Define *admission against interest* and *res gestae* and identify how these concepts apply to use of evidence in a court of law.
11. List the steps a person should follow when
    a. Confronted with a lawsuit.
    b. An incident occurs that could lead to a suit.
12. Describe how the "patient as partner in care" concept can prevent legal action.
13. Explain the concept of consumer advocacy and how it relates to the ethical duties owed to patients.

The contractual relationship between a health care provider and a patient has been described as one in which some service is provided for the patient, for which the patient pays a *fee*. A fee is a consideration, usually in money, for services. It is an essential part of a contract between two competent parties.[1,2,4-6]

Just as a contract may be express or implied, so may a fee. A fee may be stated either orally or in writing, or a fee may be implied by the actions of the parties—an assumed component of the fact that the patient requests care and the health care provider performs the services.[4-6] Few patients would honestly expect care for free. So the

issue of debate then centers on the question, "How much?"

Most court actions regarding fees relate to the patient's contention that the fee was unreasonably high. So how is a fee determined to be reasonable or unreasonable? The simplest answer is that it ought to be in keeping with the complexity of the services provided.

A more specific determination of what is "reasonable" is based on four considerations: (1) what is customary in the geographic area for the particular procedure, (2) the cost of materials and other overhead considerations (such as time) in order to provide the services, (3) the complexity of services and the skill and expertise of the operator, and (4) (some have contended) the ability of the patient to pay.[4]

Professional organizations may actually publish a list of suggested fees to which they hope their membership will adhere. However, the Supreme Court, in a case involving lawyer's fees has declared this practice to be price-fixing and therefore an illegal restraint of trade in violation of the federal antitrust laws.[3] But even without published, suggested fees, a community of professionals is often aware of the "going rate" and may not deviate from it too drastically. Despite the fact that most professions do not advertise their services and fees, patients often are aware of what various procedures cost. And if a fee greatly exceeds their idea of "reasonable," they may choose not to pay part or all of it. An unexpectedly high fee may be countered by more than just nonpayment. It may trigger a malpractice suit, particularly if there is some measure of dissatisfaction with the procedure.[4] Such a suit can present problems to the practitioner even where there is little doubt that the patient's case ultimately will fail.

Once again, the danger of an implied contract or fee is apparent. If the fee hasn't been discussed, there is a significant possibility that it will be an unpleasant surprise to the patient. Many health care providers may view the discussion of the fee as an unprofessional or embarrassing occurrence. The fact is that patients do expect some sort of a fee, and the health care provider may be able to allay their concern if it is simply discussed in an open manner at the time of case presentation.

Since not discussing the fee is risky, there are two remaining approaches worthy of consideration. One approach is quoting the fee; the other is estimating the fee. Quoting the fee gives the patient an exact indication of what dollar investment will be needed in order to receive care. There are no surprises, and the fee is either paid in a series of partial payments during or after care is completed or paid in full upon completion. Although surprise to the patient is eliminated, a surprise may be in store for the health care provider. A quoted fee does not usually allow for unexpected materials costs or for treatments not anticipated to be necessary at the time of the treatment plan. If the case involves more time, effort, or other cost, the fee legally remains unchanged when it is quoted exactly.[4]

A health care provider who has been stung by the quoted fee may decide to take the second approach, the estimated fee. In this instance, the case presentation includes an estimated fee, which is subject to costs incurred in providing the outlined care. If more effort is needed, this can be explained to the patient and the fee adjusted upward. Likewise, if the procedures progress more easily than anticipated, the fee can be adjusted downward. The estimated fee provides the patient with a reasonably accurate idea of what the cost will be, but it also ensures a measure of flexibility to cover the unexpected. Even though the estimated fee allows the provider legal flexibility, it is wise for him/her to advise the patient when unexpected circumstances necessitate a substantial deviation from the estimated figure.

In most instances a policy of expressing the fee either orally or in writing will prevent most legal encounters over fees. However, even in cases when a fee is stated and agreed to, some patients will refuse to pay. One tactic patients may take is to make a partial payment by check and label it "paid in full." In a few states, accepting the partial payment without comment may be interpreted as meaning that the balance due is not expected. So it is important to compare payments labeled "paid in full" with the actual balance due. Any discrepancy should be resolved before the partial payment is accepted by depositing the payment.[4] It is advised that the provider ask an attorney whether the state still follows the old rule allowing for discharge of the obligation by acceptance of an "in full payment" check.

In instances where the patient simply refuses to pay, the health care provider does have some recourse. The provider can issue warning letters in increasingly persistent language. If the letters are not successful, the account can be turned over to a collection agency, which continues the dunning process and which can alter the patient's credit rating.[4,5] The agency charges a percentage of the fee ultimately paid by the patient in return for its efforts. It is doubtful whether this collection fee can legally be passed on to the delinquent patient unless this practice was made known to him/her prior to the rendering of the services in question.

If the letters and the efforts of the collection agency prove to be futile, the health care provider can bring a suit of breach of contract against the patient. And the suit may be successful. However, it is important to recall that litigation is costly in time, money, and aggravation. Furthermore, given the possibility of a countersuit, legal action for fee collection should be viewed as a last resort and be used only when the unpaid balance is substantial.

It should be clear that express contracts and agreed fees are good preventive measures. Another is a clear, concise, accurate patient record. The patient record is probably the most important piece of evidence in court. If it is easily understood, meticulously recorded, and focuses on the needs of the patient and the care provided to meet those needs, the rationale and quality of care will be much easier to defend. Sadly enough, the best of care may be indefensible in court if it isn't discernible in the record. Poor radiographs, pencil entries, undated entries, missing or incomplete entries do not present a picture of quality care.

The patient record should include radiographs of diagnostic quality; the entries should be made *in ink* and be dated with the month, day, and year. All patient visits and procedures should be described. The progress of health should be discernible. A medical history, kept up to date, should be present in the chart. Before and after intraoral photographs can be invaluable when the practitioner is confronted with a malpractice suit. A well-kept record can have a very positive impact on the judge and jury. The very

fact that the patient knows the records are accurate may dissuade him/her from filing suit.

In contrast, the scribbled, incoherent, misspelled chart may smack of lack of due concern or even incompetence. By tolerating inaccurate charts, the health care provider is stacking evidence against him/herself.

There are other ways in which the health care provider can create evidence that is harmful in a court of law. One such way is for the health care provider to make some spontaneous statement during treatment that is self-incriminating. For instance, if during an oral prophylaxis, an instrument slips and cuts the tissue and the operator exclaims, "Oh, I should have had a better fulcrum," the operator has made a comment that can be used against him. This self-incriminating spontaneous utterance constitutes *res gestae*, which means "a part of the action," since the statement occurred simultaneous to the action in question.[1,5] Evidence that might otherwise be barred from court by the rule against "hearsay" may be admitted under the *res gestae* exception.

If a person makes an out-of-court statement, either spoken or in writing, which proves the opposite of what he/she is contending in court, the statement is an *admission against interest* and is admissible as evidence against the person,[1,4] again in exception to the general rule barring hearsay evidence. For example, a nurse may write a letter to a friend describing an error she made in administering a medication and explaining that she is fighting a charge of malpractice. The letter may end up as evidence against the nurse, since it may contradict what she is contending in court. An admission against interest differs from *res gestae* because it is a statement made at any time, which goes against the pecuniary or other legal interest of that person. A patient-plaintiff, of course, could make an admission against interest just as the provider could.

The use of *res gestae* and admission against interest as evidence should provide an indication of an important rule to follow if the health care provider finds him/herself in a potential legal tangle: He/she should discuss it with no one except his/her attorney and the malpractice insurance carrier.[4,5] Direct communication with the patient may prove disastrous. When an injury occurs, the patient should be informed of the injury and appropriate steps should be taken to correct it. However no incriminating explanations should be offered about the reason for the error. The problem should not be discussed with colleagues or friends, except as advised by the attorney. Any injury that could be viewed as a stimulus for a lawsuit should immediately be reported to the insurance carrier.

Express contracts and fees, accurate records, and careful responses to potential lawsuits are all useful preventive measures. But they imply a defensive approach to the legal aspects of health care delivery. While it is appropriate to be protective of one's own well-being, it is more in keeping with a service-oriented profession to conduct oneself with the well-being of the patient as the primary consideration.

The very philosophy that a health care provider provides services *for* a patient rather than *to* a patient can create a "partnership" approach to health care. Including the patient as a responsible co-determiner of the nature of health care services is probably the most significant step in preventing lawsuits and in ensuring success of treatment. Patients who feel a commitment to the care they receive by virtue of understanding their needs will cooperate more fully in obtaining and maintaining the successful treatment.

The day of the consumer awareness of rights dictates involving the patient as a partner in health care. If care is indeed patient-centered rather than procedure-centered, the health care provider might look beyond the matter of care to be provided to issues relating to the dignity of the patient, the procedures to which the patient is subjected (including the red tape of forms and multiple visits), and the quality of overall care the patient is receiving.

If a health professional or a group of professionals adopts the role of consumer advocate, patients whose rights are violated might be assisted in obtaining restitution. Patients can be informed of their rights, be provided with guidelines for determining the quality of care delivered, and be directed to legal aid, if necessary. Poor quality health care, fraud in charging for procedures not performed, and the unhelping, elitist attitudes of some health care personnel cost the public a great deal in terms of time, money, discomfort, and dignity. A commitment to changing these negative aspects of health care may in itself change the negative reputation that some believe health care has acquired in recent years.

Review questions

1. How do the two types of fees relate to the two types of contracts?
2. How is a "reasonable fee" determined?
3. A patient pays only 60% of the fee due. The physician files a breach of contract suit for nonpayment. What is a possible legal response from the patient?
4. Identify four characteristics of a well-kept patient record:
   a.
   b.
   c.
   d.
5. A spontaneous statement accompanying some injury or error is referred to as _____ .
6. A statement made by a person which conflicts with the position taken by that person in court is known as _____ .

ANSWERS

1. Contracts and fees may be implied or express (verbal or written).
2. It is based on what is customary locally, on the scope of the procedure and the skill of the operator, overhead costs, and the ability of the patient to pay.
3. He may countersue, charging malpractice.
4. a. Accurate, coherent, quality radiographs
   b. A medical history
   c. Care is related to need
   d. Progress of health is discernible
5. *Res gestae*
6. Admission against interest

GROUP ACTIVITIES

1. Have a panel discussion to debate whether fee determination ought to be based in part on the patient's ability to pay.
2. Poll professional associations to see if recommended fess are published for members.
3. Assess sample patient records for their usefulness as evidence. Design a set of records that clearly depicts care needed and provided and the progress of health.
4. Conduct a mock trial in which the patient record offered in defense is:
   a. Unhelpful, even detrimental
   b. Helpful
5. Role play instances of *res gestae* and admission against interest.
6. Read and critique one or more books written

to serve as a guide for consumers of dental care.

REFERENCES

1. Black, M. A.: Black's law dictionary, ed. 4, St. Paul, Minn., 1968, West Publishing Co.
2. Creighton, Helen: Law every nurse should know, Philadelphia, 1957, W. B. Saunders Co.
3. Goldfarb v. Virginia Bar Association, 96 Sup. Ct. 2004 (1975).
4. Miller, S. L.: Legal aspects of dentistry, New York, 1970, G. P. Putnam's Sons.
5. Sarner, H.: Dental jurisprudence, Philadelphia, 1963, W. B. Saunders Co.
6. Stetler, C. Joseph and Moritz, Alan R.: Doctor and patient and the law, St. Louis, 1962, The C. V. Mosby Co.

CHAPTER 11

Criminal charges: actions contrary to state statutes regulating practice

OBJECTIVES: The reader will be able to:

1. Differentiate between civil law and criminal law.
2. State the purpose of a state practice act, governing the practice of health care professionals.
3. Explain how the health care practitioner's professional actions are governed by the two branches of law: civil and criminal.
4. Given a series of hypothetical situations, identify whether each situation is covered by civil law or criminal law.
5. Describe the role of the "state board" in enforcing the practice act.
6. Differentiate "open" practice acts and "closed" practice acts.
7. Describe briefly how the trend toward greater scope of practice for auxiliaries is affected by the practice act.

So far the legal considerations for health care providers have been within the realm of the patient-provider relationship, described as consensual and contractual and in which certain rights and duties are reciprocal between the parties involved. Difficulties encountered in this contractual relationship are dealt with through one of the two branches of civil law: contract law or tort law. In civil law, the individual who believes a wrong has occurred files against the offender through a private attorney. The previous chapters have identified the rights and duties owed in the patient-provider relationship. The chapters offered suggestions for preventing such difficulties.

It is important to realize that the health care provider is also obligated to observe the limits defined in *criminal law*.

A 'crime' [is] punishable upon conviction by:
1. Death; or
2. Imprisonment; or,
3. Fine; or,
4. Removal from office; or,

5. Disqualification to hold any position of trust, honor or profit under the state; or,
6. Other penal discipline.[3]

Criminal law involves actions that constitute a wrong against society. Civil law is related to actions causing harm to an individual. In criminal law, the state takes action against the wrongdoer, whereas in civil law, the plaintiff (wronged individual) files suit through a private attorney. Statutory law (enacted by the legislature) forms the basis of most criminal law, with case law (which is based upon precedents established by the courts) comprising a smaller portion. Case law and statutory law are of equal importance in civil law.

It may not be obvious at first how a health care provider may commit a criminal act in the normal course of a day's professional activities. The "crime" that a provider commits is rarely the kind dramatized on television. It is usually an infraction of the state practice act (statute) covering the scope of activity of the particular provider in question.

Many health care professions are covered directly by a state practice act, which defines the practice of the particular profession and stipulates the means by which a person may be granted a license to practice as a member of that particular profession. All licensed health care provider groups are regulated by state statute.

In all states or licensing jurisdictions, there is a "state board" to administer the written word of the practice act. The state board is an agency of the state; its members are usually appointed by the governor. The primary purpose of the practice act is to protect the public from incompetent would-be practitioners of the profession.[5-7] The practice act prohibits persons from "setting up shop" unless they have specific, proved qualifications and competencies. The practice act empowers the state board to review the qualifications and competencies of applicants and to issue or deny a *license* to practice. The act also empowers the state board to suspend or revoke a license, if the practitioner violates the regulatory provisions of the act.[5-7]

Any act committed by a person in violation of the applicable state practice act is a crime against society and subject to prosecution and, upon conviction, punishment. The action is brought against the offender by "the people" in the person of the attorney general at the request of the state board.[5,6]

An illegal act need not result in actual bodily injury or property damage in order to be a criminal offense. The "harm" is considered to be the violation of the principles set down by the people through the action of the legislature.[1-3,5,6]

For instance, if a state dental practice act stipulates that dental hygienists or dentists are the only persons recognized to perform the oral prophylaxis, any other person who performs that procedure has committed a crime—even though no actual harm to the patient may have resulted. If a graduate hygienist begins to practice before he/she is issued a license, that hygienist has committed a crime. If a dental practice act empowers a dentist to delegate specific functions to an auxiliary in the office and a dentist delegates more procedures than those permitted, the dentist has committed a crime, but the person who performed the procedure has also committed a crime by aiding or abetting unauthorized practice. Any violation of the state practice act is a criminal violation. The seriousness of the violation determines what the punishment will be if prosecution results in a conviction.[1-3] The state board may issue a fine or revoke the person's license or at least suspend it for a specified time. If court action is involved, the practitioner may be heavily fined or even imprisoned, depending upon the severity of the infraction. An example of an infraction that could result in a criminal conviction is the illegal prescribing or dispensing of narcotics by a licensed professional. The court may determine that such activity should result in a more severe penalty than license revocation.

Criminal acts committed by persons governed by one of the practice acts may be reported to the state board by a patient, another practitioner, or any other person who recognizes the infraction. The state board then sends out an investigator to gather evidence necessary to determine whether an infraction has occurred. If sufficient evidence is gathered, the board conducts a hearing. In extreme cases the attorney general may be asked to begin criminal proceedings. It should be obvious from the list of possible punishments that charges of violation of the state practice act can be substantial for the person found guilty.

The responsibility of the health care provider in more recent years is complicated by the status of most practice acts. In the 1930s when many dental practice acts were enacted, frequently all provisions for practice were stated in the law (a *closed* practice act). The state dental boards were empowered to enforce what was clearly stated in the act. However, with the trend toward utilizing auxiliary personnel to support dental practice, the states' acts went through a period of change. This trend and period of change reached a peak in the late 1960s and early 1970s.[7] The changes that were enacted often provided the state dental practice act with only general descriptions of the scope of functions of dental personnel. A few functions were listed in the act as allowed and a few functions were listed as disallowed, in order to provide a semblance of a definition of the health care provider being described. In addition to the skeleton listings, many revised acts added a phrase such as, "This person may perform any other functions which the state board of dentistry determines to be appropriate," resulting in an *open* practice act. This catchall phrase and others similar to it give power to the state boards to decide what activities are appropriate for each covered health care provider.[4] Many states' laws include statements permitting the supervising dentist in the practice to delegate a wide variety of functions, according to his/her judgment.

There are many advantages to the open practice act, the most important of which is the fact that the entire state legislature need not reconsider the practice act in order to allow delegation of certain additional functions to personnel. As the times change and the need for support services changes, the state board through an official ruling can alter what is allowed to be delegated. The most liberal or open act reads, "The health care provider may perform those procedures which he/she has mastered through formal education." The state board must then identify a limit on what procedures are allowable, which it includes in its rules and regulations relating to the practice act.

The difficulty with this trend in the structure of practice acts belongs primarily to the health care provider and to the consumer-patient, whose task it is to be informed of what is or is not permitted in a particular state or licensing jurisdiction. The rules are no longer found in the published practice act. The regulations that are to accompany an open act may have been tied up in hear-ings for years after the act is passed. Or, the regulations, even though decided upon by the board, may not be published. Inquiries to different members of the same state board may result in different, in fact opposite, descriptions of what is legally allowable.[7] Yet, it is the health care provider's responsibility to *know* the law and then to obey it.[2,3]

The problem is compounded when a health care provider decides to move to another licensing jurisdiction. Aside from the usual requirement that he/she again prove competence to practice before a license is issued, the provider must begin anew the effort to determine what is or is not allowed in that state. Are all stipulations published? Is the state board in a period of indecision or disagreement? Are some published regulations not enforced at all because of the ensuing debate? What may the practitioner legally provide the patient?

The issues surrounding the practice acts in various states are complex ethical, economic, political, and legal considerations. Earlier parts of this text discuss those issues more fully. But in terms of self-protection from prosecution, it is best to request the practice act and any accompanying rules, regulations, and interpretations *in writing* and then retain them with the issued license. If a request for written clarification is refused, one choice may be to secure the aid of an attorney or to at least retain the written refusal. This may be the only defense in a criminal case. Also, it is a wise policy to read professional journals to learn of any current discussion or proposal changes or "clarifications."

As described earlier in this text, the dental practice act is one of the major considerations in expanding the scope of care a dental auxiliary may provide.[4,7] It can be a major roadblock to change, or it can be an initiating force to promote change. Regardless of its role in hindering or helping change, the individual dentist or auxiliary is legally responsible to it. And a breach of that responsibility is a criminal act.

Review questions

True or false:
1. Civil law covers those rights and responsibilities owed in the contractual relationship between a patient and the health care provider. _____
2. Criminal law covers infractions against an individual patient when harm results to the patient. _____
3. The sources of criminal law are federal or state statutes enacted by the legislature. _____
4. Dental practice acts are written and enacted by the state boards of dentistry. _____
5. The state board of dentistry enforces the state dental practice act. _____
6. In an "open" practice act, all regulations are contained in the act as passed by the legislature. _____
7. The purpose of a state practice act is to protect the profession. _____

Indicate which of the following acts is covered by civil law (contract or tort) or criminal law:

	Civil	Criminal
8. A dental hygienist places restorative materials in prepared teeth. Despite the fact that the services are performed well with no harm to the patient, the practice act does limit this activity to the dentist.	_____	_____
9. A patient is injured by a dental hygienist administering a local anesthetic. Rules of the state board permit delegation of this function to the dental hygienist.	_____	_____
10. A patient is harmed by a negligent act of a dental assistant who is scaling teeth, despite the practice act's prohibition of this activity by dental assistants.	_____	_____
11. A nurse prescribes and administers a medication. The state law prohibits the prescription of medication by nurses.	_____	_____

ANSWERS

1. True
2. False. Criminal law is an act committed against society by virtue of a violation of an enacted state or federal law or case law.
3. True. Case law is another source.
4. False. Dental practice acts are written and enacted by the legislature.
5. True
6. False. In a "closed" practice act, all regulations are contained in the enacted law. In an "open" practice act, some modifying or clarifying clauses may be made by the state board in the form of rules and regulations.
7. False. It is to protect the *public*. It also limits entry to the profession, which many view as a form of professional protection.
8. Criminal law
9. Civil law
10. Civil *and* criminal law. The patient can sue the assistant and dentist. The state can prosecute the assistant and dentist.
11. Criminal law

GROUP ACTIVITIES

1. Consult a recent compilation of provisions included in state dental practice acts and compare and contrast four of them according to:
   a. Legally permitted functions for hygienists and assistants
   b. Requirements for licensure
   c. "Open" or "closed" characteristics
2. If there is ongoing discussion for changes in the dental practice act, attend public hearings and prepare a summary of the issues addressed and how the resolution of the issues could affect the scope of your practice.
3. Conduct an "inquiry" regarding the provisions of the practice act in your area. Five or six students should familiarize themselves with the current act and its rules and regulations and play the role of the state board. The remainder of the class will play the roles of "interested consumers," hygienists, assistants, and dentists wishing to *inquire* about the provisions of the act. Questions prepared by the inquirers should reflect the role each has adopted for purposes of the inquiry.
4. Prepare a review of the literature surrounding the "best" way to structure a practice act.
5. Review the ADHA recommendations for the structure of dental practice acts.
6. Request information regarding the role of the ADHA Regional Legislative Consultants in facilitating change in dental practice acts.
7. Attend a hearing or trial in the case of a health care provider charged with a violation of the practice act.

REFERENCES

1. Black, M. A.: Black's law dictionary, ed. 4, St. Paul, Minn., 1968, West Publishing Co.
2. Hall, Jerome and Mueller, Gerhard O. W.: Criminal law and procedure: Cases and readings, ed. 2, Indianapolis, 1965, The Bobbs-Merrill Co., Inc.
3. Hall, Jerome: General principles of criminal law, ed. 2, Indianapolis, 1960, The Bobbs-Merrill Co., Inc.
4. Manual for Consultants to State Boards of Dentistry, Chicago, 1973, American Dental Hygienists Associations.
5. Miller, S. L.: Legal aspects of dentistry, New York, 1970, G. P. Putnam's Sons.
6. Sarner, H.: Dental jurisprudence, Philadelphia, 1963, W. B. Saunders Co.
7. Woodall, Irene: Changes in state licensing acts allowing for expanded use of dental auxiliaries. In Mescher, Kay, editor: Proceedings of a training workshop on adaptation of dental hygiene practice to changing concepts in delivery of oral health services, Little Amana, Iowa, 1972, Iowa Dental Hygienists Association.

PART IV

ETHICS FOR HEALTH CARE PROVIDERS

To the health care provider, the term *ethics* may have a nebulous meaning. It may carry connotations of morality, religious orientation, or a more secular approach to "right behavior." If health care providers are to be ethical or to practice professional ethics, it may be helpful for them to focus on the various interpretations of the word and on how other professionals relate it to their roles as providers of health care.

Proceeding a step further, it may be helpful to identify ways in which ethics can be practically applied in day to day activities. And finally, attention must be given to the need to cope with changing social and professional views of ethics.

CHAPTER 12

Assessment of "ethics" and its translation into codes

OBJECTIVES: The reader will be able to:

1. State at least one definition of *ethics* that is acceptable to the student.
2. Differentiate brief, simplified descriptions of the Judeo-Christian, existentialist, and behavioral approaches to ethics and identify at least one philosopher whose theory is compatible with one of each of the brief descriptions.
3. Identify and explain the basic components of the current American Dental Hygienists Association Code of Ethics.
4. Differentiate an ethical code from a "patient's bill of rights."

A very large component of philosophy consists of the various approaches to the concept and implications of ethics. While the term can be very superficially and simply viewed as "knowing and doing what is right," it has much more complex and deeply rooted meanings for people. Who "knows" what is right? Can a particular situation cause some action to be viewed as "right" that in another situation would be "wrong"? Is ethics always directed toward the needs of the "other person" or is there an element of personal integrity that prompts ethical actions? Is ethics a matter of obeying an absolute standard established by an external entity?

APPROACHES TO ETHICS

These are but a few of the complex questions that are asked again and again in consideration of ethics. The answers vary with the philosophical base of the respondent. Two of the ancient Greeks, Plato and particularly, Aristotle, in his *Nicomachean Ethics*, viewed ethics as a value to be strived for that is the basis of harmony in life and personal happiness.[4,10] The contemporary French philosopher, Jean-Paul Sartre, would scoff at such a projected view of ethics and

focus on the dilemma it poses to the existential person in coexisting with persons whose needs may not always be compatible with his own.[2,4] B. F. Skinner, a primary figure in the behavioristic movement, sees ethics as a matter of a performance discrepancy, devoid of personal value and consisting mainly of activities that have to be "learned" by a management of the contingencies.[9]

In Western culture people are almost exclusively attuned to the Platonic-Aristotelian approach, which posits that ethics is a definitive absolute value to be strived for.[6,8] Goodness is seen as an unalterable, specific "form" toward which humans endeavor to perfect themselves.

Thomas Aquinas, in the thirteenth century, Christianized Aristotelian ethics, translating the *absolute value* into the Christian God and redefining human behavior in relation to this God as *moral behavior*. The new religious view of Aristotelian ethics became the basis for the codes of behavior established by the Roman Catholic Church, the dominant theistic-philosophical forum in Western civilization at the time. The emphasis was placed increasingly on the division of body and soul—more specifically on the soul's struggle to override the body's "animality." Augustine, in the fifth century had described this division as a matter of choice—an either/or decision to travel the rough road to heaven or the seemingly smooth road to hell. The matter of choice was definitive in its polarity. Behavior was right or it was wrong. The reward was heaven or hell. God was on one side; the devil was on the other. Good and Evil were seen as the difference between light and dark. This simplistic view of behavior became known as dualism. Religious paintings depict a man deciding which pathway to follow at the fork in the road. The road to heaven could be managed by a "right soul," which was successful in meeting and fending off the body's temptation. To choose short-range pleasure, permitting the body its desires, meant the long-range suffering at the end of life on earth.

With the Protestant Reformation in the Renaissance period of the sixteenth century, the either/or approach to ethics and morality remained basically intact.[8] In fact, the matter of only two paths to follow was intensified by the fact that there was no provision for earthly absolution of sins and no provision for an afterlife to cleanse the soul of its impurities (purgatory) so that the minor offenders could move on to heaven.[1a]

The Hebrew views of ethics followed similar patterns, reinforcing the either/or, light/dark, right/wrong approach to life and ethical behavior; Hebrew teachings were one of the wellsprings of Christianity.[7,8] Both elements of the Judeo-Christian tradition focused on the ultimate authority of God as father with mankind as the sometimes erring, sometimes obedient child.

With this cultural background guiding ethical behavior, people tend to search for external guidelines for right conduct and spend a good deal of energy identifying to whom it is they report their behavior.[6] Perhaps it is this cultural need that causes people to write codes of ethics and form "ethics committees" to enforce the codes.

To present the issues and their origins in such a simplified form does them injustice. Yet these issues are at the very core of a health care provider's professional mandate to behave in a manner that is in keeping with the "service" orientation and in response to patients' trust in the provider's good judgment and high ideals. A closer look at philosophical approaches other than the dualistic approach to ethics may provide health professionals the understanding to fashion a more eclectic approach to professional personal ethics.[6]

Existentialism has its roots in contemporary Europe, where wars, economic instability, and declining reliance on the Christian God spawned a turning inward that focused on the despair of daily life and inevitable death.[2] This philosophy described humans as having no predetermined nature, flying in the face of philosophies that were built on the platonic "ideal forms." Humans, to the existentialist, are "becoming." Their nature is defined as they live.[2] The whole matter of the ethics of relationship between people, "I" and "Thou," is far more complex than the Golden Rule.

Behavioristic thinking seems to take a more pragmatic approach. The behavioral premise is that an ethical, or any other, action is the result of learning through the positive and negative reinforcements and punishments received for similar actions taken by the person earlier in his or her life. Would the professions adopt a policy of teaching ethics by means of contingency management? Would they establish a program to identify the reward sequence and system that best produces ethical responses in people and then set out to improve the ethics of the professional membership?

The question of ethics for health care providers should extend beyond a listing of right or wrong actions that the associations of health care providers define as their codes. With the obvious changes in the late twentieth century society's approach to what is or is not acceptable, morally, ethically, or pragmatically, the health care professions might do well to equip themselves with the ability to cope with change and yet retain the mandate of providing care for patients, maintaining the very highest ethical values. Patterns of acceptable or unacceptable behavior are increasingly based upon the particular situation in which the behavior occurs. Although many people still adhere to the clearcut definitions of right and wrong, many others have basically set aside most of the time-honored rules in favor of such a *situation ethics* approach. Perhaps somewhere between dogmatic delineations of proper behavior and the challenge of operating with no guidelines there is a reasonable approach.

CODE OF ETHICS FOR DENTAL HYGIENISTS

Given that we do live in a dualistic, either/or world, it is not surprising to find that the American Dental Hygienists Association has developed codes of ethics. The first was in 1926, which stood until 1962. Others were written in 1969 and in 1975.

1926 CODE
The duties of the profession to their patients

Section 1. The dental hygienist should be ever ready to respond to the wants of her patrons, and should fully recognize the obligations involved in the discharge of her duties toward them. As she is in most cases unable to correctly estimate the character of her operations, her own sense of right must guarantee faithfulness as to gain the respect and confidence of her patients, and even the simplest case committed to her care should receive that attention which is due to operations performed on living, sensitive tissue.

Section 2. It is not to be expected that the patient will possess a very extended or very accurate knowledge of professional matters. The dental hygienist should make due allowance for this, patiently explaining many things which seem quite clear to herself, thus endeavoring to educate the public mind so that it will properly appreciate the beneficent efforts of our profession. She should encourage no false hopes by promising success when in the nature of the case there is uncertainty.

Section 3. The dental hygienist should be temperate in all things, keeping both mind and body in the best possible health, that her patients may have the benefit of the clearness of judgment and skill which is their right. [1]

1962 CODE
Principles of ethics of the American Dental Hygienists Association

The maintenance and enrichment of this heritage of professional status place on everyone who practices Dental Hygiene an obligation which should be willingly accepted and willingly fulfilled. This obligation cannot be reduced to a changeless series of urgings and prohibitions for, while the basic obligation is constant, its fulfillment may vary with the changing needs of a society composed of human beings that a profession is dedicated to serve. The spirit and not the letter of the obligation, therefore, must be the guide of conduct for the professional woman. In its essence this obligation has been summarized for all times and for all men in the golden rule which asks only that "whatsoever ye would that men should do to you, do ye even so to them."

The following statements constitute the *Principles of Ethics* of the American Dental Hygienists Association. The constituent and component societies are urged to adopt additional provisions or interpretations not in conflict with these *Principles of Ethics* which would enable them to serve more faithfully the traditions, customs and desires of these societies.

Section 1. Basic Deportment. If and when a member of this Association is employed, she shall be associated with a member of the American Dental Association or with a dentist whose practice is in accord with the *Principles of Ethics* of the American Dental Association.

Section 2. Education Beyond Usual Level. The right of a dental hygienist to professional status rests in the knowledge, skill and experience with which she serves her patients and society. Every dental hygienist has the obligation to keep her knowledge and skill freshened by continuing education throughout her professional life.

Section 3. Service to the Public. The dental hygienist has a right to win for herself of those things which give her the ability to take her proper place in the community which she serves, but there is no alternative for the professional woman in that she must place first her service to the public.

The dental hygienist's primary duty of serving the public is discharged by giving the highest type of service of which she is capable and by avoiding any conduct which leads to a lowering of esteem of the profession to which she belongs.

Section 4. Government of a Profession. Every profession receives from society the right to regulate itself, to determine and judge its own members. Such regulation is achieved largely through the influence of the professional societies, and every dental hygienist has the dual obligation of making herself a part of a professional society and of observing its rules of ethics as defined by statute and ordinance in various states, territories and dependencies.

Section 5. Leadership. The dental hygienist has the obligation of providing freely of her skills, knowledge and experience to society in those fields in which her qualifications entitle her to speak with professional competence. The dental hygienist should be active in and available to her community, especially in all efforts leading to the improvement of the dental health of the public.

Section 6. Limited Practice. The dental hygienist has an obligation to protect the health of her patient by not taking upon herself any service or operation which requires the professional competence of a dentist. The dental hygienist has a further obligation to the patient of placing herself under the supervision of a dentist at all times, as prescribed by law.

Section 7. Consultation. The dental hygienist has the obligation of referring for consultation and diagnosis to her supervisor all patients, whose welfare should be safeguarded or advanced by having recourse to those who have special skills, knowledge and experience.

Section 8. Unjust Criticism. The dental hygienist has the obligation of not referring disparagingly to the services of another dental hygienist or dentist in the presence of a patient. A lack of knowledge of conditions under which the services are afforded may lead to unjust criticism and to a lessening of the patient's confidence in the dental profession.

Section 9. Advertising. Advertising reflects adversely on the dental hygienist who employs it and lowers the public's esteem of the dental hygiene profession. The dental hygienist has the obligation of advancing her reputation for fidelity, judgement and skill solely through her profes-

sional service to her patients and to society. The use of advertising, in any form, to solicit patients is inconsistent with this obligation.

Section 10. Cards, Letterheads and Announcements. A dental hygienist may not utilize professional cards, announcement cards, recall notices to patients of record, or letterheads other than as an adjunct to that of her supervisor.

Section 11. Office Door Lettering and Signs. A dental hygienist may properly utilize office door lettering and signs, providing that they are utilized as an adjunct to those of her supervisor.

Section 12. Use of Professional Titles. A dental hygienist may use the title of dental hygienist or letters of R.D.H. in connection with her name on cards, letterheads, office door signs and announcements, but only as an adjunct to those of her supervisor.

Section 13. Directories. A dental hygienist may not permit the listing of her name in other than professional directories.

Section 14. Health Education of the Public. A dental hygienist may properly participate in a program of health education of the public involving such media as the press, radio, television and lectures, provided that such programs are in keeping with the dignity of the profession and the custom of the dental profession of the community.[1]

1969 CODE

The philosophical, practical science of ethics, establishes, by reason and intelligent observation, principles to direct our human conduct. Professional conduct incorporates the knowledge of these principles into practice.

The following principles constitute a guide to the responsibilities of the dental hygienist to:

Self. The dental hygienist, supporting the laws governing dental hygiene, is individually obligated to assume responsibilities for professional actions and judgments when rendering services to the public.

The dental hygienist has an obligation to improve professional competency through continued education and research.

The dental hygienist functions harmoniously with and sustains confidence in all members of the dental health team.

The dental hygienist is obligated to report unethical practice to the appropriate authority.

Professional Organization. The dental hygienist has the responsibility to support and participate in the professional organization.

The dental hygienist participates in the study of and acts on matters of legislation affecting the dental hygienist and dental hygiene services to the public.

The dental hygienist through the professional organization participates responsibly in establishing social and economic status for the practice of dental hygiene.

The Community. The dental hygienist as a member of a community understands and upholds the laws of that community and has a particular responsibility to work with all allied health professions in promoting efforts to meet the general and oral health needs of the public.[1]

1975 CODE

Each member of the American Dental Hygienists Association has the ethical obligation to subscribe to the following principles:

To provide oral health care utilizing highest professional knowledge, judgment and ability.

To serve all patients without discrimination.

To hold professional patient relationships in confidence.

To utilize every opportunity to increase public understanding of oral health practices.

To generate public confidence in members of the dental health professions.

To cooperate with all health professions in meeting the health needs of the public.

To recognize and uphold the laws and regulations governing this profession.

To participate responsibly in this professional Association and uphold its purpose.

To maintain professional competence through continuing education.

To exchange professional knowledge with other health professions.

To represent dental hygiene with high standards of personal conduct.[1]

Limitations of codes

Perhaps the most startling contrast is between the 1962 code and the others. None of the others dwells on the protocol issues of advertising or use of professional titles. And it is only the 1962 version that makes strong statements about the "obligation to the patient of placing herself under the supervision of a dentist at all times."[1]

The tenor of this 1962 code seems to be

setting limitations rather than of opening the hygienist to an increased scope of responsibility. A case in point is Section 14. It seems strange that the section dealing with the health education of the public would serve merely as an indicator that it is permissible to appear in the public eye, but that the hygienist had best be careful that the programs are "in keeping with the dignity . . . and custom of the dental profession."[1] It is uncertain how this section relates to ethics at all.

PATIENT'S BILL OF RIGHTS

Another approach to ethics, and perhaps one more in keeping with a consumer advocate role is the "Patient's Bill of Rights" statement. Such a statement was adopted by the National League for Nursing. It includes three basic assumptions:

1. Nursing care encompasses health promotion, the care and prevention of disease or disability, and rehabilitation, and involves teaching, counseling and emotional support as well as the care of illness.
2. Nursing care is an integral part of total health care and is planned and administered in combination with related medical, educational and welfare services.
3. Nursing personnel respect the individuality, dignity and rights of every person, regardless of race, color, creed, national origin or social or economic status.[3]

The actual differences between this Patient's Bill of Rights and the various codes of ethics ADHA has adopted are not very great. The reason seems to be that in both the ADHA and NLN codes, the elements focus on the *provider* of health care ("nursing care" or "nursing personnel") rather than on the expressed wants, needs, or expectations of patients. The title, which focuses on the patient, is appropriate for the age of consumerism, but the content still clings to professional self-centeredness: How *ought* the *provider* act? A statement of wants, needs, and expectations on the part of the patient could cause each health care provider to be challenged with patient-centered-ness: How can the *patients'* rights *be met?* The latter approach seems to be more goal oriented, whereas the former is focused on behavior or actions as ends in themselves. In many ways the rights and responsibilities (outlined in Chapter 6) as an integral part of the patient–health care provider relation-ship, provide a better basis for drafting a patient's bill of rights.

It should be obvious that health care is in fact patient-centered and therefore should focus on the well-being of the patient as the primary ethical goal.

Review questions

In questions 1 and 2 match the following ethical theories with the appropriate description and then with the philosophers whose positions are compatible with the theories.

a. Behavioral
b. Existential
c. Either/or

1. *Descriptions:*

    _____ Based upon a code of rights and wrongs, with an external authority; characterized by a striving toward the "ideal" of ethical behavior, a value in which harmony and happiness are rooted.

    _____ Viewed as a learning process in which a person adopts certain patterns of action as a result of the reward system following each action.

    _____ Seen as almost antithetical to the philosophy itself since it often involves a compromise of personal need or freedom; it is a dilemma because it focuses on the "other."

2. *Persons:*

    _____ Socrates/Aristotle/Aquinas/Augustine
    _____ Sartre/Buber/Heidegger
    _____ Skinner

3. State briefly your own definition of ethics.

4. Given the four ADHA ethical codes, identify which code best exemplifies the either/or approach to professional behavior. Explain why.

5. Is the NLN's "Patient's Bill of Rights" an example of an innovative approach to codes of ethics?

ANSWERS

1. c, a, b
2. c, b, a
3. The question asks for *your* answer. Discuss yours in relation to your classmates' responses.
4. The 1962 version is probably the most either/or set of ethical principles adopted by ADHA. It consists of a series of *dos* and *don'ts* that characterize ethics as a matter of following nominal behavior routines centering mostly on tradition.
5. Clearly the three ADHA codes focus on the behavior of the health care provider. Unfortunately, despite its title, so does the NLN code. A true "Bill of Rights" lays out patients' wants, needs, and expectations. It is up to the health care provider to respond to those needs.

GROUP ACTIVITIES

1. Obtain the ethics codes of the American Dental Association or of two other health care professions. Evaluate each in terms of its either/or orientation, its emphasis on service, and its reliance upon professional judgment for implementation. Find out whether they have an enforcement mechanism.
2. Draft a Patient's Bill of Rights that focuses on patients' wants, needs, and expectations.
3. Compare and contrast your individual definitions of ethics.
4. Read *Beyond Freedom and Dignity* by B. F. Skinner and discuss how this theory relates to the whole concept of ethics.
5. Read *Irrational Man* by William Barrett and trace the origin of existentialism and how its supporters view the issue of ethics.

REFERENCES

1. ADHA Code of Ethics, 1926, 1962, 1969, 1975.
1a. Bainton, Roland H.: The Reformation of the sixteenth century, Boston, 1950, Beacon Press.
2. Barrett, William: Irrational man, New York, 1962, Doubleday & Co., Inc., Anchor Books.
3. Carnegie, M. Elizabeth: The Patient's Bill of Rights and the nurse, Nurs. Clin. North Am. 9:557.
4. Durant, Will: The story of philosophy, New York, 1954, The Pocket Library.
5. Herberg, Will, editor: Four existentialist theologians, New York, 1958, Doubleday & Co., Inc., Anchor Books.
6. Johnson, Wendell: People in quandries, New York, 1946, Harper & Row, Publishers.
7. Pegis, Anton C.: Introduction to Saint Thomas Aquinas, New York, 1948, Modern College Library Editions.
8. Sabatier, Auguste: Outlines of a philosophy of religion, New York, 1957, Harper & Row, Publishers, Harper Torchbooks.
9. Skinner, B. F.: Beyond freedom and dignity, New York, 1971, Bantam Books, Inc.
10. Veatch, Henry B.: Rational man: A modern interpretation of Aristotelian ethics, Bloomington, Indiana, 1962, Indiana University Press.

CHAPTER 13

Changing ethical standards in society: practical application of principles

OBJECTIVES: **The reader will be able to:**

1. Identify at least one way in which an individual can fulfill each of the principles of ethics, such as those adopted by ADHA.
2. Given "touchy" questions asked by patients, express a response that reflects:
   a. Sensitivity to the patient's need
   b. Respect for the limitations under which health care professionals provide care
3. Identify examples of contemporary changes in ethical standards.
4. Redefine "professionalism" in terms of responsibility to patients.

The previous chapter identified examples of ethical codes, including the principles of ethics currently adopted in ADHA. The chapter also pointed out some larger concerns regarding the ethical philosophy upon which most codes are based and suggested that an awareness of other, perhaps more contemporary ethical philosophies could be of assistance in acquiring an ethical perspective compatible with the challenge of the future. With all of the questions that remain unanswered, it may appear somewhat futile to focus for very long on the specific principles associations have set down as guidelines for ethical behavior. The goal may be rather to define and implement a new code or an entirely different approach to ethical conduct.

However, there is a great deal of merit in closely analyzing each guiding principle, as it now stands, in terms of how it can be put into action. Such an exercise is good preparation for developing a new statement of ethics, *and* it is one way to gain an appreciation for the appropriateness of each element currently identified by the membership of an association as important. The code can be analyzed for its clarity and its compatibility with reality.

Referring to the 1975 ADHA Principles of Ethics, which are not unlike the codes of many allied health organizations, and identifying how each principle can be put into practice may be useful. The first principle is: "To provide oral health care utilizing highest professional knowledge, judgment and ability."[2] Does it have any message for how well a student attempts to learn what is offered during the educational process? Is "beating the system" in order to graduate compatible with this ideal? Does it perhaps offer the student a guideline for the quality of care delivered to patients while participating in the clinical portion of the curriculum? It implies that the theoretical components of dental education have some definite relationship to the clinical components of care for people. Once the theory is linked with the practical, clinical functions, the student should take the time and energy to think about what plans for care are most appropriate and then act in the best interest of the patient.

This first ethical principle is the embodiment of the *service* orientation. It addresses itself to the well-being of the patient by focusing on the provider's need to know, think, and care. It should be easy to see how it applies to graduate clinical practice. It describes the graduate clinician as a knowledgeable, thinking, caring person who carefully assesses the patient's needs, plans care and appointments so that those needs can be met, and who delivers the care to the very best of his or her ability. The clinician avoids the monotony of repeated prophylaxes and better serves the patient by never assuming that scaling and polishing are the automatic need of any patient. Beyond that the hygienist may ensure that the full range of dental hygiene services are available and may be selected as appropriate procedures for a patient seeking dental hygiene care.

The principle implies that the dental hygienist reviews the patient's medical history and alters care appropriately. It charges the hygienist with the responsibility for sterilizing instruments and otherwise ensuring that patients are not exposed to infectious agents from other patients who seek the care of the hygienist.

It suggests that the hygienist ought to place the patient first on the list of priorities.

The second principle of ethics reads, "To serve all patients without discrimination."[1] The intent of the principle is to encourage the dental hygienist to put aside any personal prejudices against other persons based on their race, color, sex, ethnic origin, age, size, or other characteristic.[3] It is wishful thinking to say that people no longer have prejudices. While prejudices are not as blatantly expressed today, low expectations of certain people or stereotypical ideas of what certain people value still exist in the mind sets of many people.

The degree to which these prejudices affect the availability or the quality of care people receive is of great concern to the membership of the profession. Frankly stated, refusing care to a patient on the basis of his/her personal characteristics is unethical. Offering a lower standard of care is also unethical.

The ethical health care provider views the *needs* of the patient as the basis for offering care.

Once the patient is accepted for care, the health care provider is mandated "To hold professional patient relationships in confidence."[1] This is the third ADHA principle of ethics. Keeping details of care provided to patients in confidence is not only an ethical duty; it is a legal duty.[3] Casual statements about the nature of a patient's problems, information contained in the medical history, or any other information obtained about or from a patient in the course of treatment must be kept in strict confidence.

Sharing the progress of the day's appointments with a fellow worker over lunch can be quite an embarrassment, and perhaps a legal one, if the conversation is overheard. Analyzing patient data, such as evaluating a radiographic series or study models, in a public location where passers-by may see the name on the chart or even be able to read chart entries is a breach of confidence.

The only occasional exceptions in the ethical *and legal* mandate regarding confidentiality are cases of child abuse,[2] venereal disease, or tuberculosis which are discovered in the course of treatment.[3] These may be expected to be promptly reported since they pose a severe public risk. However, it is best for a provider to consult an attorney for information about the precedents in the particular state in which he/she practices. Expectations concerning disclosure of such information vary from state to state; knowledge of the appropriate procedures to follow for reporting such cases is important.

Perhaps this whole concept of determining what to do when one finds himself or herself in such a predicament is a true test of appropriate judgment and due caution that are integral to ethical behavior.

"To utilize every opportunity to increase public understanding of oral health"[1] addresses itself to the *teaching role* of the dental hygienist. This charge relates to the need for the dental hygienist to be "spreading the word" about dental health and the means to attain it. This applies to the one-to-one educational process that occurs in the patient–health care provider relationship. It also refers to educating larger groups of people through community activities. What does this ethical principle say about the practitioner who does not choose to include patient education procedures in his/her clinical routine? Is this principle an ethical matter or is it more a proclamation of the scope of practice of the dental hygienist? Perhaps it does suggest that ignoring this phase of clinical practice is a matter of ethics as well as definitions.

The Principles of Ethics take a stand with regard to *professional isolation* when they make it an ethical mandate: "To cooperate with all health professionals in meeting the health needs of the public."[1] In an era when the scope of practice of the dental hygienist has been defined as extending into hospitals, nursing homes, and health maintenance organizations, it is probably a logical sequel that cooperation with the various health care providers in those and other settings would become a responsibility of the dental hygienist. The ADHA membership has made it an ethical principle. Cooperation is intended to extend to dental auxiliaries and dentists, as well as to medical personnel, in coordinating efforts to meet people's needs. It asks that the team approach be extended to its logical boundaries.

It may seem obvious that it is only proper "to recognize and uphold the laws governing this profession."[1] However, in this era of change in the utilization of dental auxiliary personnel, there is a steady trend to implement what seem like logical changes in patterns of utilization *before* the laws are actually modified to permit those changes. Auxiliaries prepared educationally to perform various services legally allowable in one state may be tempted to provide the needed service in states where the law says "no." Employing dentists may ask an auxiliary to learn and perform functions that the law does not permit, or the employer may decide to substitute on-the-job training for the legal requirement of formal education in order to more quickly prepare support personnel for an expanded role.

The ADHA believes that regardless of the state of flux of many laws, regardless of the person's skills or convictions, the individual must practice within the limits of the law.

If the individual is convinced that the law should be changed or that the scope of responsibility of the dental hygienist should be addressed, the professional membership of ADHA urges the individual "to participate responsibly in this professional association and uphold its purpose."[1] The most effective way to facilitate change is to participate in a group with similar goals and objectives. Unity, strength, and logic are the keys to change. If the Association does not appear to have all or perhaps any of the keys, then the place to direct energies is within the Association first. Scattered, individual pleas for change have little impact in the long run. But the concerted efforts of dedicated individuals within the framework of an organization can have far-reaching, tangible impact. The support network of the organization tempers wild-eyed idealism, disseminates ideas for membership discussion and possible action, develops the working knowledge of the members, channels energy into productivity, rejuvenates those who have fought for earlier causes, and creates a sense of belonging and accomplishment. Real change has occurred as a result of Association effort. And each Association member has the opportunity to help mold future changes.

The ADHA challenges the provider "to maintain professional competence through continuing education."[1] Hygienists who have the keenest awareness of the need to make *education* a lifelong process are those who were educated in the late 1960s. A decade of technological advances and legal redefinition of practice has created a competency gap for graduates of that era who may have been unable to keep pace with the changes.

Dental hygiene is one of the professions that has experienced substantial change in scope of practice. Functions taught in the 1970s often were not included in the 1960s curriculum. Technological and research discoveries have been great, as well. In order to remain "competent" the health care provider must keep up with the present. Continuing education is one way of accomplishing this.

Closely related to the continuing education principle is the mandate, "to exchange professional knowledge with other health professions."[1] *Sharing knowledge* is another way to keep up to date. It is an informal way of learning and a critical aspect of the societal nature of the professional association. A clinician who rarely ventures beyond the operatory walls is at a distinct disadvantage in terms of sharing experiences, techniques, ideas, and dreams. It should be clear by now that there is a great deal to be learned from nurses and the other allied health professions.

And finally, the profession asks the hygienist to strive "to represent dental hygiene with high standards of personal conduct."[1] The example that comes immediately to mind is a faculty person admonishing a student wearing a uniform to stay out of bars when attending a professional meeting. There are other concerns, however, that seem peculiar to the tempo of the times and probably better reflect the intent of this last principle of ethics.

In these times of tumultuous change and with the constant battering of "old morals," few are shocked to consider members of one of the health professions engaging in premarital sex, experimenting with hallucinogenic drugs and chemicals, drinking alcohol to excess, choosing to live openly with a member of the opposite sex with no intention to marry, or "associating with those who do." One theory is that the only difference between 1957 and 1977 is the degree of openness. It is fair to say, however, that a 1957 ethics committee might have made some effort to discipline a provider who was found to have been involved in any of the listed activities. Today's ethics committees wonder if it is any of their business. So might the provider's lawyer.

Personal matters seem to have come to rest right back on the individual. Matters of personal decision cannot readily be assumed by anyone else for that individual. The ADHA does, however, address the issue through its stated principles and does hold that personal conduct often does reflect on the profession.

Actually the ADHA is probably more concerned about personal conduct issues that affect the patient's well-being rather than matters unrelated to the provision of health care.

Perhaps one of the most serious problems in contemporary society that relates to the professional ethics of the health care provider is the matter of fraud. With the tremendous dollar volume of the third-party payments for health care (medical and dental insurance), a few "professionals" apparently acquire payments for procedures never performed or performed so poorly that they might as well have never been done. It is important to note that the fraud is perpetrated against the insurance carrier, but the real victim is the consumer. Fraud in insurance payments is a significant factor in the determination of premiums. The consumer pays for the fraud through the higher and higher premium charges. This issue of personal conduct, which is also a legal one, seems to be worthy of the attention of a professional association. Can the profession set up a "watchdog" system to monitor for fraud and then report the instances to the insurance carrier? Organized dental hygienists in at least one state, appalled at their employers' outright theft, did create such a system and reports were made that led to reports to insurance carriers and appropriate investigatory action.[1a]

Another ethical problem relates to the refusal of some health care workers to provide care for patients receiving federal benefits for health care (Medicaid or Medicare). The intention of such financial assistance is to permit patients to seek the health care provider of their choice and to be the recipients of adequate care. But some dentists do not wish to bother with the protocols involved or may have preconceived notions of the attitudes such patients will have regarding health care. In any case it can be difficult for a patient receiving public assistance to find a dentist who will even see him/her. Access to health care is a bigger problem than just providing funds for payment.

Some dentists may believe that patients who need federal assistance are suffering from low motivation and would be incompatible with their ideal of a practice consisting of "highly motivated" patients who immediately see the need for a comprehensive reconstruction of the dentition and who have been religiously practicing prevention on cue. In the 1960s there seemed to be a trend to "classify" patients according to their "dental I.Q." Class A patients were top. Class B patients might make it someday, and Class C patients were the "uncaring" group who either had to move up the category ladder or go somewhere else. It was some dentists' view that a practice of all Class A patients was *the* goal. That probably isn't a bad goal, but it was sometimes achieved by eliminating the people who were classified otherwise as soon as the dentist could afford it. This is a clear case of stereotyping, which is also a questionable ethical practice.

Being a health care provider or a student preparing to enter a health field does carry with it an enormous responsibility to individual patients and to society. Patients depend on the provider's skill and caring attitude. They entrust the provider with their bodies. The enormity of that responsibility should be at the very core of professional, ethical behavior.[4]

Review questions

1. List five of the current ADHA Principles of Ethics and write out one practical implementation for each.
2. Identify one major contemporary ethical issue that is a problem in the health professions.

ANSWERS

1. Compare your five principles with the 1975 code in the previous chapter. Save your written suggestions for inclusion in group discussion.
2. a. *Fraud*, wherein health workers fill claims for payment by insurance carriers for either poorly performed services or services never performed. Often, higher than usual fees are charged the patient covered by insurance.
   b. Refusal to treat patients who are entitled to Medicaid or Medicare benefits.

GROUP ACTIVITIES

1. Address the question, "What is professionalism?"
2. Conduct a role play session in which students playing the part of patients ask "touchy" ethical questions of group members playing the part of health care providers. Discuss the ramifications of the spontaneous responses the group members gave to the questions.
3. Have a representative of a third-party payment organization speak on the incidence of fraud and how it can be combated.
4. Share, in a discussion format, your individual responses to how you could implement each of the principles in the 1975 ADHA code.

REFERENCES

1. American Dental Hygienists Association Principles of Ethics, 1975.
1a. Michigan Dental Hygienists Association, Board of Trustees, minutes of meeting, 1974.
2. Miller, Sidney L.: Legal aspects of dentistry, New York, 1970, G. P. Putnam's Sons.
3. Motley, Wilma E.: Ethics, jurisprudence and history for the dental hygienist, ed. 2, Philadelphia, 1976, Lea & Febiger.
4. Purtilo, Ruth: The allied health professional and the patient, Philadelphia, 1973, W. B. Saunders Co.

PART V

PRACTICE MANAGEMENT

Health care providers do more than minister to the needs of people. They function as an integral part of a system—a health care system. The health care system relies upon efficient management for its effectiveness. It is a business management matter to determine how to provide care in the most efficient, cost-effective manner, within ethical and legal limits.

In an era when the scope of responsibility of dental auxiliaries is increasing, the appropriateness and potential of the dental auxiliary as a manager emerge. The individual health care provider has the responsibility to wisely manage his/her utilization of time, energy, supplies, and procedures so that more care can be delivered to more people at the lowest cost and with the very highest quality of service and with the greatest impact on raising and maintaining health.

One way in which these management skills can be developed is through the application of basic group communication theory in practice. There has been a great deal in the literature about the concept of team health care of delivery, but there has rarely been a thorough analysis of how the team forms and how it can function effectively to improve the cost benefit and quality of care as a result of group problem solving and decision making.

Most of the literature about team dental care seems to follow a rather traditional, hierarchical model in which the dentist is the "captain" or "quarterback." Some male physicians and dentists do attempt to draw an analogy between team health care and football and describe leadership patterns in terms of highly directive, dentist-centered activities.

It is not clear that this authoritarian model is the most appropriate one for health care. The alternative is a democratic style leadership, which allows "group" formation. Active (feedback) listening; shared responsibility in identifying problems, gathering data, decision-making, and implementing change; and opportunity for leadership to be assumed by any member of the team in meetings centered around a given person's area of responsibility and interest—these are the keys to developing a team that will feel a sense of commitment, loyalty, and involvement.

In order to be part of such a team, it is crucial to understand the key elements of practice management. This portion of the text describes those elements.

CHAPTER 14

Appointment scheduling

OBJECTIVES: The reader will be able to:

1. Explain how appointment scheduling affects the efficient utilization of time.
2. Compare the advantages and disadvantages of walk-in nonscheduling for delivery of care and structured appointment scheduling as approaches to management of the resource of time.
3. Describe at least two approaches to patient scheduling that are attempts at minimizing the impact of appointment cancellations.
4. Identify the advantages and disadvantages of the two approaches.
5. Describe the impact of single operatory and multiple operatory practice settings on patient scheduling.

Time is a primary resource in the management of the delivery of health care. It is a factor that, managed effectively, can have a tremendous impact on the quantity and quality of care delivered, on the sustained energy of the health care providers, and therefore on the economic success of the practice. Time is not easily stored. It is constantly moving, presenting itself for productive use and moving on whether or not it has been effectively used.

The dollars spent on mortgage or rent are actually dollars spent to purchase time in a facility where health care takes place. Money, spent on salaries of personnel, purchases the time of those people as well as their services. If the time spent in the facility by those personnel is productive (services being provided for a fee that is collected), there is some income to pay for the overhead costs of rent or mortgage and salary. The facility may also be providing care for patients enrolled in a prepaid plan and who have presented themselves for services. If patient demand for care to which they are entitled cannot be met because of poor time utilization, dissatisfaction with the plan may cause patients to drop the plan or to choose an-

other provider group. Ultimately, this results in fewer capitation payments to the practice and, therefore, less income. The skill of time management has as its goal the maximum, continuous utilization of each unit of time so that the quality of care is not compromised, so the providers are able to comfortably work at capacity, and the income of the office exceeds total overhead.

The scheduling of appointments is the primary method of managing time. Together with other factors, including utilization of auxiliary personnel and planning space and motion, appointments scheduling can have a significant impact on the system of providing care.

The usual pattern of health care delivery is to have the facility open for a stated number of hours each week, at which time patients may appear for care. The greater the number of hours the facility is open per month or per week, the greater the value received by the facility for the rent or mortgage paid, either in fees collected or in ability to accept additional patients in a prepaid capitation plan.

In a fee-for-service structure, if a health care provider is ill, or if a patient does not appear for treatment, rent or mortgage is still paid, but income is not received for the time purchased. The more time that passes without a fee-for-service activity, the less net income is available for the provider, not only because no income was received but because the costs of having the facility open continue. In an effort to combat this time crunch, some providers arrange to have services continually available to patients by keeping the facility staffed more hours per week and per month.

In simple language the economic health of a practice depends upon a full appointment schedule.[2] Time becomes money. Personnel whose responsibilities include patient scheduling may have a better appreciation of this fact when they tally up the day's receipts after a blizzard has closed down the transportation system in the city, stopping many patients from being able to appear for their scheduled appointments.

In a practice in which a significant percentage of the patient population participates in a prepaid plan, the facility relies upon the efficient utilization of time so that a maximum number of persons may receive care. The day to day scheduling will have less effect on overall income generated than in a fee-for-service arrangement, since in a prepaid plan an agreed upon premium is paid to the practice regardless of whether the patient-participant seeks care. The goal is to schedule efficiently so that a high demand for services from the patient-participants can be met, keeping satisfaction with the program high.

The challenge is to design a system of appointing patients that maximizes the utilization of time and minimizes the trauma of broken appointments or catastrophes that necessitate closing the facility or a portion of its operation.

Appointment scheduling is a system that matches the patient's time with the provider's time and that keys alloted time with needed time. The system divides the full day's time into reasonable blocks of minutes and ensures that the appropriately skilled

provider is available for the services and that the space will be available for the procedures to be performed.

The most restrictive or inflexible form of patient scheduling is the one-operatory facility, where a patient cannot be escorted to a treatment area and prepared for the health care provider until the previous patient leaves and the operatory area is cleaned. A one-operatory practice limits the usefulness of auxiliary personnel for providing preparatory and therapeutic procedures for the patient.

Two operatories for each direct patient care provider increases the efficiency of the facility. With a little finesse, three operatories can function well for two providers, provided all operatories are equipped for the provision of care by either of the health care providers. For instance, in a dental setting, a dental hygienist, dentist, and two chairside assistants may use three operatories to maximize the scheduling of patients of both direct patient care providers. As the hygienist is completing treatment for one patient, the chairside assistant is preparing the operatory not in use for the acceptance of the next patient. As the first patient is discharged, the hygienist moves to the newly occupied room, while the chairside assistant prepares the newly vacated operatory for the dentist's next patient. Scheduling becomes a matrix of times, since this utilization of operatories functions best when patients for both providers are not arriving at the same time. Fifteen-minute intervals might be the most useful approach to this kind of scheduling.

In Fig. 14-1, each box represents a patient appointment, which is composed of one or more 15-minute units. The areas marked by broken lines preceding and following appointment times indicate the time needed for support personnel to prepare the operatory and greet and seat the patient and then the time needed for support personnel to provide postoperative care and to assist the patient from the room.

The sequence of events for each of the two operators can be seen by following the arrows

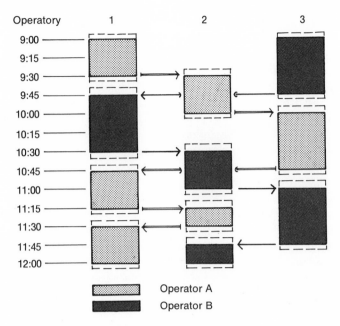

Fig. 14-1. Conceptual appointment matrix for a three-operatory facility with two direct patient care providers. Double arrows trace the path of Operator A; single arrows trace Operator B.

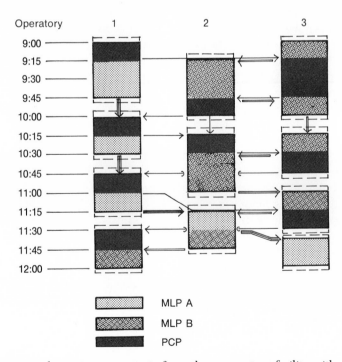

Fig. 14-2. Conceptual appointment matrix for a three-operatory facility with one primary care provider (PCP) and two mid-level practitioners (MLP A and MLP B). Single, double, and triple arrows trace the paths of PCP, MLP B, and MLP A, respectively.

from appointment block to appointment block. Maximum utilization of operator time can be facilitated by utilizing three operatories that allow support personnel to seat and dismiss patients and prepare the operatory without delaying the direct patient care providers. This is best facilitated by simply ensuring that appointment blocks do not stop and start simultaneously for both providers.

The graphic illustrates that with a three-operatory system and two direct patient care providers, 6 hours of provider productivity are (at least conceptually) assured during a 3-hour period. In a two-chair facility two operators would each have their productivity decreased by the time needed to seat and dismiss the patient. This delay time during which the operators wait for their next patient can be considerable if there is a large number of appointments scheduled during the alloted time.

With the addition of multiple direct patient care auxiliaries, the schedule becomes more complex. (See Fig. 14-2.) The team of providers may make it possible to schedule two or more patients during a given appointment time as long as space is available for the patients. While one provider is preparing the patient by administering anesthesia or recording blood pressure and medical history data, another provider is caring for another patient. Functions delegated to auxiliary medical and dental personnel make it possible for physicians and dentists to limit most of the care they provide to those complex procedures that require their expertise. With this distribution of services among a team, appointment scheduling can be more a function of who is available when and how long. Any given patient's appointment may involve the coordinated efforts of two or more personnel.

This more complicated patient scheduling matrix in a dental setting may require a restorative therapist or expanded functions hygienist on the staff so that during the time anesthesia is administered and the actual restoration is being placed, the dentist can be in a different operatory performing those services restricted to the dentist. The more complex the scheduling matrix, the more important it is to analyze who is going to be doing what in what location for how long. Separate vertical columns in the appointment book may mark the activities of the treatment rooms. Blocks are then marked in for each column to identify when a certain patient is receiving care in each of the available operatories. If it is apparent that a provider will be free for 15 minutes (usually considered one unit of time) between anesthesia and placement of restoration, it may be possible to schedule a radiographic survey, a plaque control evaluation, or study model impressions for another patient during that time. The goal is to maximize the utilization of all available personnel in delivery of care.

To understand this appointment matrix it may be helpful to follow each of the practitioners through the course of a day. The single line arrows describe the path of the primary care provider (PCP), such as a dentist or physician, from patient to patient. The graphic shows which person provides each component of care for each patient. Likewise, it may be helpful to notice that most appointments involve consecutive delivery of services from two different providers. The 11:15 A.M. appointment in operatory 2 involves two mid-level practitioners working together to provide care—with one assisting the other. The other exception is the 11:45 A.M. appointment in operatory 3, which calls for the services of only one provider.

The stream of activities can be carefully coordinated with all providers knowing where they should be at what time in order to keep the system functioning. Or it can be a case of fulfilling last minute identified needs based more on luck than planning. The former "systematized" approach may be more productive and less crisis ridden, but unfortunately human behavior often precludes this clockwork mechanism. The latter approach is certainly not dull, but it may result in dissatisfied, waiting patients and frenetic providers. So it is up to the keeper of the schedule to attempt to operate a finely tuned system or to sort out all the problems and complaints associated with the "do what you can with who's here" approach.

Regardless of the sophisticated system of appointment scheduling that the "keeper" follows, there will be some broken appointments. Again, it is this person's responsibility to minimize broken appointments. There are several approaches that can be taken to reduce broken appointments.

One procedure for minimizing lost time, which is directly related to the appointment book, is the way in which patients are scheduled. Some offices simply do not schedule appointments. This practice is more prevalent in physicians' offices, where patients call in descriptions of their difficulties, and the office personnel suggest they come into the office that day. The patients simply wait their turns after those other patients who felt the need to visit the physician that same day. The rationale for that procedure for scheduling (or nonscheduling) in physicians' office is that it is difficult to delay a patient's need until an appointment is available and that the patient will probably be just as glad to be in the office waiting as at home doing the same. Having an open schedule and many ill patients makes for maximized time utilization.

However, many physicians have shifted to appointment scheduling—perhaps as a way to end the office-call routine sometime near 5:00 P.M. each day, since the nonscheduled day can run until 8:00 P.M. just as easily as it can end at 3:00 P.M. A day scheduled by appointments has a reasonably certain ending time, and it is more compatible with a greater emphasis on preventive care, which can be scheduled in advance. Dental offices have typically used the scheduled day, since the majority of dental needs are not urgent, painful situations, particularly in a prevention-oriented practice.

Some offices schedule at least one extra patient per day, at a time when the presence of the "extra" will have the least trauma on the daily schedule if all patients should appear. For instance, there may be a time period when several short appointments can be blocked into a 45-minute period. Scheduling one extra short appointment may not be too devastating since the provider may be able to make up 2 to 3 minutes per patient scheduled during the time and have ample time to see the extra patient. However wise it may seem to simply schedule the extra patient or two in the daily schedule, the operator may begin to feel as the airlines do when all passengers for a flight, booked 111%, appear for their seats. There is little that can be done if there is no place to seat the patient and no available operator to provide the service to be rendered. Usually what happens on an already grey day is the arrival of an emergency patient or a patient with a mismarked appointment card simultaneous with the arrival of the extra patient. If the scheduler of appointments has no inclination toward facing such a dilemma, it may be wisest to avoid overbooking as a solution and try a different approach.

Some practitioners of the art of appointment scheduling have a list of readily available patients who do not mind appearing for services at a moment's notice.[1,2] Patients who live near the health care facility are handy to keep in mind, along with a brief description of their treatment needs, so that they can be evaluated in terms of how well their needs align with the available time that day. If 15 minutes into a 90-minute appointment elapses with no patient arriving, a quick call to the nearby patient may provide the facility with a procedure to perform for at least 30 to 60 minutes of the appointment. One way to make being "on call" attractive to patients is to offer them a reduced fee for appearing on such short notice. Certainly, the reduced fee does lower the anticipated income for the procedure, but it does provide the practitioner with productive time and some income for the units of time. This system works particularly well when there is a few hours' notice rather than minutes' notice of the available appointment time, since "on call" patients are more often able to rearrange their schedules with a little lead time.

Confirming patients the day before or the day of the appointment often provides the keeper of the schedule with extra lead time on cancellations and does improve the chances that patients will show up.[1] At least it reduces the incidence of patients who do not appear because they failed to check their calendars for date and time. The cost in this procedure is the time it takes the office personnel to call all the patients for the next day and the cost of the telephone calls themselves. If such a procedure significantly improves the appearance rate of patients, the costs involved may be comparatively minor, especially when telephone costs are not directly related to the number of calls placed.

Another tack is to indicate on the appointment slip that a charge will be made if the patient does not supply adequate notice prior to cancelling the appointment. Most health care providers use the threat but seldom carry it through. Patients are angered by this practice, particularly if they usually are present and on time for their appointments.[2] To assess a "no show" fee may trigger some court action and be more costly than it is worth in the long run.

A prime way to prevent broken appointments is to follow two simple rules at the time the appointment is made.

The first rule is to be certain at the time the appointment is made that the patient *wants* the appointment at the time for which it is being made. A show of hesitancy about the time is the first sign that the patient will not be there when the appointment time arrives. An awareness of nonverbal and verbal responses to suggested dates and times will help avert many broken appointments. It is simply not possible to coerce a patient into agreeing to an appointment he/she cannot keep. The best method is to ask the patient what time is convenient within the office hours of the practice and schedule the appointment accordingly.

A second rule is to ensure that adequate time is allowed for laboratory work to be completed, with results back in the office prior to the appointment. And adequate time must be available and allowed for the performance of procedures planned for the visit.

There is nothing more frustrating for a patient or a health care provider than to have to cancel an appointment at the last minute or to have to provide less than complete care because of a scheduling error. It is loss of income for the provider because of the wasted time. It may be a loss of income for the patient who had to leave a job. It certainly is an energy depleter for both because of the element of anticipation followed by the letdown.

A few other hints for appointment scheduling may prove helpful. The day, date, and time of the appointment should be said aloud to the patient and while writing it on the appointment card and in the appointment book. Saying it aloud minimizes writing errors and serves to solidify the correct time on the patient's memory. Writing errors can be disastrous, since the patient doesn't show when expected and does arrive at an unexpected time. The keeper of schedules may have less than ideal control over patients who forget appointments or over the weather and its surprises, but he or she does have control over the care with which appointments are made.

Patients and care providers usually have little patience with errors in scheduling. And with any awareness of the hourly cost of operating the health facility, care providers will expect errors to be minimal if not nonexistent. They expect that every effort will be made to fill openings, regardless of the untimeliness with which the openings occur. Care is not being provided unless patient and provider have a time to meet. And unless care is provided efficiently and consistently, the operation of the facility will be on less than stable economic ground. Time is a most critical element in the operation of a practice setting.

Review questions

1. How does appointment scheduling affect the efficient utilization of time?
2. What is one advantage of walk-in (nonscheduled) health care? What is one disadvantage?
3. List two ways in which the effects of patient cancellations can be minimized in scheduling.
    a.
    b.

True or false:

4. a. Having one operatory and one care provider permits almost no flexibility in scheduling. _____
    b. Three operatories and two care providers increase scheduling flexibility. _____
    c. Teams of care providers with multiple operatories permit greatest flexibility and the most complex appointment scheduling. _____

ANSWERS

1. Appointment scheduling is a system that matches the patient's time with the provider's for the time needed in an available space in the facility. It ensures the continuous flow of provision of care, minimizing "lost" time.

2. Advantage: There is no need to worry about "late" patients or patients who fail to appear. Disadvantage: It can lead to late hours or unevenly distributed arrival times of patients and it is somewhat antithetical to preventive practice.

3. a. Schedule extra patients on the book.
   b. Have a list of people on call available for last minute appointments (usually at a lower cost).

4. a. True
   b. True
   c. True

GROUP ACTIVITIES

1. Plan a day of appointments for a multi-operatory team health care facility, using a matrix of providers' times.
2. Role play the procedure for making an appointment for a patient focusing on:
   a. Patient's response
   b. Entry in book and on appointment card
   c. Assessment of time needed
   d. Availability of laboratory services prior to appointment
3. Estimate the financial losses to a health care delivery setting as a result of a day without patients because of a local flood.

REFERENCES

1. Ehrlich, Ann B. and Ehrlich, Stanley F.: Dental practice management: The teamwork approach, Philadelphia, 1969, W. B. Saunders Co.
2. Goldberg, M. J., editor: The business of dental practice, Stamford, Conn., 1969, Professional Publishing Corporation.

CHAPTER 15

The management of time and motion

OBJECTIVES: The reader will be able to:

1. Define time and motion management.
2. List the objectives of time and motion management.
3. Describe a system for evaluating various operations for their effective and efficient utilization of time and motion.
4. Evaluate various operations for their efficient utilization of time and motion.
5. Identify at least four benefits of an efficient program of time and motion management.
6. Identify the primary considerations in motion economy.
7. Evaluate facilities design in terms of motion economy and traffic flow.
8. Identify how traffic flow, use of auxiliaries, and such factors as sound and illumination impact the efficient utilization of resources.
9. Correct various inefficient operations so that time and motion are used more efficiently.
10. Design a floor plan for a dental operatory to accomplish conservation of personnel time and energy and accessibility of equipment and materials.

The efficient utilization of the resources of time and personnel has been addressed in earlier chapters in terms of appointment control and team management. However, within each appointment time and for each person on the health care delivery team, there is a microcosm of time utilization, motion complexity and frequency, and stress factors that can be studied.

SYSTEMS APPROACH TO MANAGEMENT OF TIME AND MOTION

The study of time and motion is often termed work simplification. Its ultimate goals are to provide the highest quality care with the most efficient utilization of the resources available to the team for the ultimate benefit of the practitioners in terms of fatigue reduction, longevity in practice, and increased income.[3] An additional important benefit is the reduction of the cost and fatigue factors of procedures for the patient.

The objective is to increase overall produc-

tivity. However, this is not accompanied by hurrying through the procedures at breakneck speed. Time and motion management seeks to reduce delaying factors and improve the usefulness of energy spent.[3] It is a systems approach to what happens in the facility, who performs the procedure for how long a time and where the procedure takes place, viewed in terms of increments of activity.

The systems approach analyzes a given person's activity in a given procedure for a given period of time to determine:

1. The number of motions made
2. The function, distance, and complexity of each motion
3. The amount of time needed for each motion
4. The surrounding environment that has an impact on the procedure's efficiency, such as:
   a. Illumination and color of area
   b. Sound control

A reasonable sampling of time and motion

focuses on each functioning person's contribution to a given health care procedure.[3] In a child's physical examination procedure for instance, the analysis would focus on the support personnel who usher child (and parent) to the examining room; weigh and measure the child; record blood pressure, pulse, and respirations; and provide injections or other medications and the physician who provides the main components of the examination. Each of these providers would be assessed in terms of the total numbers of motions carried out. Each motion would be categorized as a *transportation* motion, an *inspection* motion, an *operation* motion, a *storage* motion, or as a *delay* (waiting for something else to happen).[3]

Then each of those motions would be categorized in terms of complexity. Motions involving walking from one area to another are most complex. The entire body is physically moved from one area to the other, drawing upon the energy of the person. Walking from the door to the examining table then to the sink, 6 feet away, and back to the examining table is an example of how complex movements are related to transportation motions.

A slightly less complex movement would be walking to the examining table, being seated, swiveling on the stool to the sink (hopefully located much closer), and swiveling back to the table. The swivel from one position to another involves less energy and less stress than walking to a position 6 feet away.

Stretching to reach supplies and twisting at the waist are only slightly less complex movements. They place considerable stress upon the body and can result in extreme fatigue if they comprise a large portion of the day's activities, particularly if those positions are held for long periods of time. Holding an infant on an examining table while twisting around to reach supplies is an example. Supporting a child for 10 minutes while leaning awkwardly from the end of the table is another.

Simply bending at the waist is less complex than bending at the neck. The "hanging" or "drooping" head can place considerable strain on the neck muscles, which can cause genuine pain. The bending at the waist seems to be more easily maintained for long periods, particularly if the spine is kept straight and an abdominal support can be used to limit the acuteness of the angle and to ease the stress of leaning forward. Placed just below the rib cage, the abdominal support facilitates body posture and balance.[4]

With the body in a basically static position (such as seated in an operator's stool at the side of a dental chair) with good posture and balance, other movements can be assessed in terms of complexity.

Arm movements can become the point of focus. The greater the distance of arm movement and the more arm muscles involved, the more complex the movement. Movement from mouth to instrument tray is more complex than moving the instrument from the lips to the teeth. Reaching up is more complex than reaching downward. Lifting a foot to a pedal is more complex than sliding it to the side.[4]

With this general classification of movements it is possible to quantify overall motion. Most complex motions may be assigned a value of five with the least complex motions assigned a value of one. With an analysis of the function and complexity of each person's movements during a given operation, it is relatively simple to compute which types of functions require the most frequency and energy. Review Table 1.

It appears that the nurse's aide does make several body movements associated with transportation, storage, and delay. They may relate to the job description of the aide who perhaps ushers patients to the rooms, prepares and stows equipment, and waits (delay) until his/her services are needed by the physician or the nurse.

One goal for improving the efficiency of the nurse's aide may be to reduce the number of transportation, storage, or delay movements or to make them less complex. If a tortuous twisting motion is necessary to stow a piece of equipment, it may be possible to

Table 1. Number and complexity of movements of nurse's aide during 20-minute pediatric examination

| | Movement | | | | | |
	Most complex 5	4	3	2	Least complex 1	Computation
Transportation	8					$8 \times 5 = 40$
Inspection			20			$20 \times 3 = 60$
Operation				6		$6 \times 2 = 12$
Storage		5	3			$(5 \times 4) + (3 \times 3) = 29$
Delay	2				5	$(2 \times 5) + (5 \times 1) = 15$
	$10 \times 5 = 50$	$5 \times 4 = 20$	$23 \times 3 = 69$	$6 \times 2 = 12$	$5 \times 1 = 5$	Total 156

improve access to it to make the stowing less of a strain. Perhaps the two "most complex" delay movements identified on the chart involve wandering out of the examining room while awaiting the arrival of the physician or during a lull in the activity.

This simple chart of movement and its complexity does provide one level of information (number and complexity of motion) that can be helpful in improving motion management. However, it does not provide any indication of distance for each movement, nor does it indicate how much time was spent completing each movement. Tables 2 and 3 add those two dimensions. With the factor of distance added, it should be apparent how much energy is expended in transportation, storage, and delay compared to direct patient care functions. Of the energy spent, most of it involves walking to and from the examining room.

The dimension of time magnifies transportation and delay movements even more. This analysis should prompt the manager to reassess how this aide is being utilized or at least to do additional analysis of this person's productivity and usefulness. If well over half of the procedure's time-cost is spent running up and down the hall, stowing supplies, and waiting for something to happen, a readjustment of responsibility may be in order so that the "unused" portions of time are spent performing some productive activity. Or if it is time for facility remodeling, the study may suggest an alternative design that minimizes the distance and time spent moving patients in and out of examining rooms.[1-3]

ANALYSIS OF TRAFFIC FLOW

Another function of a time and motion study can be to analyze the amount of traffic flow at any given point in the facility.[1-3] Usually worn carpeting or stairs indicate heavy traffic areas just as well, but a quantifiable method can be used by collecting information about (1) the number of times a person passes a certain point, (2) the number of people who pass that point in a given period of time, (3) the purpose of each person in that

Table 2. Number, complexity, and distance of movements of nurse's aide during 20-minute pediatric examination

	Movement				
	Most complex 5	4	3	2	Least complex 1
Transportation	8 × 50 ft				
Inspection			20 × 12 in	6 × 12 in	
Operation		5 × 6 ft	3 × 12 ft		
Storage					
Delay	2 × 50 ft 8 × 50 ft × 5 = 2000 2 × 50 ft × 5 = 500 2500	5 × 6 ft × 4 = 120	20 × 1 ft × 3 = 60 3 × 12 ft × 3 = 108 168	6 × 1 ft × 2 = 12	5 × 6 in 5 × .5 ft × 1 = 2.5
Factor	2500	120	168	12	2.5

Table 3. Number, complexity, distance, and time of movements of nurse's aide during 20-minute pediatric examination

	Movement				
	Most complex 5	4	3	2	Least complex 1
Transportation	1 × 50 ft × 30 sec 3 × 50 ft × 2 min 1 × 50 ft × 1 min 22 sec 3 × 50 ft × 27 sec				
Inspection			10 × 12 in × 3 sec 4 × 12 in × 2 sec 6 × 12 in × 4 sec		
Operation				6 × 12 in × 1 sec	
Storage			3 × 12 ft × 5 sec		
Delay	2 × 50 ft × 4 min	5 × 6 ft × 10 sec			4 × 6 in × 6 sec 1 × 6 in × 10 sec
Factor	800.25	6.1	3.92	.12	.29

location, and (4) how long each is there. This can be a most helpful study in cost effectiveness if the busiest traffic is next to the area of the facility where the work requiring the most concentration is supposed to occur. A case in point is the records center of a health care facility where insurance forms are completed; correspondence is opened, answered, and filed; and fees are collected.

A continual stream of people, perhaps including the "delayed" nurse's aide in the previous example, may hamper the efficiency or quality of the work performed in that area. Location and relative privacy of various components of a health care facility do indeed have a significant impact on the efficiency of the operation.

Therefore, the overall floor plan of a facility is a major contributor to the efficiency of the operation.[1-4] Location of equipment and supplies in any given examining room is also important, but on a smaller scale.

There are several guidelines that facilitate analyzing and planning the efficient location of components.

1. *Frequently used equipment, supplies, or areas should be located as close as possible to the persons using them.* Examining rooms used constantly in a facility should be located near the patient's reception area. Private work areas such as laboratories or desk space that are not intended for frequent patient use should be located away from the patient reception area. Frequently used equipment such as suction mechanisms or handpieces in a dental operatory should be located where they are most accessible to the operator's use in providing dental care. Less frequently used equipment such as pulp testing or ultrasonic scaling devices may be stowed farther from the immediate area.

2. *Bottlenecks of activity should be avoided by permitting adequate space for traffic flow in heavily used areas.* In a large group practice a source of heavy traffic flow may be the central sterilization area. If ten office personnel typically are converging on the area to deposit or accept instrument trays, the process will be better facilitated by an open access. If all ten must wait in line at 2 feet of counterspace, there may be considerable delay time for each person just to drop off or obtain instruments. Likewise, crowding the operator's and assistant's working space into a corner of an operatory while considerable space is "wasted" at the other end of the examining room may cause a sense of claustrophobia for the workers as well as injured persons and broken equipment as the personnel squeeze into their respective positions near the patient. Also crowding the operating area near the chair often precludes having a left-handed operation, which will be necessary if a left-handed operator joins the staff.

3. Generally speaking, *counter space should be 2 inches below the person's extended arm.* This minimizes upward stretching (complex) motions to reach instruments or supplies. Logically enough, if these items are to be reached from a seated position, measurements for counterplacements should be made from the perspective of the seated person.

4. Maximum utilization of floor space can be accomplished by *locating frequently utilized areas or focal points of activity in the center of the space rather than at the periphery.* A classic example is the reception area with the chairs and tables lining the walls with several square feet simply being looked at and walked across by the patients. Positioning chairs and tables throughout the room gives it a more inviting appearance and permits greater utilization of the space. Careful positioning can create a smooth traffic pattern that minimizes patients moving in front of each other and that escapes the "waiting room line-up" atmosphere. Another example is the laboratory area that has work space, once again, only at the periphery of the area. Kitchens are often designed this way, also. The person using the area may at first be impressed by the overall size but then finds him/herself crossing

the wide open space while moving from one piece of equipment or area of supplies to another in order to complete a procedure. A better approach is to place an island area in the large space, which permits the user to have access to frequently needed space or equipment by simply turning around. For instance, if a sink is needed often for a large percentage of the procedures to be performed, it can be placed in the island area for ready access regardless of the location of other operations.

5. *Use of moveable partitions and other barriers can create a more sequestered environment* for activities that must be positioned near a heavy flow of traffic but that also require concentration or privacy. Personnel working with patient records need to be near the patient record files, which often are located at the patient reception area, a necessarily heavily trafficked spot. A partition can separate, at least visually, the workers from the traffic.

With these five guidelines in mind it is possible to review a floor plan and a study of traffic flow and generate modifications in the design, which can have significant impact on the utilization of time and energy.

Refer to Fig. 15-1 and begin an analysis of the location of each component and the overall design of the facility in terms of traffic flow. By using the five guidelines it is relatively simple to detect several traffic and space utilization problems.

The "frequently used" operatories are located near the back of the facility, whereas the laboratory, which requires little if any access to the source of patients, is located close to the reception area. Therefore, patients are constantly ushered past the laboratory on their way to the appropriate operatory. The providers or other personnel have to pass by all the operatories and all the arriving patients as they move to the laboratory. And the noise usually generated by laboratory equipment can be quite fatiguing and annoying.

The sterilization area is located at the far end of the facility. Fortunately there are only three operatories that require supplies from that area. If there were more, the location of "central" sterilization would present quite a bottleneck by virtue of its remoteness and the narrow pathway in front of it, which would be a doubling-back point for people who received supplies to move back to an operatory. Also, its location across from the facility's private desk area could pose a serious distraction for personnel attempting to concentrate.

Then, of course, there is the reception area and the business area, which receive the heaviest traffic. The reception area has furniture lining the walls so that the patients sit and look out an open area. Persons sitting on the couch against the wall near the door may be in the awkward position of attempting to avoid tripping persons moving into the facility. People will be passing in front of them for as long as they are seated on that couch.

There is little if any privacy or space for persons who need to concentrate on forms, records, and receipts.

Although the linear design of the facility severely limits the number of ways in which space can be utilized, several relatively simple changes in design could result in less annoying traffic and better access to the most heavily used areas. Consider the remodeling suggestions in Fig. 15-2. By simply changing the access to the lavatory and moving the locations of the private office area and laboratory, the traffic flow and noise control can be greatly improved. Plumbing and basic structures such as supporting walls and mechanical spaces can be left unaltered. All traffic must continue to flow up and down the same aisleway, but there should be fewer head-on collisions since personnel and patients do not need to encounter each other as often, now that their respective areas are more separate.

Personnel moving to the lab need not pass by all operatories and arriving patients. Patients moving to the private office area for case presentations and consultations need not travel the full length of the corridor. And

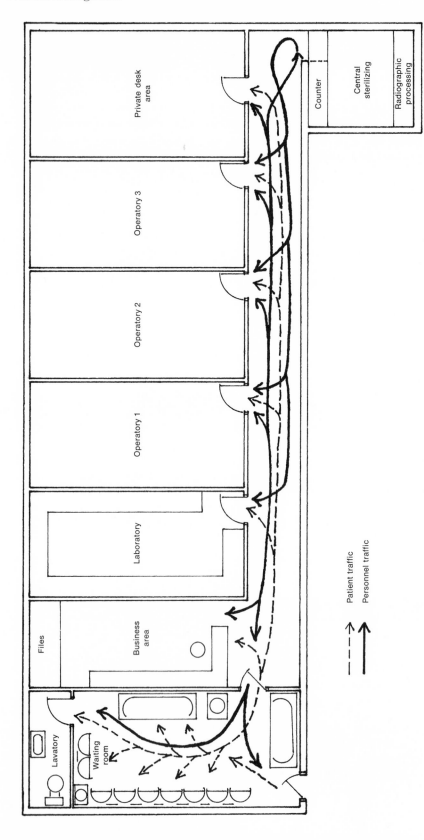

Fig. 15-1. Design of space causing traffic problems.

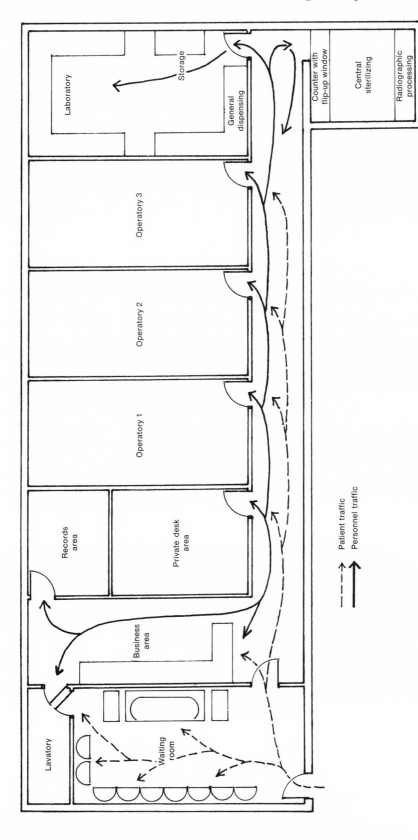

Fig. 15-2. Moderately improved traffic flow (simple modifications).

it is no longer directly opposite the noise of the central sterilization area.

With even greater effort and cost, traffic flow can be enhanced even more significantly. Fig. 15-3 shows how two portals of entry can be made to the operatories by reducing the unused space at the ends of the operatories and by creating a second hallway for personnel traffic.

The business area now has a partitioned section for paperwork requiring concentration. Consultations can be scheduled for this area as well, allowing personnel to have a private area at the rear of the facility. And the reception area no longer has a hazardous or boring seating arrangement.

With relatively few modifications, the floor plan has created a more open environment, too. Instead of high walls and hinged doors, operatories are basically open on one side except for attractive, smooth-operating folding "walls" that can be closed to ensure privacy. These expanding walls allow easier access for handicapped patients and permit easier movement of equipment.

Fig. 15-4 depicts one of the facility's operatories prior to redesign. The storage area in the lower left corner contains most of the supplies used for each dental appointments, but it is positioned too high for easy access by the seated assistant or operator. The one sink is located at the opposite corner of the room at standing height. The assistant and operator must stand in line to use it prior to the beginning of care. And then there will be a squeeze play to fit into the corner space alloted to the seated assistant and operator. If it is necessary for the assistant to leave the operatory, there will be another scramble and squeeze. The storage under the counter where the sink is located is accessible to the operator with a rather restricted swivel on the chair.

What is most obvious is the limited space allocated to the operating team. One probable reason this is such a common problem in facility design is that space is measured with the patient's chair in an upright position, rather than in the fully reclined position it

will be in during the appointment. As the chair reclines, the center of activity is increasingly moved back from the site of the chair base, so what appears to be plenty of space is quickly lost as the operator, assistant, and instrument tray cart center around an area approximately 3 feet back from the chair base. The high intensity light, used to illuminate the oral cavity, is often positioned for use over the chairbase, making it a common problem that the light cannot reach to a point directly over the supine patient.

Even with slightly decreased square footage to allow for the second aisleway, it is possible to reposition equipment in the operatory to improve space utilization and access to equipment. See Fig. 15-5 for the improved design. Two sinks at "seated" height are installed to facilitate the team beginning procedures with minimal delay. Supply storage and counter tops are lowered and more accessible. More working area is provided for the seated team. The dental light is track mounted on the ceiling so that it can reach the mouth even when the patient is in the supine position. The patient enters from one door; the operating team enters from the other.

With the improved floor plan and operatory design, the number of footsteps (and therefore time and energy) are reduced. People are less likely to be trying to occupy the same lifespace at the same time. Concentration (and productivity) will improve as a result of increased privacy. And the relative positions of space should improve the comfort of the office. It will appear less cluttered, cramped, and busy and yet be more productive.

Sound control may be better since the lab is away from the operatories. Folding walls that absorb sound rather than reflect it will also lessen noise. And there should be fewer instances of people running into each other and tripping over obstacles, thus reducing those elements of stress considerably.

In the operatory setting the complex movements of moving to and from the sink, twisting to reach, and stretching upward to-

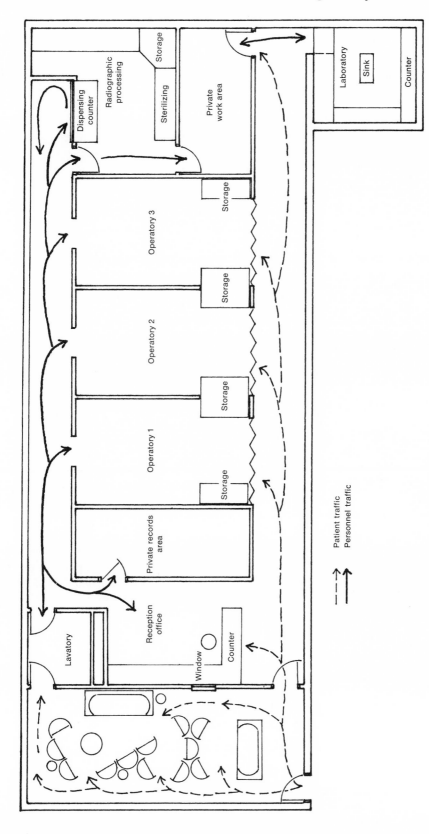

Fig. 15-3. Significantly improved traffic control (structural modifications).

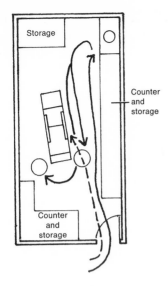

Fig. 15-4. Typical operatory unit.

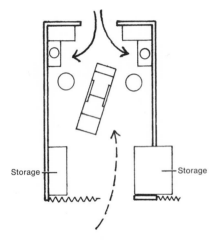

Fig. 15-5. Modified operatory unit.

ward supplies are replaced by simpler swiveling motions.

ENVIRONMENTAL FACTORS

The color of the rooms can be brightened or modulated as needed. Studies indicate that yellows and oranges warm the atmosphere, bright red causes the blood pressure and anxiety to rise, and blues cause people to cool off and slow down. Green seems to provide the right element of comfort, but it soon becomes boring. Many color experts find that green used as a basic color is readily accepted when accented with red or orange.

The general rule is to use cool blues in sunlit rooms and warm yellows and orange in rooms with no natural light or where windows face north.

Colors can have a significant impact on the patient's perception of the practice and thus can affect their willingness to return. Colors can also affect the productivity of the team members, who become less productive if they feel bored, stressed, or cold.

Another environmental factor that affects productivity is overall room light. Dimly illuminated areas cause eyestrain, fatigue, and headache. The ratio of overall room light to the intense intraoral light should not exceed one to four. So it will not help to simply brighten the intraoral light to make up for low room lighting. This ratio should be kept in mind when removing fluorescent bulbs as an energy saving effort. Removing too much candlepower may greatly reduce efficiency as well as consumption of electricity.

With even a rudimentary understanding of how to assess energy factors such as complexity of movements, frequency of movement, distance traveling, space needs, noise and color control, and proper illumination, it is possible to assess a health care facility and recommend modifications that can reduce stress and improve productivity. Such factors are of tremendous importance when any facility is being designed. Careful review of traffic patterns, accessibility of supplies, and equipment and space needs should precede construction, or the providers may find themselves in a shiney, new, miserably inefficient facility.

Review questions

1. What is time and motion management?
2. List four benefits of an effective program of time and motion management:
   a.
   b.
   c.
   d.
3. If a person is charged with determining how efficiently a given procedure is performed, how could the analysis be designed?
4. What impact does color have on efficiency?
5. In an analysis of a dental care procedure, the assistant is observed making frequent twisting motions to reach instruments on the tray located over the patient's lap. The operator is continually rising and moving to a cabinet several feet away to obtain additional supplies. Offer brief suggestions to improve the efficiency of the operation.
6. Generally speaking, "personnel only" areas should be located (near/away from) patient care areas.
7. Privacy can be given to personnel who must concentrate in heavily trafficked areas by using _____ .

ANSWERS

1. Time and motion management is a systems approach to analyzing who does what, where and for how long, which focuses on minimizing delay and maximizing the efficient utilization of energy.

2. a. Reduction of fatigue
   b. Increased productivity
   c. Longevity in practice
   d. Reduced cost to patient and provider

3. Each person who participates in the procedure is analyzed for number, function, complexity, distance, and time required of motions. The factors of energy expenditure are then reviewed so that changes in design and timing can be made to reduce the energy factors, especially in nonproductive function categories. Sound control, illumination, and color factors are also reviewed.

4. Yellow and orange create warmth; blue is cool. Red raises blood pressure and anxiety. Green can be boring except when appropriately accented.

5. Locate the tray in front of the assistant. Move storage areas within easy reach of operating team.

6. Away from

7. Moveable partitions

GROUP ACTIVITIES

1. Use a movie camera to film a health care procedure, exposing the film at one frame per second. Analyze the film for frequency and complexity of movement as well as for distance of movement. Institute motion economy measures and refilm the procedure. Compare the two films.
2. Analyze the traffic patterns in a variety of practice settings. Suggest remodeling and equipment placement changes to improve time and motion.
3. Design an "ideal" operating or examining room floor plan that would maximize efficiency of movement.
4. Analyze room colors for the moods or feelings they create.

REFERENCES

1. Hilborn, L. Bruce, Campbell, Edward M., and Hall, William R.: Facility design and equipment considerations for the team practice of dentistry, Dent. Clin. North Am., **18**:873.
2. Jerge, Charles, R., and others, editors: Group practice and the future of dental care, Philadelphia, 1974, Lea & Febiger.
3. Kilpatrick, Harold C.: Work simplification in dental practice, Philadelphia, 1974, W. B. Saunders Co.
4. Simon, William J.: Clinical dental assisting, New York, 1973, Harper & Row, Publishers.

CHAPTER 16

Logistics for a prevention-oriented practice

OBJECTIVES: The reader will be able to:

1. Briefly describe the primary objective of a prevention-oriented health care delivery setting.
2. List the characteristics of a prevention-oriented practice.
3. Contrast a prevention-oriented practice with a traditional approach to health care delivery.
4. Describe and implement two different approaches to a recall program for health maintenance.
5. Explain how third-party payors view prevention in terms of reimbursement for service.
6. Project how prevention could be systematized so that fraud can be minimized.
7. Project how prevention could be systematized and structured with contingencies that enhance the patient's willingness to participate and reduce dental disease.

Health care periodically rediscovers the concept of prevention of disease. Despite the fact that the health providers of ancient times described an approach to caring for patients that emphasized the control of disease and the establishment of a personal hygiene routine that would prevent disease, the literature over the ages has contained numerous "new" prevention approaches to peoples' need for a healthy existence. A specific example of a recent resurgence of prevention was the formation of the American Society for Preventive Dentistry (ASPD), which occurred in the late 1960s. Establishing an annual meeting and a journal, the society appealed to dental health care providers to (once again) focus on retaining healthy teeth rather than on monitoring peoples' teeth over the years as they one-by-one succumbed to caries or periodontal disease.

The ASPD challenged the profession to concern itself less with therapy and more with prevention. Speakers who traveled the association circuit, proselytizing prevention, pointed out candidly that the people who were now toothless owed their fate to the dentists who extracted them. One particularly candid speaker accused dentists of "slickin' 'em" and charged that such a practice was hardly in keeping with the "health" aspect of the prevention.

The emphasis was on "If you've got 'em, floss 'em." Removal of plaque became the daily recommended dose of prevention, and nutritional counseling became a far more common part of "patient education." Dental hygienists found this trend rather amusing as they recalled all their efforts to have toothbrushes, floss, and time available for recall patients to learn prevention.

After more than 10 years of revival, prevention is fortunately still an important part of many modern dental practice settings. However, this trend is not universal. It is difficult to make prevention a financially sound component of the delivery of health care. If prevention is to be honestly addressed and if efforts are genuine, the primary goal should be to put oneself out of business. As a result of a full program of prevention, people should no longer need to rely upon dentists for therapy. After all, if prevention works, restorative care is not necessary. Committing oneself to the concept of eventually outmoding the need for income-generating care is not often taken very seriously after the ballyhoo of a fresh approach to the daily routine has worn off. To the pragmatist, prevention must be a paying proposition if it is to be implemented.

PAYMENT FOR PREVENTION

In some ways, it may be the dedicated hygienist who caused prevention to be a money "loser" for the practice. Most hygienists have rarely specified a separate fee for patient education (or "control" as it is called in the current jargon). Historically, it has been a part of the prophylaxis appointment. Patients became accustomed to having it as a part of the package, with a toothbrush and a new sample roll of floss included for good measure.

With the advent of dentistry's new awareness of prevention, charging a fee for the sixteenth-revised-edition of the prevention approach became nearly impossible. It is not easy to begin charging a fee for what has been "free." New gadgetry was introduced, with specially colored (red) sinks separate from the dental operatory so that a control therapist could have a more clearly distinct opportunity to discuss prevention. Multiple appointments to measure plaque and hemorrhage indices for patients were introduced, with a fee specifically attached for all the attention. Some practitioners recommended charging high fees because it caused the patient to "realize the importance of" the control appointments. It was not uncommon to find a fee of $250 to $500 attached to such a sequence of care.

It may be easily argued that it is far better to pay hundreds of dollars to keep one's teeth rather than hundreds of dollars to lose them. However, it did become an ethical issue among providers whether such high fees could be justified for a procedure that used minimal supplies, very little space, little time, and the services of an auxiliary, who in some instances had little or no formal preparation in controlling dental disease.

Regardless of who is providing the patient education, it is still difficult to make it a paying proposition. Several approaches have been taken in attempting to underwrite its cost. The first, mentioned previously, is to simply charge large amounts of money, with the hope that the patient will accept the fee as reasonable and the procedure somehow as magical, and therefore worthy of its high cost.

A second approach is to bury patient education in the cost of other procedures, such as the oral prophylaxis or the oral examination appointment. Instead of charging for only the actual scaling and polishing or for the actual oral examination, a charge is assessed for the time and supplies used in the control portion of the appointment. In other words, patient education is not really specified as a separate cost item, but there is some dollar allotment in the total fee to cover its being provided for the patient. This causes the business manager to begrudge prevention's inclusion in the daily schedule a good deal less. It is no longer a "free" service. In a time of rapid inflation, such as that experienced in the early 1970s, increasing fees to reflect that added factor was a realistic solution to the problem, since fees were rising anyway. Burying the patient education fee also makes it a good deal easier to obtain third-party reimbursement for the procedure. Health insurance carriers will often cover the cost of the oral prophylaxis but are wary of covering such nebulous procedures as "control appointments." It is far too easy to fake such delivery of care, and the third-party payment system has difficulty being certain that prevention has any measurable impact on the patient's health.

A third approach to receiving a fee for prevention is to sell the patient dental "insurance" or a "guarantee" based on their continued participation in a control program in the office. In other words, the dentist charges a substantial fee for the oral examination, oral prophylaxis, and control sequence. The patient is informed that if he/she returns for frequent assessment of oral health conditions and if the oral hygiene index indicates that plaque is being regularly removed, then the dentist will provide at little or no cost any restorative or other therapeutic work necessary once control has been established. So the patient may pay for initial restorative and other therapy, but as long as the patient is under control and follows the recommended sequence and interval of control appointments, no cost will be incurred if additional disease appears. The dentist in this case is saying that he/she believes in prevention and is guaranteeing that the practice of prevention will indeed prevent dental disease. The patient has the added bonus of pleasant dental visits and a much greater likelihood of keeping his/her teeth for a lifetime.

This system does have its loopholes. The patient can feverishly brush and floss just before the control appointment, placing the control therapist in an awkward position with regard to accusing the patient of playing the system. Specific, defensible, observable criteria must be spelled out in advance for the patient regarding how compliance will be measured. The oral hygiene index or other measures to be used should be explained in detail, so the patient is aware of how prevention of disease can be measured. The patient needs tools to self-assess progress between the control visits, also, so that the recall visits are minimally authoritarian in nature. The visits should be an objective verification of how well the patient wishes to practice control and comply with the insurance arrangement. The visits can provide additional instruction and motivation for the patient, if the assessment indicates that less than adequate efforts (or at least results) are evident.

A dental auxiliary's basic education includes great emphasis on the prevention of dental disease. What that education should also include is a method for integrating patient education or prevention into the daily operation of the practice setting, so that it is a reasonably successful endeavor economi-cally, logistically, and in terms of actual patient benefits.

For instance, knowing how prevention can bring in revenue to the office is a helpful tool to have when introducing prevention into a practice setting. A full discussion of the options and the risks of each approach may result in a system that is acceptable to the person responsible for the fiscal operations of the practice, to the provider of preventive care, and to the patient. The three approaches offered previously provide a good baseline for determining how a practice can "afford" prevention. The key to each is to determine how much the procedure costs in time, supplies, expertise, and other resources and then to determine how costs can be covered in fees.

Once the mechanism for payment is generally defined, it is appropriate to determine just what prevention will consist of. Will it be something more than teaching the patient how to brush and floss? Will patients be selected for such care, or will it be an integral part of every patient's care in the practice?

One approach to prevention that tends to make the provider's intentions apparent to the patient is the practice of having the patient establish successful control before the oral prophylaxis is even begun. This works particularly well for patients who have been relying for years on the periodic scaling of the teeth as their answer to the threat of "pyorrhea." Intraoral photographs of the tissue and all the calculus and stain before control is begun will serve as a baseline to which "after" photographs can be compared when the patient is on control and the calculus is still present, usually standing free from the gingiva because of the reduction in pseudopockets as the inflammation decreases. Seeing the calculus present, but the tissue healthy, places the importance of having teeth scaled in proper perspective.

The oral prophylaxis has become a point of debate with regard to its appropriateness for children as well. Self-administered prophylaxis with the child or groups of children brushing the fluoride paste onto the teeth seems to have replaced the rubber cup polish and garmer or tray-style fluoride treatment in many practice settings. Again, the emphasis is on the patient's minimal need for professional therapeutic care and on the patient's ability to improve his or her own health with a few simple hygiene procedures.

Awareness of other oral conditions and general health conditions seems to be increasing among the practitioners of prevention. Not only is plaque under attack, but so are poor nutrition and deglutition problems associated with abnormal oral habits. Nutrition focuses on a balanced diet and on food selection and preparation; it is no longer limited to a discussion of carbohydrates in the diet.

Prevention now includes anti-smoking campaigns. Prevention-oriented practices have agreed that the risks of smoking are as great if not greater than the risk of plaque-ridden teeth. The entire well-being of the patient is under the watchful eye of the practitioner far more than it used to be, when "white teeth" were the focus of oral hygiene care.

Perhaps the most integral element in all of the procedures that are found in a prevention-oriented practice is the new emphasis on communications skills and psychology. Health care providers are seeking out the wisdom and handy techniques of transactional analysis in assisting patients to control their own dental disease. And there is a new emphasis on the management of contingencies in assisting patients in achieving control. Continuing education seminars and workshops for health care providers often include such topics. Articles describing how such techniques can be implemented on a day-to-day basis are far more prevalent in the journals and newsletters of the dental and medical professions.

THE RECALL SYSTEM

A prevention-oriented practice still recognizes the value of a reliable recall system for ensuring that patients return for regular evaluation and preventive care. This is a more traditional component of dental and some medical practices, but if often operates at less than perfect efficiency. How can the patient be prepared and scheduled for regular recall appointments with minimal direct cost to the practice (in terms of postage, telephone costs, or personnel time)?

There certainly is no way to establish a recall system that is free of costs. But some systems are more expensive than others.

One method is to simply schedule the patient for an appointment in the month in which the recall is due. For instance, a patient completing treatment in June may be scheduled for a recall evaluation visit in October. One way to operate the scheduling of that return is to make an appointment for October before the patient leaves the office in June. The advantage to this method is that no separate attempt at communication is necessary to make the appointment and the patient is guaranteed a time in the month when recall is needed. The obvious disadvantages are: (1) the patient may totally forget about the appointment by the time October arrives, necessitating a confirming phone call; (2) the appointment book is boxed in for months ahead, making vacations, attendance at professional meetings, and other plans very difficult to manage; the patients scheduled during those times will all have to be called and rescheduled; (3) if the recall becomes increasingly heavy, there may be no time to schedule new patients receiving extensive therapy over a series of appointments.

A second approach is to simply place a postcard addressed to the patient in a file box at the time of the June visit. The file box is divided by months, so the recall postcard would be filed behind October. When the second week of September arrives, all the postcards filed for October are mailed. The postcard reminds the patient of the need for the appointment and suggests the patient call to arrange a time. The advantage is that the procedure is really quite simple to implement. All that is really required is the addressing of the postcard at the last visit and the mailing of the cards at the appropriate time. The expense in this case is in postage. A monthly recall of 200 persons is somewhat costly. And every practice always has a number of patients who forget to call or call during the lunch hour or who simply do not make the effort or take the time to schedule the appointment. While it is certainly a reasonable argument that it is the patient's responsibility to ensure that he/she schedules needed appointments as suggested, it is a logistical fact that a great many patients will be lost from the recall system each month if there is no follow-up to the postcards. Some practices send out postcards and retain a list of recall names and phone numbers. As the patient calls in, the person responsible for appointment management checks the name on the list. After 2 or 3 weeks have lapsed, those patients who have not called for an appointment are contacted by phone to inquire about making an appointment. Or they are sent a second mail reminder. The follow-up phone call technique is probably more efficient in terms of having patients actually scheduled for appointments.

Forgetting the entire postcard system and relying on the telephone for initial and follow-up contact for recall is a third approach to the system. In this method the person who manages the appointments calls the people whose cards are placed in the file behind the current month. Or they may work a month ahead of time, calling November recalls as early as October 15 for appointments. Telephone contact is the most certain way to schedule recall appointments. A person on the telephone with the office personnel is more likely to seriously consider an appointment than one who is casually reading the day's mail. Where each call is charged as a separate cost unit by the telephone company, this cost factor is important because of the outrageous phone bills that result, particularly if the patient is again called to confirm the appointment the day before it is to take place. However, it takes a great deal of time and patience to call patients repeatedly (no answer, not at home, not ready to make appointment) until an attempt is successful.

Somehow a balance must be established between the patient's responsibility for his/her own health maintenance and the responsibility the health care provider owes the patient in terms of ensuring the appointments are available and that some effort is made to initiate the recall visit.

One other handy procedure that can facilitate the logistics of a recall system is to keep a separate alphabetical file of patients, with a file card for each patient upon which is entered the date of the next recall appointment and the time the appointment is scheduled. This facilitates answering patient's questions about when their next appointment is in the month to come. Otherwise a great deal of of time can be spent scanning the appointment book in search of the patient's name.

Other key information can also be provided on the alphabetical file card, including the components of patient education that have been provided for the patient in an effort to control dental disease and promote health. If a plaque index score is available, it might be entered so the provider has some indication of the progress of the patient at a quick glance. The amount of time usually needed to care for the patient may also be entered on the card so that an appropriate length of time can be scheduled for the recall. Some practitioners advocate entering comments regarding the patient's cooperativeness. However, judgmental kinds of entries, such as, "This patient does not care one hoot about his oral health," or "Do not give this patient oral health instructions; he is beyond motivating," can be devastating both in terms of subsequent providers' prejudicial approaches to the patient and to the patient himself if he should see the remarks. However, with a cautious eye to the objectivity of entries made on the cards, the "alphabetical file" of cards can provide concise, crucial information regarding the patient.

The "best" system provides for direct contact with patients, ensures some follow-up mechanism for straggler patients who are late for their recall, and provides a reasonable data base for managing appointments. It may prove to be the most costly approach in terms of initial overhead and the most profitable approach in terms of patients retained in the practice, adequately scheduled time for individuals' appointments, and in terms of positive, caring communication with the patients.

Prevention in itself can be a very rewarding mode of operation. However, it does require some soul-searching in terms of abandoning our profession's notions about how the provider is needed. The provider needs to ask "why" about every component of care provided and to pinpoint how the need for restorative or other corrective care can be headed off before it starts—with the patient assuming primary responsibility for prevention and using the professional as a resource.

It is unfortunate that federally funded and private enterprise third-party payment systems have such great difficulty accepting prevention as a reimbursable service. Full-scale prevention could greatly reduce the need for the far more expensive therapeutic services, thus saving the underwriters of reimbursement many dollars. The underwriters agree with the benefits of prevention but cannot identify a system to cope with the fraud possible in such an approach to care.

Review questions

1. What is the primary objective of a prevention-oriented health care delivery setting?
2. Is a prophylaxis every 6 months an indicator that prevention is fully operative in a practice?
3. Identify three ways in which prevention can become a paying proposition:
   a.
   b.
   c.
4. List three characteristics of an ideal recall system:
   a.
   b.
   c.
5. How do third-party payors view prevention in terms of its being a reimbursable service?

ANSWERS

1. The primary objective is to make oneself dispensible because disease *is* prevented and therapeutic services are therefore not needed.
2. A prophylaxis at regular intervals may be one component of prevention. If it stands alone, it may be a primary indicator of supervised neglect.
3. a. Charge a sizeable direct fee for the "control" hoping the patient will then attach more merit to the procedure.
   b. Charge a sizeable fee and "guarantee" the success of control by providing at no cost any subsequent therapeutic care—as long as the patient demonstrates compliance with the control program.
   c. "Bury" the cost in the overall cost of services provided at the appointment.
4. a. Involves direct contact with the patient
   b. Ensures follow-up for stragglers
   c. Provides data base for managing appointments
5. Often they do not reimburse for prevention because of its susceptibility to fraudulent practices.

GROUP ACTIVITIES

1. Design and implement a recall system for a health care facility. Or design two separate systems and analyze them in terms of overhead costs and patient return rates.
2. Attend a dental meeting where one of the circuit-riders of preventive dentistry is the speaker.
3. Poll patients regarding the amount of preventive dentistry they perceive they are receiving in their health settings.
4. Ask individual hygienists what they do each day to prevent disease. Ask them how they know disease has been prevented.
5. Invite a representative from a third-party payor organization to discuss how prevention is reimbursed (if at all) and how fraud could be perpetrated by practitioners if prevention were fully funded. Design a system that eliminates fraud in implementing prevention.
6. Describe in detail all those features that characterize a truly prevention-oriented practice.

CHAPTER 17

Multi-handed dental care delivery

OBJECTIVES: **The reader will be able to:**

1. Define the concept of four-handed dentistry and its sequel, multi-handed dental care delivery.
2. Explain how time and motion economy relate to the concept of multi-handed dental care delivery.
3. Specify those elements of time and motion management that are necessary for maximum productivity in the delivery of chairside dental care.
4. Explain how four-handed dentistry can be generalized to four-handed dental hygiene and expanded function dental auxiliary practice as a measure for improving productivity.
5. Provide possible explanations for the rarity with which chairside assistance is available to dental auxiliary practitioners who provide direct patient care.

DEVELOPMENT OF FOUR-HANDED DENTISTRY

Until the 1960s, little had been done to evaluate the practice of dentistry in terms of time and motion economy. A few inventive dentists had tinkered with equipment design and with sit-down dentistry using an assistant,[4,6] but for the most part, dentistry was a stand-up operation with two hands accomplishing almost all tasks related to the actual delivery of care. It was not uncommon for a patient to be amazed at the contortions a dentist could accomplish in order to see the areas of the mouth needing care.[4,6] Neck and back spasms and varicosities of the legs were listed as primary occupational hazards of the profession. And yet, dentistry continued to function with the patient upright, with minimal support staff, and with minimal attention paid to the stress and strain placed upon the dentist's body during the delivery of care.

One definite gain for dentistry from the "demand for care" scare of the 1960s was a new focus on how the practice of dentistry could become more productive.[1] Included in this focus was a careful examination of how time and motion were used during various procedures. Time and motion films were made of various procedures where no assistant was used, where the assistant's role was primarily to mix cements and change burs, and then where the assistant assumed a far more active role in the delivery of the service. Attention was paid to the relative position of the patient, operator, and assistant with time and motion evaluation again used to focus on the most efficient approach to the delivery of care.

What was painfully obvious from these studies was that stand-up dentistry with little or no support services from an assistant involved large numbers of tremendously complex motions on the part of the dentist. The longer the distance of motion traveled, the more time spent in the operation. The more frequently the motions were made, the longer the procedure lasted. And the more complex the motions, the more fatigued the operator at the end of the appointment.

The basic guidelines for the management of time and motion were first applied to the dentist in order to minimize repetitious motions and the necessity of traveling long distances. The same guidelines were applied to the dental assistant. Initially it was believed that the assistant should stand at the same side of the chair that the operator was occupying, using a two-handed instrument passing technique. The operator would reach back to pass the used instrument to the assistant, the assistant would grasp the instrument and remove it from the operator's hand, and then the assistant would place the next needed instrument in the operator's waiting hand with the other hand. In other words, the assistant's right and left hands were occupied with instrument passing, which was somewhat limiting in terms of what the assistant could do to further assist the actual procedure. To facilitate these primitive attempts at reducing time and motion, the operator was encouraged to follow a predictable order of instrumentation and the assistant was expected to develop an acute awareness of what the operator might want next. "Anticipation" was the magic quality each assistant hoped to acquire.

Along with these first efforts at using chairside assistants came several other fundamental procedures that could reduce time and motion. One was to use prepared trays of instruments.[1] Any given dental procedure should have a prepared tray of exactly what would be needed for the procedure to be completed. This would reduce the complex activity of delving into the storage drawer for another instrument. Trays at first were cluttered with every possible instrument that could be needed, in an attempt to reduce the drawer delving. But eventually it became apparent that the only way to find an instrument when it is needed is to reduce the array of possible instruments and decide on which ones are really necessary. Rarely used instruments were relegated to the storage drawer again to be used only in those instances when they were essential to the procedure's success.[1] The use of double-ended instruments became more popular since they could be paired to minimize instrument exchanges and they were one step closer to minimizing tray clutter.

Equipment designers then developed tray set-up systems where a set-up could be used, scrubbed, and autoclaved on the same tray and returned to a storage area for reuse without having to be disassembled and reassembled in the sterilization center. Trays could be color-coded for specific procedures, so that they could be readily identified and easily returned to their proper storage area and selected for use. Next, the relative position of instruments on the tray became important. Frequently used instruments were located in the most accessible area of the tray, and often the instruments were placed on the tray in the usual sequence of their use.[4]

Then the position of the tray in relation to the operator, patient, and assistant became a focal point. Usually the tray had been located somewhere over the patient's lap, and often quite high in relation to the seated operator. Reaching for instruments required a twisting motion for the chairside assistant, which is stressful if it recurs throughout the appointment and the day's schedule. When the efficiency experts decided that the assistant as well as the dentist ought to be seated, the assistant's position was relocated at the other side of the chair, and the tray was placed in front of the assistant, often on a mobile cart along with a storage drawer and other frequently used equipment, such as an amalgamator and mixing supplies. The assistant could now reach instruments directly in front of him/her and had better access to the oral cavity for assisting the dentist in the provision of care.

With the invention of the high speed handpiece, the time required to complete the preparation of teeth for restoration was drastically reduced. But with the high speed handpiece also came a flood of water used as a coolant and irrigating mechanism. Someone was needed to evacuate the water from the oral cavity since the passive suction of the saliva ejector could not accomplish the task effectively. With this new function assigned to the chairside assistant, one hand could be used to evacuate, but only one hand remained for the transfer of instruments. Thus, necessity invented the one-handed instrument transfer. Assisting a right-handed operator, the chairside assistant uses the left hand to accept and pass instruments and the right hand to aspirate fluids and perform other functions that may or may not require a surgically clean hand. The left hand, having been scrubbed, touches only those items that will contact the oral cavity or the operator's surgically clean hands. The right hand, following the scrub procedure, may touch clean —but not sterile—chair buttons, the overhead light, the amalgamator, and the unsterilizable hose of the aspirator without fear of introducing foreign microorganisms to the patient.

The picture of the efficient dental operation now includes two seated persons, in addition to the patient, with a prepared tray of only necessary items with double-ended instruments, with the tray placed in front of the seated assistant for ready access. The instruments are transferred to the operator with one hand while the other hand assists the operator in the preparation of materials, the evacuation of fluids, and the adjustment of various items of dental equipment. Not only has the operation taken on a smoother, more efficient appearance, but the likelihood of introducing some other patient's diseases to the patient is greatly reduced. The operator has virtually no reason to contaminate his/her hands with foreign bacteria, and the assistant is able to ensure that instruments entering the oral cavity are indeed contaminated only with the patient's own microorganisms.

TIME AND MOTION MANAGEMENT IN MULTI-HANDED DENTISTRY

With a predictable order of instrumentation, the operator can expect that this four-handed dentistry approach will improve the productivity of the staff by at least 50%.[1] It will probably take 50% to 75% as long to perform the same procedure; there will be less stress on the patient; and the operator and assistant will have minimal stress in completing the procedure.[1,4]

There are certain key elements in four-handed dentistry that are virtually essential to this or a higher level of productivity:

1. The use of prepared trays, with only necessary items included on the tray and positioned in a logical order and location
2. The operator and the assistant properly seated on opposite sides of the chair at the head of a fully supine patient
3. The use of high speed equipment and high volume suction devices
4. A one-handed transfer technique for instruments, with only the assistant taking and replacing instruments
5. Standardization of operating procedures to eliminate guesswork in instrument transfer, instrument selection, and timing in the preparation of materials[1,3-6]

In order for these principles to be followed, both the operator and the assistant must know how to observe and carry them out throughout the provision of care. An operator who reaches past the assistant for instruments or who changes procedures and instruments on a whim not only can be a frustration to the properly trained assistant but also the monkey wrench in the efficiency of the operation.

A little planning can produce the standardized prepared trays and procedures. And there are few dentists who do not have modern, efficient, high speed equipment with which to function.

Perhaps the most frequently underestimated and thus violated principles in practice are the importance of proper seating and relative positioning and the necessity of a smooth instrument transfer. The properly seated operator should have feet flat on the floor, thighs parallel to the floor, and back straight. It should not be necessary for the operator to have a curved spine or a drooping neck, if the mouth mirror is used correctly to obtain indirect vision and adequately reflected light. The stool must provide full support for the weight of the body, and ideally it includes a body rest that can be

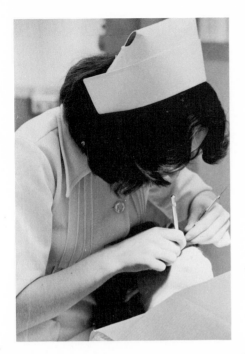

Fig. 17-1. Operator with mouth mirror positioned too far back in the mouth, necessitating forward incline at neck.

used behind the operator or as additional support under the rib cage in front of the operator.

Fig. 17-1 is a familiar sight when observing an operator who has not yet learned to use the dental mirror optimally. The back is curved forward, and the neck is stretched in an effort to see the lingual surfaces of the teeth on the maxillary quadrant closest to the operator. Simply by moving the mirror out to the anterior teeth and handling it differently, the operator will be able to see the lingual surfaces of those teeth while maintaining a reasonable posture. (See Fig. 17-2.)

Notice that the patient is in a full supine position, with the mouth positioned at the height of the operator's elbows when the arms are kept close to his/her sides. Fig. 17-3 shows the frequent error of positioning the patient at the height of the elbows when they are spread for flight. Beginning operators may complain that they cannot see

unless the patient is high, but usually this brings the patient much closer to the face of the operator than the recommended 12 to 14 inches[4]; failure to see often is attributed to the weak sight of the operator or to the slowness with which the use of the mouth mirror is mastered. The operator's eye physician can correct his/her focal length so that it is at the recommended 14 inches.

With the patient in a full supine position and the operator correctly seated on the stool (see Fig. 17-4), it is a relatively simple matter to adjust the position of the assistant. The assistant's eye level should be 4 to 6 inches above the eye level of the operator in order to enable the assistant to see the field of operation without interfering with the activities of the operator.[1,5,6] Most efficiency experts recommend that the assistant have a foot support that enables the thighs to be parallel to the floor, since a downward angle of the upper legs against the chair edge can reduce circulation. An abdominal rest or body support is also a helpful feature on the assistant's stool since it provides better balance as the assistant angles slightly forward in the chair.

The cart is then positioned in front of the chairside assistant for ready access, and the prepared tray of instruments and supplies is located on the cart. The cart also includes high volume suction devices and an air/water syringe to facilitate visibility of the area of care.

The usual way in which the relative positions at the chair are described refers to the patient's head location as the center of a clock.[1,6] The right-handed operator is often positioned between 9:00 and 12:00 at the right side of the patient with the assistant sitting at a position between 3:00 and 1:00. (See Figs. 17-5 and 17-6.) The exact location of the operator and assistant is largely one of comfort, and it is often modified by the constraints imposed upon positioning by the size of the operator and assistant, the size of the patient, and the area of the mouth receiving attention. Generally speaking, the positions most frequently assumed by the team may be

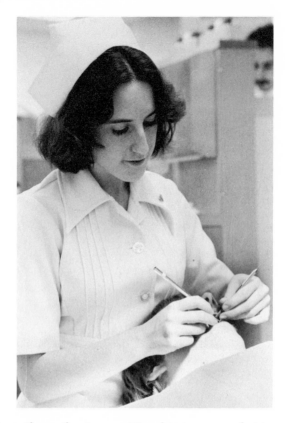

Fig. 17-2. Operator with mouth mirror positioned to ensure good vision of the area with no stressful incline at the neck.

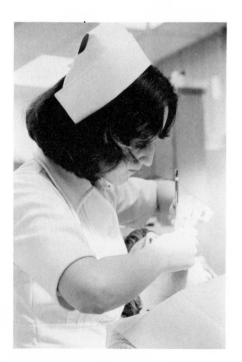

Fig. 17-3. Operator positoned with patient too high, causing upper back and arm fatigue.

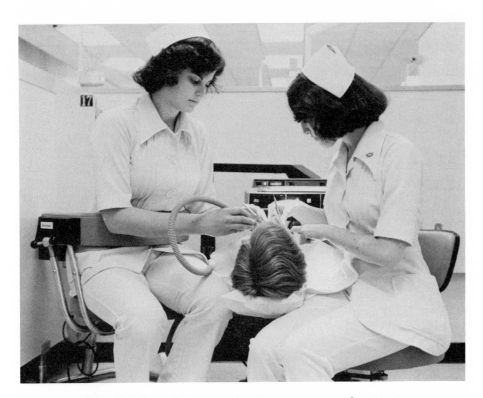

Fig. 17-4. Properly positioned patient, operator, and assistant.

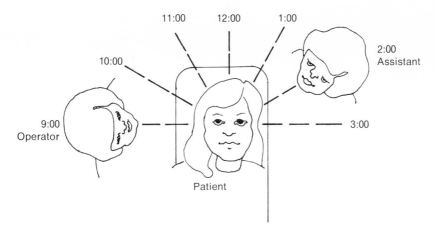

Fig. 17-5. Right-handed operator seated at approximately 9 o'clock with assistant at 2 o'clock.

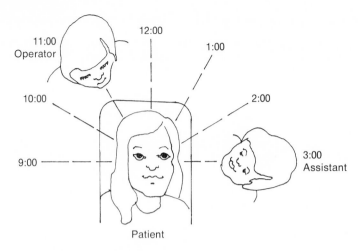

Fig. 17-6. Right-handed operator seated at 11 o'clock with assistant at 3 o'clock.

described as a front position (somewhere between 9:00 and 10:30) or a rear position (somewhere between 10:30 and 12:00). The corresponding front and rear positions for the other side of the chair are from 3:00 to 1:30 and from 1:30 and 12:00, respectively.

Many procedures, especially those involving restorations for single teeth or a single quadrant, can be performed from start to finish from the rear position by the operator and the front position by the assistant.[6] The operator positioned at the rear of the chair, straddling the back of the chair with the patient's head located at approximately heart height has the best fulcrum opportunity and leverage for intraoral procedures. The view for the assistant is ideal, and instruments can be safely transferred in front of the patient over the chest area, with virtually no loss of eye focus on the part of the operator. The operator simply rocks outward from the mouth on the established fulcrum as a signal for the next instrument transfer; the assistant grasps the instrument to be removed and replaces it with the next instrument. The operator, still maintaining the original fulcrum, rocks back into the mouth to the next phase of the operation, without having to move the eyes, arm, back, head or any other part of the body except the hand and wrist. This is

a classic example of motion economy, safety in instrument transfer, and smoothness in operation. The procedure can develop a graceful rhythm with practice.

There are numerous texts that teach the basic principles of instrument transfer, including multimedia approaches to the process, using slides, film loops, in-class practice sessions, and workbooks. Both the chairside assistant and the operator should practice instrument transfer techniques so that this important phase of the procedure can operate smoothly.

For most dental restorative procedures that involve single teeth or quadrants, the positions in relation to the patient are fairly constant and the need for instruments can be easily standardized. However, in procedures that include contact with all surfaces of all teeth, such as the oral prophylaxis or root planing, an efficient approach to the procedure must also address itself to minimum numbers of complex body movements (such as moving from front to rear positions and back again) and an order of instrumentation that reduces the need to change instruments or positions. Also, the position of the patient should be at lap height rather than heart height to maximize leverage and vision.

The object is to provide care for as many

Table 4. System of positions (patient in supine position)

Area of operation	Patient's head position	Operator's position	Fulcrum	Vision	Use of mirror
		Positioning for the right-handed operator			
Mandible					
Right buccal	Left	9:00	Occlusal	Direct	Retract tongue
Left lingual	Left	9:00	Occlusal	Direct	Retract tongue
Right lingual	Right	9:00	Occlusal	Indirect	Retract cheek; indirect vision and illumination
Left buccal	Right	11:00	Occlusal	Direct	Retract cheek
Anterior lingual	Straight*	11:00	Incisal edge	Direct	Reflect light; retract tongue
Anterior labial	Straight*	11:00	Incisal edge	Indirect	Indirect vision; retract lip
Maxilla					
Right buccal	Left	9:00	Occlusal	Direct	Retract cheek
Left lingual	Left	9:00	Occlusal	Direct	Reflect light
Right lingual	Right	11:00	Occlusal	Indirect	Indirect vision; reflect light
Left buccal	Right	11:00	Occlusal	Direct	Retract cheek
Anterior lingual	Straight*	11:00	Incisal edge	Indirect	Indirect vision; reflect light
Anterior labial	Straight*	11:00	Incisal edge	Direct	None
		Positioning for the left-handed operator			
Mandible					
Left buccal	Right	3:00	Occlusal	Direct	Retract cheek
Right lingual	Right	3:00	Occlusal	Direct	Retract tongue
Left lingual	Left	3:00	Occlusal	Indirect	Retract cheek; indirect vision and illumination
Right buccal	Left	1:00	Occlusal	Direct	Retract cheek
Anterior lingual	Straight*	1:00	Incisal edge	Direct	Reflect light; retract tongue
Anterior labial	Straight*	1:00	Incisal edge	Indirect	Indirect vision; retract lip
Maxilla					
Left buccal	Right	3:00	Occlusal	Direct	Retract cheek
Right lingual	Right	3:00	Occlusal	Direct	Reflect light
Left lingual	Left	1:00	Occlusal	Indirect	Indirect vision; reflect light
Right buccal	Left	1:00	Occlusal	Direct	Retract cheek
Anterior lingual	Straight*	1:00	Incisal edge	Indirect	Indirect vision; reflect light
Anterior labial	Straight*	1:00	Incisal edge	Direct	None

*Patient is asked to turn the head slightly as the operator moves from cuspid to cuspid in the anteriors.

surfaces as possible in the mouth before having to change positions, instruments, or the ends of the instrument. Changing positions takes time and energy. Also, it is logical to have an efficient order of instrumentation so that the assistant can anticipate what the next needed instrument will be.

It is possible to combine these goals very nicely and generate a system of positions at the chairside and an order of instrumentation that minimizes the number and complexity of movements and that can be easily remembered by both the operator and the chairside assistant.

The system of positions can be seen in Table 4.

Access to each area of the mouth is made relatively easy through the combination of the operator position; the patient's head position; the use of the mouth mirror for retraction, reflection of light, or indirect vision; and the dental light. Beginning operators initially have difficulty obtaining access to the lingual surfaces of the mandibular quadrant closest to them and the buccal surfaces of the maxillary quadrant closest to them. Areas of indirect vision cause some difficulty until working with a reverse image is mastered. But with practice, this sequence of positioning makes it possible to obtain a solid fulcrum for each area of the dentition and also facilitates minimizing instrument changes.

Moving from buccal-to-lingual-to-lingual-to-buccal-to-anterior surfaces is easily remembered and is a compatible procedure for using the universal explorers, the contra-angled sickles, the universal curettes, paired hoes, paired files, and Gracey curettes. For instance, if one end of the contra-angled Jaquette sickle can be used on the maxillary right buccal, that same end can be used on the maxillary left lingual. No position change is necessary and no instrument change is necessary for the operator to complete these two areas of the dentition in sequence. The Gracey #11-12 curette can be used on the mesial surfaces of posterior teeth. The end that adapts to the mandibular right lingual also adapts to the mandibular left buccal. One position change is necessary but no instrument exchange must be accomplished for these phases of the arch to be completed. The arches are separated for purposes of an order of instrumentation because it is often a logical division point for services involving the entire mouth. Generally it is better to *complete* one area entirely than to do an incomplete procedure for all teeth.

Many operators encourage creativity in positioning and expound at great length regarding how the operator ought to experiment with many approaches to an area until the approach feels comfortable. The only difficulty with this theory is that often the position the operator settles into includes a twisted neck, a doubled-up body, minimal use of the patient's ability to turn the head, and a fulcrum location that defies control of the instrument. A sequence that can be demonstrated to facilitate ease of instrumentation and minimal body changes and instrument transfers is probably the best choice, as long as the operator is given ample opportunity to correct old contortion habits and to assess the ease with which the operation can proceed. A quick tour through a clinical facility that encourages individual preferences first and standardization second in patient and operator position may provide a very interesting array of body positions and approaches to adaptation of the instrument in use.

Following an order of instrumentation may at first sound like old-guard regimentation. But once again, if the system is designed with economy of motion in mind and if it facilitates the use of a chairside assistant, it may be the best approach to the operation. Continuing the tour through the "creative" clinic may show operators reaching past assistants to rifle through the instruments while the trained assistant yawns and looks bewildered at what is happening. The procedure is unpredictable and therefore unassistable.

CHAIRSIDE ASSISTANCE FOR DENTAL AUXILIARY PRACTITIONERS

There are several helpful hints for utilizing a chairside assistant during the typical dental hygiene procedures of the oral prophylaxis and root planing. An obvious one is the use of the assistant in instrument transfer. This person may also mark charts while findings are being called off by the operator. Aspiration during scaling, planing, and polishing procedures makes it unnecessary for the patient to engage in several hundred cuspidor sit-ups during the appointment, and reduces chair time considerably. In fact, the very first rule in reducing chair time is to eliminate the cup-rinse procedure practices of ancient times and at least use a water syringe to rinse areas, even if it is necessary for the patient to empty into a high volume suction funnel attachment or, if absolutely necessary, the cuspidor.

Also, the chairside assistant can use a wide tipped syringe to spread a layer of prophylaxis paste ahead of the area currently being polished, so that the rubber cup does not have to enter and exit the mouth to obtain additional paste for each tooth.[7] During the polishing procedure, the assistant is aspirating with one hand and spreading paste with the other. Some practitioners actually delegate the polishing procedure entirely to the assistant, moving to a second operatory to perform those procedures requiring the skill of a dental hygienist. However, the polishing procedure does move rather rapidly with a four-handed operation, and the amount of time required for the procedure to change hands may not accomplish much in improving the productivity of the team.

The chairside assistant can place periodontal packs after curettage has been performed and remove the packs prior to the dental hygienist's inspection at a subsequent visit.

Many dental hygienists who manage one or more assistants as control therapists may make suggestions for altered plaque control or nutritional procedures and delegate the actual instruction to the chairside assistant/ control therapist.

Hygienists who administer local anesthesia, place rubber dams, and then restore the area prepared by the dentist use the chairside assistant in the same manner the dentist would if he/she were performing the entire procedure without the aid of an expanded function restorative auxiliary.

Despite the fact that dental procedures can be 50% more productive if they are performed with the aid of a chairside assistant, the concepts of four-handed dentistry have been slow in transferring to the practice of traditional or expanded dental hygiene and even to the practice of expanded function dental auxiliaries. While the dentist employs full-time chairside assistants and other "roving" personnel to facilitate a smoothly operating, productive care delivery system, it

is rare that the dental auxiliaries who provide direct patient care have the same benefits. In fact, a review of most dental offices shows that the dental hygienist, for instance, is often relegated to outdated equipment, which precludes adequate positioning at the chair and forces the hygienist to strain, reach, twist, and even stand as the dentist did in decades past. Productivity is equally important in the dental hygiene phases of care, especially when the recall is heavy and the hygienist finds him/herself limited to a continuing stream of oral prophylaxes and a limited opportunity to practice any of the newer functions permitted hygienists in many licensing jurisdictions.

An inefficient practice in the dental hygiene component of the office is just as much of a financial weak spot as it is in the dental components. The patients are unduly stressed; the hygienist is likely more fatigued than is necessary at the end of each appointment; fewer patients can receive care in a day; and the overhead cost of the facility is constant regardless of the less than optimal income generated because of the inefficiency. Time and motion studies show that a hygienist performing oral prophylaxes, radiographic surveys, root planing, curettage, fluoride applications, study model impressions, and other such functions can increase productivity by 90% if a full-time trained chairside assistant is made available for the hygienist. Seeing nearly twice as many patients, the hygienist is still not as fatigued after working with an assistant as when the usual number were seen without the aid of an assistant.[7]

Why is it that four-handed dental hygiene practice is so unusual? Perhaps it is because hygienists are not properly prepared in their educational programs to use a chairside assistant, so attempts at such an approach to practice are viewed with hesitancy or awkwardness. Hygienists have rarely been included in the federally funded TEAM programs to learn how to use a chairside assistant and other support staff. Dental students in TEAM programs have not always had educational experiences in utilizing a hygienist, and from that it is safe to conclude that they did not have experience in how to facilitate the efficient operation of a dental hygienist.

In addition to this pragmatic hypothesis, it is also possible to speculate that dentists do not hire assistants for hygienists simply because "it isn't done." In continuing education sessions on the efficient practice of dental hygiene, the suggestion that a chairside assistant is a major step in improving productivity is often met with incredulous laughter on the part of the participants. The frequent phrase is, "He'd never hire me an assistant. Why would he want to hire a servant for his handmaiden?" While it is possible that there is some attitudinal bias that prompts the dentist to provide outmoded equipment and no assistant for the dental hygienist, it is also quite likely that the hygienist may have never asked or that both the hygienist and the dentist need to assess the impact a chairside assistant will have on productivity.

Just as health care providers who are unknowledgeable in the overhead factors of a business operation tend to focus on the income generating power of their own work, they often take into account only the overhead cost of the chairside assistant and not the actual increase in productivity (and thus income) that will result from the employment of the support person.[2] Dentists first confronted with the prospect of paying out dollars for an assistant when the concept of four-handed dentistry was beginning to grow in the 1960s were probably just as hesitant to take the step. However, once the first step was made and the productivity rose while the stress level dropped, the investment in the chairside assistant was regarded as essential.

Perhaps the dental hygienist will be able to overcome this barrier by acquiring a full understanding of how a well utilized assistant can improve productivity and then by agreeing to a trial employment of such a person. Some hygienists have been able to make their point by hiring an assistant out of their own salaries. The reduced fatigue and the "point made" justified the outlay of funds. Hygienists working on a percentage or commission basis could offer to accept a slightly lower percentage of the income if an assistant is employed. The resultant increase in productivity will more than replenish the lowered percentage, and again the point is well made.

The reluctance to employ chairside support personnel for expanded functions dental auxiliaries, which is perhaps not as frequent as it is in relation to dental hygiene, can be overcome in a similar fashion. Special configurations of how the assistant-for-the-auxiliary is utilized in the daily operations of the facility may be necessary if the expanded functions auxiliary is by design the one assisting the dentist while preparing the tooth. The chairside assistant may be involved in a procedure in another operatory until needed by the expanded functions auxiliary or he/she may have a role as a third pair of hands during the total procedure. With a little inventiveness and a careful analysis of how time not spent at the chair could be productive in other ways, the chairside assistant can be an asset in the efficient operation of the restorative procedures and in other ways in the health care facility.

The crucial rule is that if a chairside assistant is hired on a trial basis, the person must be adequately prepared to perform efficiently and the auxiliary using the chairside assistant must be able to work efficiently with that person, if productivity is expected to improve immediately.

The gradual shift in the discussion of the efficient operation of dental procedures has been from the limited "four-handed" concept to the limitless "multi-handed" concept which can use, eight, ten, twelve, or more active care-providing hands in the delivery of the services the patient needs. The dentist, the dentist's chairside assistant, the expanded function auxiliary and his or her assistant, and any laboratory personnel or roving assistants who facilitate chairside operations in several operatories comprise a team approach to health care. Each person with specific competencies is able to contribute those skills to the smooth operation and productivity of the practice.[1,2,5] The real skill lies in knowing how to assess whether productivity is indeed optimal in terms of time and motion and then to identify how the operation could be modified to better utilize the resources of time and personnel available. In an era when the cost of health care is rising so very rapidly, this element of economy may be a significant factor in providing the greatest amount of quality care possible with the least amount of expenditure of resources.

Review questions

1. What is four-handed dentistry?
2. List five elements of time and motion management that are necessary for maximum productivity:
   a.
   b.
   c.
   d.
   e.
3. Explain briefly how four-handed dentistry can be generalized to four-handed dental hygiene and expanded function dental auxiliary practice for purposes of improving productivity.
4. Provide one theory explaining why chairside assistance is so rarely available to dental auxiliary practitioners who provide direct patient care.

ANSWERS

1. Four-handed dentistry refers to an approach to dental procedures that utilizes the two hands of the dentist and the two hands of the dental assistant in performing the intraoral procedures with a minimum of complex and long-distance movements and with minimal stress for the operator and assistant, for the purpose of increasing productivity.

2. a. The use of prepared trays, with only necessary items included on the tray and positioned in a logical order and location
   b. The operator and the assistant properly seated on opposite sides of the chair at the head of the fully supine patient
   c. The use of high speed equipment and high volume suction devices
   d. A one-handed transfer technique for instruments, with only the assistant taking and replacing instruments
   e. Standardization of operating procedures

3. The same basic principles of four-handed dentistry can be employed for improving the productivity of auxiliaries who provide direct patient care. Procedures such as the oral prophylaxis and root planing, which require access to all surfaces of all teeth, require a specific sequence of positions for optimal access and a sequence of activity so that movements can be minimized and the steps in the procedure can be anticipated by the assistant.

4. One theory is that the dental auxiliary practitioners rarely have the opportunity to learn to adequately utilize support personnel for their own practice efficiency. Another theory is that it is somehow not compatible with the dentist's perception of staffing patterns, such as "providing a servant for the handmaiden."

GROUP ACTIVITIES

1. Assess patient, operator, and chairside assistant positions in a health care facility in terms of how closely they adhere to four-handed dentistry guidelines.

   Offer suggestions for improvements.
2. Take instantly developed photos of operators' positions and analyze them in terms of body stress.
3. Poll local hygienists regarding the vintage of their equipment and the ease with which it can be adjusted to sit-down practice.
4. Film a dental hygiene procedure, such as the prophylaxis, at one frame per second when no chairside support is utilized. Film the same procedure at one frame per second when support is available. Contrast the two films in terms of total time spent, and the number, distance, and complexity of motions.
5. Interview a variety of dentists regarding their reasons for employing or not employing chairside assistants for auxiliaries who provide direct patient care.

REFERENCES

1. Cooper, Thomas M: Four-handed dentistry in the team practice of dentistry, Dent. Clin. North Am., **18:**739.
2. Green, Edward J.: Selection, hiring and training of dental auxiliaries, Dent. Clin. North Am. **18:**771.
3. Hillborn, L. Bruce, Campbell, Edward M., and Hall, William R.: Facility design and equipment considerations for the team practice of dentistry, Dent. Clin. North Am., **18:**873.
4. Kilpatrick, Harold C.: Work simplification in dental practice, ed. 3, Philadelphia, 1974, W. B. Saunders Co.
5. Simon, William J.: Clinical dental assisting, New York, 1973, Harper & Row, Publishers.
6. Wolfson, Edward: Four-handed dentistry for dentists and assistants, St. Louis, 1974, The C. V. Mosby Co.
7. Woodall, Irene: Time and motion studies of dental hygiene functions, Kalamazoo, Mich., 1970-1973, unpublished findings.

CHAPTER 18

Financing health care

OBJECTIVES: The reader will be able to:

1. Identify at least three sources of income related to the provision of health care.
2. Identify overhead costs in operating a health care facility.
3. Explain how each item of overhead is affected by the efficiency of the operation of providing health care.
4. List and explain four ways in which employees in a health care facility may receive remuneration for the services they provide.
5. Identify the advantages and disadvantages of each method of remuneration and select a method that is most compatible with his/her own personal goals.
6. Summarize ways in which cost effectiveness and overall productivity can be measured in a health care delivery system.

The previous chapters have emphasized how time and motion management, management of personnel, and the application of basic legal and business principles can impact the overall operation and productivity of a health care delivery system. The more wisely and efficiently the system operates, the more care will be delivered to the patient, hopefully with a higher level of quality and a greater positive impact on health levels.

Along with the increase in the delivery of care is the increase in the amount of monetary income received. In a fee-for-service system, there is no question that improved efficiency increases income, and if the fatigue levels are reduced, as indicated in previous chapters, the quality of care should be an additional benefit, since the personnel will have the energy to provide quality services. Increased income through sound management practices may enable the provider to stabilize rising fees and perhaps even reduce fees charged the patient.

More efficient management may make it possible to accept a greater number of patients in prepaid capitation plan, thus increasing income.

The long term productivity of the practice can be more cost effective because people may be more willing and likely to appear for scheduled appointments. Each time a patient changes health care providers, a certain amount of delivery time is lost as the patient is "established" in the practice. Many evaluation and assessment procedures will have to be repeated, especially if the patient is reluctant to request that the results of such earlier effort be forwarded to the latest health care provider for evaluation. Longevity of patients in practice is in itself a health care economy since it is now possible to extend attempts at modifying behavior toward the practice of prevention over a longer period of time and with a more planned approach to motivation development. Every patient who is able to control his own disease decreases the overall need for treatment and is therefore an economy factor in the nationwide or worldwide effort to establish health.

Therefore, it is possible to see not only the narrow range economic impact of successful management technique for all resources but also the broader range of impact of such techniques. More dollar income is generated for the particular practice; costs of services to patients may stabilize or be reduced; patients are more likely to reduce their own disease; and there is minimal duplication of services since patients tend to remain within a given health care practice.

FUNDING OF HEALTH CARE

Focusing again on the specific practice setting, it is appropriate to identify how health care is funded since the source of funds may have a significant impact on the care delivered and the financial well-being of the practice. In dental care delivery patients often pay directly for the services they receive. Two other sources of income becoming more prevalent in dentistry are the private and government-sponsored third-party payment mechanisms.[1,3]

In fee-for-service systems, the patient receives a statement of what is owed and is expected to pay in cash either at the completion of the care or within 30 days of that date, if the patient is granted such credit by the practice management. The primary source of complication related to this source of income is that it may take some time to receive payment. Patients may delay payment for some months or make smaller payments over a period of several months. Some may refuse to pay at all. Collection from individually paying patients is therefore a major concern to the practice. Regardless of how much care is delivered in an economically sound manner, the practice will not survive if payments cannot be collected.

When third-party payors are involved, as in insurance companies that reimburse for services rendered, the usual problems of collection are modified. The provider of care must be concerned about whether the care provided meets the guidelines and specifications of the carrier. Is the service covered under the policy? Is this particular family member included in the coverage? Are the requests for payment reimbursement accurately and completely prepared? Does the carrier require that the patient records be examined prior to reimbursement for this type of procedure? And ultimately, how long will it take for the carrier to process the forms and actually complete the payment? While ultimate reimbursement may be more certain when specific guidelines are followed, there are more involved and precise procedures that require additional personnel time. Great care must be taken both before and after the provision of care to ensure that *all* protocols are met. Otherwise, delays can be considerable, causing income to be slow in arriving.

It is important to recognize the difference between government-funded reimbursement programs and privately operated insurance programs. The former programs often are restricted to certain segments of the population. The elderly, children (especially the handicapped or orphaned), and socioeconomically deprived persons are more often included in government assistance programs. Both federal and state governments have supported such programs in the past in order to make care available to persons who could otherwise probably not afford the "luxury" of health services.[3] In accepting patients receiving assistance, it is important for the office personnel to review the government guidelines regarding what services are allowable and what dollar allotments are available for reimbursement for such services. There may be special restrictions that the patient is unaware of, which could cause embarrassment and perhaps nonpayment if those services are accepted by the patient and then cannot be funded by the government agency reviewing the procedures provided.

A classic and recurring example of procedures rarely funded by such agencies is orthodontic care. This aspect of dental care is still often viewed as primarily cosmetic by laypersons who write the laws to fund health services.

The private insurance carrier is not federally supported. Either the patient himself or the company for whom that person works pays a premium to the insurance company, which then insures that that person will have health care paid for when it is needed. Health care insurance was for many years restricted to general physical illness and did not in many instances cover the cost of dental care. The reason for its exclusion from private insurance coverage is quite simple. It may cost the insurance carrier a great deal to pay out claims when over 90% of the population is likely to have need for health care. The prevalence of dental disease is so much higher that it could be difficult for the carrier to collect sufficient premiums to pay for all the care delivered and still make a reasonable profit. The prevalence of periodontal disease alone, which includes over 90% of adults, can account for a large percentage of the health dollar especially when costly periodontal surgery is involved.

Despite the potential cost, many insurance carriers have added dental care to their available packages. This trend was magnified when the large labor unions successfully negotiated to have dental care coverage available to workers and their families as a fringe benefit. To a large extent, insurance coverage for such care is handled as a fringe benefit rather than as a direct cost carried by the patient.

When handled as a private enterprise, there is less likelihood that coverage will be applicable only to certain age or socio-economic groups. However, it is still important to determine whether the fringe benefit package extends coverage to all members of the family or only to the person employed by the company providing the benefit. The guidelines should be assessed for what services are or are not covered by the benefits, and the amount of reimbursement allowable should be evaluated for its compatibility with the practice's usual fee schedule. If only 50% of the cost of a planned procedure will be reimbursed by the carrier, the patient should be aware of that fact and choose to pay the difference or decide some other plan of treatment. Otherwise, the embarrassment referred to previously may occur and

the provider may even find him/herself with an excellent opportunity to provide 50% charity work.

With the advent of national health insurance, which has been the focus of debate in the federal legislature for nearly a decade, patients will have the majority of their health care paid for by the government, probably under a system similar to that used for Medicare benefits for the elderly. If it is indeed regulated and implemented by the government, social security taxes will rise if this is the funding mechanism finally agreed on, for all employed persons, thereby providing the "premium" for services to be available to the public seeking care. This trend is often referred to in the literature as "socialized medicine" since care would be available to all persons regardless of whether they are paying the premiums or not. The large bulk of the working public would carry the burden of those people unable to work or find work. The term refers to the new enforced "social consciousness" of the public, which makes dollars for care available for more people and reduces the "free enterprise" element of the provision of health care. Under the current free enterprise system, people who can afford to pay their own premiums or their own fees (or who are employed where such premiums are a part of a fringe benefit package) have care available to them. Persons who cannot afford care do not receive it, unless the providers of care choose to donate a portion of their time and talent to charity.

It is fair to say that many of today's health care providers categorically reject the idea of socialized medicine, partially for ideological reasons but also because it is likely to have a significant impact on their economic well-being. There will be less opportunity when under federally funded programs for providers to charge fees for the care delivered based on the ability of their clientele to pay. Patients will be able to receive care under a more predictable and standardized system—probably regulated by the government.

The finally drafted and approved legislation for national insurance may or may not include dental care. Several versions have included it, at least for children, but the majority of proposals introduced to the legislature have not included broad dental care benefits. The government may very well decide to focus on the life and death aspects of health care rather than on the dental needs of the public. Also, there is some possibility that a private insurance carrier may implement the legislation, since this will help answer many people's concern that governmental control is too far-reaching when it initiates, implements, and regulates all funding for health care. If it is ever made law, the mechanisms associated with regulation of the law will be of significant importance to the income of a health care delivery facility, since the majority of services provided may be reimbursed by this one mechanism.

There is a third method for financing health care. In addition to private and government insurance programs, there are prepaid capitation plans in which a range of services is provided to persons enrolled in the program in return for a set amount of money paid to the provider per enrollee. Fees are not collected per service from the enrollee, except for those services for which the contract specifies copayment by the patient. Income to the practice is more predictable in a capitation plan, and it is based on the number of enrolees (not services provided.)

OVERHEAD COSTS OF THE HEALTH CARE FACILITY

What happens to that income once it is received by the facility? As mentioned earlier, a significant portion will be spent to pay personnel, to purchase or rent the facility, to pay for utilities, equipment, and

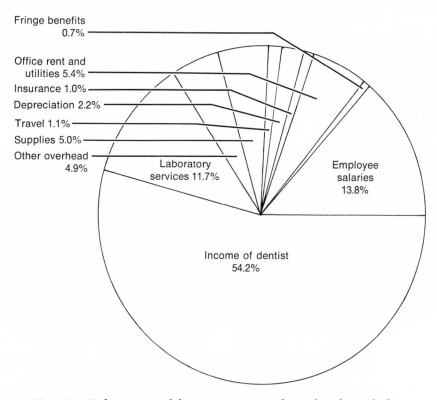

Fig. 18-1. Disbursement of the income generated in a dental care facility.

supplies, to pay taxes, and to purchase contract services such as laboratory testing or construction of ordered prostheses. With each category there is a multitude of costs that often is not apparent to the casual observer.

Fig. 18-1 is a graphic description of the way in which the dental health income dollar is disbursed. The percentages are representative of the results of a number of assessments made of the cost of operating a dental care facility.[5,6] It shows that approximately one half of the gross income is the salary of the dentist. The percentage of profit or salary for the dentist will vary with the provider's ability to wisely manage the resources in the office. The efficiently run office may have a considerably smaller percentage going to overhead costs.

Salaries and benefits

In the category of personnel salaries, the upfront cost of paying the person is obvious. If a salaried person earns $150 each week, then that clearly is a cost of $150 dollars to the practice. It may appear to be less than that to the employee, since the actual paycheck will be considerably less than $150. Amounts covering income tax (federal, state, and even local), social security, and other costs are deducted by the employer before the check is written to the employee. The usual guideline is that a person works 1 day per week "for the government" (20% of effort) and this amount is deducted from the check. However, it is important to understand that it is not the employer who is keeping that 20% deduction. The employer deducts it from the paycheck and forwards it to the government.

In addition to the obvious gross salary amount that the employer pays the employee, there is another less obvious 10% to 25% or more of the salary that the employer is paying. Social security deductions from paychecks are matched by the employer. In other words, if $15 is subtracted from a person's weekly paycheck each week to pay for social security, the employer must pay $15 of the practice's income too, so that a total of $30 is sent to the government for the social security benefits of that employee each week. Worker compensation and unemployment insurance are also costs subtracted from the practice income.

Other benefits included in the 10% to 25% of gross salary suggested here include money spent for health or life insurance that the employer pays for the employee. It may include the cost of free health care in the facility (which costs the practice lost income dollars since no other patient can be receiving care during that time and since it may cost the practice the amount of related laboratory services paid for by the practice). Lab coats or uniform service may be provided to the staff person, costing additional weekly dollars. And factored into the weekly salary is the cost that the practice will incur if that employee loses days because of illness or bereavement or when the employee attends professional meetings or takes a vacation. The cost of replacing the person on the days he/she is away from the office is absorbed by the practice while the "missing" employee's salary is continued. Even if no replacement is hired for those days, the working power of that person is lost, reducing the efficiency and subsequently the overall productivity of the practice on those days.

The percentage of additional cost to the employer for benefits will of course vary with the benefits the employer is offering. Some employers may have a profit sharing plan. Some offer a retirement plan, where money set aside by the employee is matched by the employer, at least in part. So the cost-conscious employee should be aware of the actual costs involved in the employment of an individual as well as the amount listed on the periodic paycheck.

Facility maintenance

Personnel costs are the largest component in the cost of delivering care, especially in team practices where multiple pairs of hands are available to provide services. Second to personnel costs is the cost of laboratory services and then the cost of renting or purchasing the facility. Rent in a commercial building is often based on the square footage of space utilized. The cost may range from a few dollars per square foot to amounts of $10 or $20 or more. The actual amount will of course vary with how much is included in the lease in services, such as remodeling, utilities, or maintenance. An operatory that occupies 100 square feet, which is not an uncommon size, would cost $500 each year to rent, if the cost were $5 per square foot. If the operatory is located in a fashionable high-rise building in the center of an urban area, it may cost the employer a good deal more. It may be more apparent now why it is necessary to assess how well utilized each operatory is for every unit of time each day, and it may be a bit more apparent why an employer is not terribly anxious to expand the size of the facility until it is certain that the expansion will generate additional income.

Related to the size of the facility and the number of usable operatories is the cost of utilities. The cost of lighting and water can be considerable to a commercial enterprise. The rates may be higher than they are for residential areas. Of course, adequate lighting and readily available water are necessary for most health services; what is important to remember is that they are expensive and should be conserved wherever possible. Perhaps this is one of the reasons the flushing cuspidor is rapidly disappearing from the practice of dentistry.

Equipment and supplies

For every operable examining or treatment room there is the equipment that must be purchased in order for the space to be functional. In the case of a dental operatory, the bare essentials can cost several thousand dollars. The very stool the chairside assistant sits on can cost $500 if it meets the specifications recommended by most time and motion experts. The cost of a single dental instrument is often $10 or more. Plumbing and electrical service must be brought to the room, often requiring special hookups because of the electrical demands of the equipment and the access to water necessary in a well designed operatory. The markup for dental equipment has been estimated to be up to 200%. That means that the employer purchasing the equipment pays three times as much for the equipment as it cost the manufacturer to make it.

The cost of marketing the equipment at numerous dental meetings accounts for a large percentage of that markup. It requires thousands of dollars to design, produce, and staff a display booth, plus the amount to rent the space for the display. While the display setup can be attractive, informative, and perhaps a pleasant source of "free" items, the cost is factored into the amounts charged for equipment and supplies being displayed and purchased by the health care provider. Since the cost of equipment affects the overhead of the office, it is ultimately factored into the cost of the care the consumer, the patient, pays for. The cost of health care is therefore driven upward by the marketing necessary for manufacturers to display their wares.

The cost of care goes up with the installation of a single operatory, therefore, not only because of the increased rent and remodeling but because of the tremendous cost of equipment. This can be quite a drain on the income side of the health dollar.

Supplies for health care delivery are similarly highly priced. Gauze squares, napkins, cotton rolls, anesthetics, mercury, needles, suture material, and a myriad of other materials must all be paid for out of the health dollar that comes into the office.

Insurance

And then there is the cost of insurance. Malpractice insurance, at exorbitant rates, is necessary if the provider is to protect himself or herself against the cost of legal damages that may be incurred if a patient wins a judgment against the provider in a court of law. As mentioned earlier, the rise in the frequency of malpractice actions has caused the insurance carriers to increase the cost of premiums substantially. Some physicians, who are feeling the increased cost far more than dentists so far, have considered foregoing malpractice insurance since it costs *thousands* of dollars annually, particularly in high risk practice areas. Others have chosen to abandon health care and begin a new career rather than pay premiums that may reduce profit by 50%. For those who choose to stay in practice and protect their livelihoods, the cost of malpractice insurance is no small item to be scoffed at. This element may increase in states where expanded function auxiliaries are delegated complex procedures to perform, particularly if actions increase against the employer and the auxiliary for negligence. The rule of agentry, remember, causes both the provider of care and the employing dentist/physician to be liable for negligent acts.

Most other items of consideration in determining the overhead of the office will vary with the efficiency with which the office is managed, but the cost of malpractice insurance will rise despite efficiency measures and perhaps not even be obtainable if the providers are on the losing side in a civil action. Prudence in actions toward patients and an ever-present awareness of the needs and expectations of the patient suddenly become apparent as another element to be considered in terms of economy. To fail to recognize those wants and expectations may result in a court action that is financially devastating, negating the effort expended to keep the day-to-day operation financially secure. Good communications skills can be as essential to the financial well-being of a practice as its time and motion economy.

Other forms of insurance are necessary, also, including fire, theft, and personal liability for any harm to a patient, which is unrelated to actual delivery of care.

REMUNERATION FOR HEALTH CARE PROVIDERS

With an understanding of the overhead costs and the ways in which health care is paid for in a health care facility, it is possible to assess how appropriate salary levels can be determined. In fact it is possible to determine what system of remuneration will be best for the provider of health care.

There was a time when the scarcity of dental hygienists resulted in the profession being one of the most highly paid for women. In 1965, when there were 58 programs in the United States preparing dental hygienists, demand for dental hygienists in dental practices was greater than the supply. As a result, dental hygienists could command a respectable salary. When I graduated in 1965, the usual salary in a large city in the Midwest was $20 per day. This was considered a reasonably high salary for a person with 2 years of college education who had the advantage of working in pleasant surroundings with a reasonable measure of dignity and esteem associated with the scope of practice. That figure rose to $50 per day before the decade was history but has really not risen much since that time. The supply of dental hygienists has increased with the number of programs that opened in the late 1960s and early 1970s. And despite the fact the dental hygiene services' fees have risen with inflation, the comparative gross income of the dental hygienist has not risen proportionately.

It is easy to conclude that the salary of dental hygienists is more a function of their availability than their contribution to practice. The situation is not really dissimilar for dental assistants. Again, their salary has been a function of their availability rather than their contribution to the economic well-being of the practice. Dental assistants have been prepared formally in dental assisting programs. Those who chose to be certified and join the American Dental Assistants Association have chosen to continue their formal education and earn additional credits toward continued competence. However, there is no legislation to ensure that dentists hire these well-educated persons. On the contrary, dental practices have been free to hire untrained personnel for similar roles and provide on-the-job training suited to the specific needs of the practitioner. Because untrained women have been readily available, dentists often have opted to hire the persons who possess no formal credentials and pay them lower wages.[3a] Women who had been employed for 20 and 30 years for dentists were earning $65 to $70 per week, gross, in 1974 and were afraid to ask for more because they might lose their jobs. Women formally prepared could hardly hope to compete with such a dedicated, poverty-stricken market, and they likewise settled for horrendously low wages.[3a] Despite the fact that the economic studies in dentistry show that the chairside assistant and the proficient office manager contribute significantly to the productivity (income) of the practice, dentists continue to pay low wages and offer few fringe benefits to the women serving as dental assistants.[3a]

There is little that can be done to combat this inequity, particularly when so many seem so content to live with the problem nationwide. The American Dental Assistants Association and other groups of organized assistants have faced this problem head on and are pouring their energies into solving it.

It appears that the solution may lie in educating the dental assistants who are willing to do something about the problem and who are willing to face the risk of losing their jobs. The education in this case is not a matter of how to better perform dental assisting procedures. The Association tackled that issue long ago and is continuing its efforts in that direction. Rather the new educational emphasis is on determining their worth in the practice. Questions such as: How do my efforts contribute to the productivity of the practice? What effect would my absence have on its productivity? What percentage of this productivity should I share with my employer based on overhead costs and his/her personal income needs? The ultimate questions may be: What level of income is minimum survival wages for me? What level am I willing to accept?

This is a new approach to income for women who for years believed they had to

settle for whatever was offered. Assertiveness in requesting a living wage was uncommon, and it was easy enough for the employer to refuse to increase the salary because there was always another high school graduate looking for a job who could fill the position after a period of on-the-job training. Assertiveness for dental hygienists was a bit easier some years ago, because they had almost all the "cards." After accepting a position at a reasonable salary, they may have discovered that frequent raises were a myth. Many moved on to other jobs, since the only way a raise could be had was to change jobs. Hygienists often acquired the stigma of being job-hoppers or prima donnas who were only interested in money and were somewhat lacking in commitment. Dental assistants, strapped by the low salary regardless of where they worked, developed an understandable resentment toward well-paid dental hygienists. Dental hygienists often did not display an appreciation for the effort expended by the assistant and undervalued the assistant's contribution. Hygienists were loners in their own operatories, keeping their own hours. Mutual lack of appreciation has kept the two categories of dental auxiliaries apart until recently when common goals and problems have served to solidify the two professions as never before.

The stabilized salaries that dental hygienists now earn and the new assertiveness that dental assistants have acquired have begun a trend to equalize the salaries the two workers earn. One element that has really precipitated this change is the delegation of additional functions to dental assistants. Once a dental assistant is trained to perform expanded functions, it costs the dentists a good deal more to change personnel each week. Retraining takes time. And in states where the expanded functions dental assistants must be formally prepared and certified or licensed, the same scarcity that caused the salary of the dental hygienist to rise has caused a similar rise in the salary of the dental assistant. This trend is not sweeping the nation so that dental assistants are now in the upper echelons of the business world. However, it does make a change, or a trend, that bodes well for the dental assistant.

Regardless of whether the auxiliary is a dental hygienist or a dental assistant with or without expanded functions, there are basically four means by which the person may receive remuneration for services provided. (See Table 5.)

Probably the most common method, especially for the dental assistant, is straight *salary*. A predictable weekly wage is paid to the person for having appeared for work and for having performed as the employer expected or contracted for. Usually this arrangement allows for continued salary even if the person is ill or on vacation. There may or may not be fringe benefits in addition to this, depending upon the individual arrangement with the employer. At the time of the employment interview, or after the person has been offered a position in the practice, the employer and employee agree upon the wage and the fringe benefits. They continue until the person is granted an increase or until the work relationship ceases.

An alternative approach is to be paid a *commission* for services provided. This method is relatively common among dental hygienists who work part-time. Hygienists earn a certain percentage of gross receipts for the day. Or they receive a certain percentage of the cost of each procedure. For instance, there might be 50% commission on prophylaxes provided, but only a 30% commission on radiographic surveys exposed. Generally speaking, the daily take-home pay for the dental hygienist on commission is higher than that of the salaried person. However, if a patient cancels or if the hygienist is ill or wishes to attend a professional meeting, no income is generated for the employer or the hygienist during those nonproductive times. Fringe benefits are not

Table 5. Methods of remuneration

Method	Risk level	Potential income level	Fringe benefits	Method of calculation
Straight salary	Lowest	Usually lowest	Often provided; includes illness and bereavement days, vacation	Fixed amount each pay period regardless of number of services delivered
Salary plus commission	Slightly higher	Slightly higher	Few included in most employment settings; little or no allotment made for days lost due to illness, vacation, etc.	Fixed amount (low) regardless of services delivered; percentage of billable services is added; amount fluctuates with productivity
Commission	High	High	Few, if any, included; no allowance for days lost	Amount earned is a percentage of billable services delivered; amount varies with productivity.
Full responsibility for financial success (gross receipts minus overhead)	Highest	Highest	None, except those provided to all staff by virtue of incorporation of the practice	Collect all income from billable services; pay overhead costs to employer of persons providing services, rent, etc.; amount fluctuates with productivity and economy of resources

as likely to be provided for the commission worker as for the salaried person.

It is important to recognize that there has been a continuing diatribe against the hygienist who chooses to work on a commission basis. There actually has been debate on the floor of the House of Delegates of the American Dental Hygienists Association concerning whether commission as a method of remuneration ought to be condemned.[4] The chant associated with this thinking has been that the hygienist on commission must be in a tremendously tenuous position, ethically, if each procedure performed is viewed as a money-making procedure. Some believe that the commissioned hygienist probably envisions dollar signs in the eyes of each patient and undoubtedly rushes through procedures so that more patient procedures (more dollars) could be realized. Somehow the salaried hygienist has been viewed as being more ethical, since he/she was guaranteed the same salary regardless of how much was accomplished.

Dentist-employers wishing greater productivity and more accountability on the part of the hygienist for patients-called-for-recalls and confirmed for appointments opted for the commission approach. And many hygienists have found this approach to be rewarding not only financially but in terms of assuming additional responsibility in the success of the practice.

A third system, which combines salary and commission, is more palatable among those persons who have attacked commissions and some of those commissioned hygienists who have suffered financially from winter blizzards closing down practices on their work days. *Salary plus commission* ensures the hygienist a minimum wage. Perhaps the guaranteed minimum is $30 per day, substantially lower than the usual gross earnings for a hygienist, but certainly better than nothing at all. The hygienist is then paid, in addition, a certain portion of the daily receipts that may exceed the baseline salary. In other words, if the hygienist were to calculate earnings on the basis of 40% of the daily income and one day's income is $200, the hygienist would earn $80 for the day. But suppose the receipts one day were only $60. Despite the fact that 40% of $60 is $24, the hygienist would earn her guaranteed minimum of $30. This procedure is a more secure an approach to income, since there will never be a time when the hygienist starves. But usually this procedure is accompanied by a lower percentage of earnings. The risk factor (*no* income) associated with straight commission is usually counterbalanced by the substantially higher take-home pay when the day's appointments are full and the procedures provided were many.

There is one other system that probably exists more than organized dentistry or dental auxiliaries realize. There are some auxiliary practitioners who literally operate their own practices within the confines of a dental practice. The patients seen by the hygienist are considered his/her own, with referrals made to the dentist in the office as needed. The hygienist receives all the income from daily receipts and pays the dentist for a share of the rent, utilities, insurance, and other overhead. In this instance the auxiliary has *full responsibility for financial success.* This really is only one step away from a hygienist hiring a dentist to perform dental work for the patients for which he/she provides preventive services. Each state law must be carefully examined to determine if a dental hygienist would be precluded from doing this very thing. It does require, however, a willingness to expend capital to establish a practice and to establish continuing responsibility for the practice and the personnel employed by the hygienist. The law in most instances simply requires that the dentist "supervise" the dental hygienist, which in most definitions is interpreted to mean physical presence in the dental facility.

The particular method of remuneration that the auxiliary selects should really be based upon the goals that individual has. If the auxiliary would really rather not worry a great deal about whether a patient arrives for an appointment or not and would rather have a predictable, albeit smaller, wage, then salary is the method of choice. It is particularly helpful for personnel who have just graduated and who have not yet built up any reasonable speed in delivering services.

The experienced practitioner might find commission, or salary plus commission, more attractive, particularly if he/she rarely needs sick days and is able to save sufficient money to finance vacations and professional trips. Surely the commission route does foster a sense of fiscal responsibility that many auxiliaries are sorely lacking. The irony of this move is that the idea of earning income on a fee-for-service system may just become comfortable for auxiliaries when national health insurance and other prepaid systems are initiated, perhaps placing dental providers on a more predictable income schedule, approximating "salary."

MEASUREMENT OF COST EFFECTIVENESS

Cost effectiveness can be assessed in two different, and hopefully complementary, ways. One is to assess the number of procedures performed as compared to the outlay of resources. The second is to assess the actual quality of the procedures or "health effectiveness" of what was provided in relation to the resources expended. Dentistry probably does better in assessing itself in terms of the economic efficiency. With a little help in time and motion management, most practices could improve the efficiency with which resources are allocated. But it takes far more skill to definitively demonstrate that health has significantly improved as a result of dental care. The fact that nearly everyone has some form of dental disease is the proof of this. Any periodontist who hourly faces the questions, "How could I have this periodontal disease you describe, when I have faithfully visited my dentist every 6 months for the last 20 years? What went wrong?" has a reasonable idea how effective or efficient dentistry has been in eliminating dental disease.

Do dental hygienists assess themselves in terms of plaque-free, sound teeth remaining in the dentition? Or do they assess their performance in terms of the number of calculus-free surfaces and bright shiny teeth at the end of each prophylaxis? What of the public health dentist or dental hygienist, or the public health physician or nurse? Have they really significantly affected the health of the population? Or can they simply say that they were able to carry out several educational programs within the state budget provided? While there is considerable merit in assessing efficiency in terms of resources utilized, the bigger challenge lies in assessing how the health of the people really changes as a result of our efforts. Perhaps the whole crux of the ineffectiveness of our health care system is the profession's preoccupation with counting diseases and treatments rather than with measuring how health improves and is maintained.

Review questions

1. List three ways in which a health care delivery practice receives income (sources):
   a.
   b.
   c.
2. List five overhead costs in a health care delivery facility:
   a.
   b.
   c.
   d.
   e.

True or false:

3. Rent for a facility for delivering health care is often calculated by the square foot. _____
4. The gross salary of the personnel in the office is the total cost of employing those persons in the facility. _____
5. If a practice is operated inefficiently so that fewer patients are seen, how would that affect overhead and income?
6. How can improved patient-provider communications have a long term effect on overhead?
7. List four ways in which employees in a health care facility may receive remuneration for their services they provide:
   a.
   b.
   c.
   d.
8. What are the two kinds of efficiencies that are evaluated in assessing cost effectiveness:
   a.
   b.

ANSWERS

1. a. Direct fee for service from the patient
   b. Third party payment from private insurance carriers and governmentally funded programs
   c. Prepaid capitation plans
2. a. Personnel costs
   b. Rent or mortgage
   c. Utilities
   d. Supplies/equipment/laboratory fees
   e. Insurance
3. True
4. False. Social security is matched by the employer and other fringe benefits should be calculated.
5. Rent and salary costs continue while income drops.
6. Improved communications may cause patients to return for further care and may reduce malpractice threats and help stabilize malpractice insurance costs.
7. a. Salary
   b. Commission
   c. Salary plus commission
   d. Accept full income of services provided and pay employer for overhead incurred.
8. a. Economic efficiency (how efficiently resources are utilized in the delivery care)
   b. Health (how effective was the service provided)

GROUP ACTIVITIES

1. Review the dental and medical benefits of four insurance carriers who reimburse for such services. Assess what services are covered, what the companies' policies are with regard to determining how much is reimbursed, and whether a mechanism for assessing the necessity and quality of the service exists.

2. Evaluate the series of national health insurance proposals that have been introduced in the federal legislature. Determine which ones include dental benefits. Discuss why a dental political action group would go on record favoring a national health insurance proposal that does *not* include dental benefits.

3. Examine the socialized health care systems of four countries. Read descriptions of the effectiveness of the care delivered in those countries and the impact the socialization has upon the health of the public and on the esteem of the health professions.

4. Interview several dental auxiliaries regarding the methods by which they are paid. Ask them why they have chosen those methods of remuneration as opposed to others that could be followed.

5. Debate the statement, "A hygienist who works on commission will not last long in practice before his/her ethical principles will be compromised and patients will be no more than dollar signs." Is this true of dentists who practice on a fee-for-service basis?

REFERENCES

1. Fein, Rashi: Health manpower: Some economic considerations, J. Dent. Educ., **40**:650.
2. Firetag, Roberta: Can you exist on your salary? The Action Committee for Dental Assistants.
3. Jerge, Charles R. and others, editors: Group practice and the future of dental care, Philadelphia, 1974, Lea & Febiger.
3a. Leibowitz, Teri and Cupkie, Patricia: Salary survey results, Dental Assistant, **44**:29.
4. Motley, Wilma: Editorial: Remuneration, J. Am. Dent. Hyg. Assoc., **45**:148.
5. Professional Management: Establishing a dental practice, San Francisco, 1974, Bank of America National Trust and Savings Association.
6. University of Pennsylvania, Department of Dental Care Systems, Philadelphia, 1977, personal communication.

PART VI

SELECTING A PRACTICE SETTING

How can a health care provider best put to use his/her personal and professional skills? Based on personal values, what employment situation will prove to be the most challenging, lucrative, secure, or stimulating for an individual?

It is important for a provider to identify his/her priorities in seeking and accepting employment, since it is unlikely that all of them will be met in any one employment opportunity in the marketplace of available positions, and since there is greater variety of settings available for consideration. Once the priorities are established, the positions open can be assessed in terms of how the provider's priorities are compatible with the settings, and how many will be forfeited if employment is accepted in any of the settings.

In addition to establishing priorities, it is important that a health care provider follow a reasonable approach to the employment-seeking process so that a reasonable number of job offers will indeed follow the interview.

This portion of the text is offered as assistance in improving those skills that will help the health care provider find and secure employment, even in the relatively limited market of the late 1970s and early 1980s that is frequently confronted by graduates of allied health programs.

CHAPTER 19

Alternative roles for direct patient care dental auxiliaries

OBJECTIVES: The reader will be able to:

1. Identify the practice settings in which direct patient care dental auxiliaries are most frequently employed.
2. Provide two reasons why the variety of practice settings for dental care providers should expand beyond the usual sites.
3. List at least eight alternative practice settings or roles that a direct patient care provider (including auxiliaries) could assume in delivering care.
4. Explain how alternative practice settings may call upon the educational preparation and the willingness to assume responsibility to a greater degree than traditional settings and roles.
5. Cite sources of information available regarding employment opportunities for dental auxiliaries desiring placement.
6. Survey the community for potential employment situations for direct patient care dental auxiliaries.
7. Outline a plan for increasing actual availability of employment opportunities in the community, which would be suited to the expertise of direct patient care dental auxiliaries.

HORIZONS OF DENTAL HYGIENE PRACTICE

The majority of dental auxiliary students and applicants for positions in dental auxiliary programs describe the role of the dental hygienist and assistant in terms of routine provision of dental hygiene and assisting services in private dental offices. Usually, such applicants have had their contact with dental hygiene and assisting within the confines of a private practice setting and see this site as the place for such personnel to seek and find employment. This is understandable since the vast majority of active dental hygienists and other auxiliaries are employed in private settings in general dentistry (80% to 90%) with fewer than 10% employed in specialty practices. The remaining 1% or 2% practice in one or more of the available "al-

ternative" practice settings.[13,22] It is important to note that the basis for these figures is a 1968 national survey and a 1971 survey in the state of Connecticut, during a time when the American Dental Hygienists Association was first formulating position statements regarding the scope of practice of the dental hygienist and encouraging dental hygiene to find its role in public health, hospital, penal and geriatric institutions as well as in the more traditional settings. The recent literature in the journal of the American Dental Hygienists Association (*Dental Hygiene*) demonstrates that hygienists are finding employment in alternative settings,* but no current data are available to measure that trend. It is likely that the vast majority still are lo-

*See references 2, 4, 7, 9, 15, 18, 21.

199

cated in private practice settings. No data are available with regard to dental assistants, but there is no reason to suspect that they would be significantly different.

If the job market for auxiliaries (particularly those with formal education and skills in providing intraoral services under minimal supervision such as the dental hygienist) is typically located in private practice, why should there be any reason to alter that fact? The reason is that the scope of activity and responsibility of auxiliaries in private practice is defined by the employer-dentist. In some practice settings, the dentist is willing to define the practice of dental hygiene in its broadest scope, calling upon the extensive basic and behaviorial science background of the hygienist in providing a broad range of clinical and educational services for patients. For hygienists fortunate enough to locate such a position, the potential for the delivery of care is translated in the actual provision of care for that segment of the population. So the employer who optimizes the resources available can provide a setting most attractive to the health care provider and most beneficial to the consumer-patient as care is more readily available and as it begins to focus more distinctly on prevention.

However, many dental hygienists find most of their educational background shelved when entering private practice, having most of their activity limited to the oral prophylaxis, preparation of radiographic surveys, and cursory patient education as defined by the employer-dentist. With the advent of control therapists, some hygienists have relinquished their roles in the education of the dental patient. For these persons, the position of dental hygienist has assumed a more task-oriented flavor. The educational preparation for a broader scope of care and responsibility exists for the dental hygienist, but it is rarely called upon. Others, less educated and perhaps more malleable, are given responsibility while the hygienist's role becomes even narrower.

As other direct patient care dental aux-

iliaries are created and educated to enter the work force, this dilemma may be theirs as well as the hygienist's. Presently, however, the hygienist is still the person most often labeled overeducated for what he/she actually performs in practice. (This chapter addresses that group's need specifically with the note that its applicability may spread.)

The basic need for expanding the horizons of dental hygiene practice is related to the fact that the profession's efforts over the past nearly 70 years have not produced a tremendous amount of reduction in the incidence of dental disease. This may be the result of the limited numbers of hygienists practicing for such a large portion of those years, but it may also be because the practicing dentists have not always agreed with Dr. Alfred C. Fones' perception of the role of the dental hygienist.[19] Hygienists have needed dentistry's collective support in the actual implementation of those services, particularly since they have been assigned to a role of being under dentists' supervision. Since it is apparent that support has been less than adequate in the private practice setting, it may be wise to expend a great deal more effort in creating and filling prevention-oriented roles in the community.

Effective utilization of dental hygienists, utilization that would permit them to reach a greater number of people, people of all ages, would include employing the present and expanded skills of the dental hygienist in a variety of social and medical settings.[11]

This call to action may have some impact on the profession and on the people needing the care if funding can be provided to create the positions within health care centers so that prevention can be introduced and made to work.

There is no need to bemoan the rising ratio of hygienists to dentists, if more than individual dentists are viewed as employers. The ratio that will be important to evaluate will be that of hygienists to population, since what will be crucial to evaluate is the availability of the hygienist to serve the needs of the community, rather than the needs of the private solo practitioner.

ALTERNATIVE PRACTICE SETTINGS

There are opportunities for dental hygienists other than in solo practice private dental offices. There are group practices, hospitals, centers for the mentally and physically handicapped, geriatric centers, penal institutions, day care centers, health maintenance organizations, area health planning programs, home consultant programs, and other public health agency programs. There is opportunity in the armed services, and opportunities can be created in various short-term governmentally funded programs in rural or inner-city areas where care is being provided to people who otherwise would not have it.

Hygienists can be employed in public school systems to provide education and intraoral services. They can be employed as consultants both for larger health programs[7] and in individual homes.[9] They can be employed on college campuses in health facilities to care for simple dental emergencies and to refer the students to dentists who are on retainer.

Of those mentioned, the setting most similar to the solo practice is the *group practice setting* where one or more hygienists are able to assume a variety of clinical and educational roles depending upon the structure of the practice and the variety of services provided within the group.[2] Hygienists may emphasize periodontal services depending upon their background or they may choose work with pedodontic patients. There may be an opportunity to practice interceptive orthodontics or to provide the first steps in endodontic treatment. The scope of practice will vary with the type of group practice, but it is far more likely to provide variety and an opportunity for growth since there is more than one pair of hands relegated to the performance of the oral prophylaxis. In a well organized preventive program, the need for oral prophylaxis appointments may decrease so that other kinds of preventive, restorative,

and therapeutic services can be performed by the dental hygienist.

Hospitals can also provide ideal settings for the expertise of the dental hygienist, both in the outpatient clinic and the inpatient components of the hospital.[4,8,10,21] The full array of medically compromised persons may be included in the patient pool, causing the dental hygienist to draw fully upon his/her background in oral medicine and the basic sciences.[4] The care provided to the patients will need to be modified to meet their particular needs, involving premedication, special precautions during instrumentation, "creative" positioning of the operator and patient, and careful followup of procedures to ensure that no complications have arisen. The hospital-based hygienist has a unique opportunity to become a full member of the "total health team" working with physicians, nurses, nutritionists, and other allied medical personnel in establishing optimal total health for the patients for which the hospital provides care.[14] The hygienist may be responsible for continuing education programs in oral medicine for the community's dental personnel, inservice training to the hospital personnel in oral hygiene procedures and the identification of oral disease, and planning and implementing educational programs for patients, providing information related to the oral implications of their particular health problems.

Centers for the physically and mentally handicapped offer similar opportunities for dental hygienists,[15,21] particularly since dental care is so infrequently provided to these groups. The dental hygienist can serve as the resident dental health educator and can provide preliminary examinations and preventive maintenance for the patients, with persons needing more sophisticated care being referred to the dentists designated to provide such care. A similar approach can be used in the *care of the elderly patient*, both on a home visit basis and in nursing homes, where the dental needs of patients in advanced ages are sorely neglected. Patients with few remaining teeth and with prosthetic appliances still need preventive care, including oral examinations, oral prophylaxis, prosthesis evaluation, and repair of broken appliances. A definite need in nursing homes is to have dentures and partial dentures marked so that their owners can be identified when the appliances turn up in the laundry.

Penal institutions for adults and those for adolescents can utilize the services of dental hygienists, also. A strong preventive program could eliminate much of the cost of providing restorative and other reparative dental treatment to persons under detention. The social awareness skills of the hygienist may be put to the test in such a situation, since the perceived needs and the value systems of the inmates may be quite different from those encountered in the suburban dental office. In large institutions a dentist may be employed by the state to provide the therapeutic components of care, but others with smaller financial resources may be able to employ a hygienist to provide screening and preventive services and to refer cases to dentists for definitive diagnosis and treatment.

Child care centers may wish to form a cooperative in employing a dental hygienist to provide dental health education, screening, and preliminary treatment for patients along with a referral program. Dental hygienists may also be used as consultants in educating the teachers and as aides to teach and evaluate oral health practices in their groups of children.[18]

The functions of a dental hygienist in a *health maintenance organization* are basically similar to those of the hygienist in an outpatient clinic of a hospital. This growing practice mode may provide a tremendous source of employment of hygienists if dental care benefits continue to be included in such plans.[20] Area health planning agencies and programs may use the planning and educational skills more than the clinical skills of the dental hygienist in evaluating practice sites for their efficiency, potential productivity, and modified staffing patterns. The dental hygienist may participate in the design of educational programs and serve as a pro-

gram implementor for community education efforts. He/she also may be involved in preparing applications for the funding of planned programs and in the subsequent direction and evaluation of those programs. In such a community planning agency there is a great opportunity to use a variety of skills and to inject a large measure of creativity in designing programs, facilities, manpower patterns and in assessing costs and financing.[7]

Home consultant programs can include nutritional counseling, muscle training for preventive orthodontics, plaque control, and bedside care for persons unable to travel to a health care facility. This program can be affiliated with visiting nurses programs, social work programs, and community action programs, such as "meals on wheels."

Many *state and county public health agencies* have vigorous programs for the prevention and treatment of dental disease, depending upon the degree of commitment and the energy of the staff and upon their success in obtaining tax and grant monies to support the programs. The activity of such programs is not restricted to health education alone; it includes clinical services.

One step removed from the mainstream of the provision of educational and therapeutic care for people are the areas of *education* (preparing health professionals for patient care roles) *and research*. With 200 dental hygiene education programs in operation,[5] there is a great need for qualified administrators and faculty to operate those programs. Educational programs must be of a quality that ensures that their graduates are prepared to enter service in any of the previously identified employment settings.

There is (currently) a less obvious demand for *research hygienists*, but there is a definite role to be played in the clinical and laboratory supervision of data gathering, in the actual provision of clinical services being researched, in the selection and supervision of support personnel, in the preparation of applications for funding, and in subsequent evaluation and report writing procedures.[17] Hygienists with a strong background in research design and management coupled with a strong background in basic sciences may be able to join research efforts that could lead to improved clinical procedures and even to the discovery of the vaccine or mouthrinse that eliminates dental disease, or at least one of its forms.

Regardless of the setting, hygienists with advanced preparation can function as *practice managers*, as *supervisors* of people, and as *policy-making administrators*. The career ladder can exist for the clinical dental hygienist if the scope of activity is seen as greater than that usually permitted in the solo private practice dental setting.

EMPLOYMENT OPPORTUNITIES

The dental literature has warned that the era of the solo dental practice is declining and that the provision of care in the future, if it is to be economically sound and if it is to include provisions for quality assurance, will be conducted in group practices.[12] The dental hygienist, so often associated with the solo dental practice, would be wise to prepare for the advent of a greater scope of practice and responsibility in the future.

In addition to the changing trends for the delivery of care, the nation seems to be directing itself, once again, to the importance of prevention. In the 1976 Carnegie Report the fifth urgent recommendation reads:

In the light of accumulating evidence that mortality rates in the United States are excessively high chiefly because of unwise personal habits and high accident rates, major emphasis should be placed in the coming years on the development of more effective programs of health education. Health professionals also need to be trained to place greater emphasis on educating patients to play a more active role in their own care and treatment.[3]

If the federal government decides that it is appropriate to develop a prevention program that can be measured for its effectiveness in reducing and eliminating disease and that can be funded with minimal fear of fraud, the dental hygienist may be a person in great demand in the delivery of health care services. As one of the very few allied health professions whose primary area of expertise is acknowledged to be prevention and who also possesses a growing number of clinical skills, he or she may be in great demand in the decades ahead.

For the person wishing to practice dental hygiene in an alternative setting, the initial efforts at finding such employment may be frustrating. There are not many alternative positions open compared to those in private practice settings—or at least they are not as apparent. One good place to find positions available to interested dental hygienists is the placement file at schools of dental hygiene. Very often unique opportunities will be listed in those records. The classified section in the professional journals is a good resource. It may be possible to convince an employer advertising for a dentist that a dental hygienist will be able to serve the purpose as well—and for less cost. The American Dental Hygienists Association has a faculty registry service where persons interested in teaching positions and programs interested in faculty submit their qualifications. State associations may sponsor a statewide placement service. And local components of the professional association often have persons responsible as registrars of available employment openings.

Even the area newspapers may provide some ideas for potential positions. A quick scan of the hospitals or nursing homes that are advertising positions available may provide some leads regarding whom to contact in personnel in order to state the case for a position within the institution. It is important to be aware that most funding for nurse's positions and other allied medical staff is derived from the third-party payment mechanism. The services these people provide are funded by reimbursement from insurance companies and the federal government. Few hospital services are on a fee-for-service basis with the patient paying directly. The administrator may point out that patients may resist preventive dental care because they will need to pay for it directly. Unless the hygienist can show how his or her services can be funded, the chances for being employed are reduced greatly. Even an awareness of this economic fact may score points with the personnel manager. One approach may be to work through the local dental society and the dentists on staff at the hospital in determining the potential role of the hygienist and likewise the ways in which the position could be funded. Some positions may be more readily available for dental hygienists if they can begin slowly (on a part-time arrangement) and then build up until they are full-time components of the staff of the facility. Or the hygienist could agree to work on a commission basis, as fees for services are collected. This may challenge the hygienist to develop his/her entrepreneurial skills and build a sound program of dental care within the hospital environment with little financial risk realized by the hospital administration.

If federal programs are announced to fund dental care delivery within hospitals and other such institutions, the dental hygienist interested in such employment might approach the health care facility, volunteering to prepare such an application while employed on a part-time basis. Once (or *if*) the funding is granted, the dental hygienist may be in a prime position to assume the position described in the grant application.

For instance, federal money to support programs where teams of health care providers work together for purposes of more greatly coordinated care were announced in 1976.[6] Educational institutions such as medical and dental schools could qualify, but teaching hospitals might also be able to receive such funds under similar grants. Therefore, an awareness of recently announced federally funded programs can be a helpful basis from which to work in finding employment in alternative settings.

Often private foundations will fund such efforts. With the support of the health care facility, a dental hygienist might approach such a foundation with a draft of a proposal to integrate dental and medical care for persons in an institution where such comprehensive services are not currently available. Listening carefully to the goals of the foundation in funding such projects, the hygienist may rewrite the proposal to meet their specifications.

Creativity, good communications skills, good timing, an awareness of funding procedures and a wise use of the local dental society's support could result in innumerable positions opening to hygienists that call upon the educational background and skills far more than current patterns of utilization.

The concept of prevention is a foreign one in the minds of many people, since the total health emphasis in many communities is on treating disease that is causing pain or threatening life.[1] This emphasis is largely the result of the cost of health care, which precludes regularly scheduled dental and medical visits and because of the lack of availability of care even when money is provided.[1] The dental hygienist who manages to become employed in a neighborhood health facility or in an active public health agency may find that prevention *can* be implemented, certainly with numerous frustrations, but at least there is opportunity to initiate and conduct a full-scale educational and therapeutic program to eliminate and prevent dental disease.

While the professional association is expending energy to produce these positions, the greatest effectiveness probably lies in the political skill of the local component and the individual, assertive dental hygienist. The opportunity is there for the bright, energetic hygienist to find rewarding employment where some measurable good can be obtained in the provision of health care services for people. But it does require more than a passive role in the job market.[16]

Review questions

1. Approximately _____% of active dental hygienists practice in general dentistry private practices.
2. Approximately _____% of active dental hygienists practice in settings other than general and specialty practices.
3. List eight alternative practice environments or settings in which dental hygienists may provide services to the public.

    a.

    b.

    c.

    d.

    e.

    f.

    g.

    h.

4. What kinds of educational preparation may be more greatly utilized in alternative practice settings? (Refer to at least three categories.)
5. Where can a dental hygienist interested in alternative practice settings find information that could lead to such employment? (List four.)

    a.

    b.

    c.

    d.

ANSWERS

1. 90%
2. 1% or 2%
3. a. Group practices
   b. Hospitals
   c. Centers for the mentally and physically handicapped
   d. Geriatric centers
   e. Child care centers
   f. Armed services
   g. Health maintenance organizations
   h. Home consultant programs
   (Others include public school systems, area health planning agencies, and community action programs.)
4. Basic sciences, behavioral sciences, and communication skills may be better put to use. Depending upon the degree to which clinical skills are utilized in private practice, this area of expertise may be better utilized, also.
5. School placement services, classified ads in journals and newspapers, ADHA faculty registry, state and local component placement services.

GROUP ACTIVITIES

1. Contact local hospitals, nursing homes, day care centers, and other institutions for the availability of positions for dental hygienists. Identify all employment opportunities in the community that could be available to dental hygienists to provide care to the population if money were available to fund such positions.

2. Design an informational program to demonstrate to each category of alternative practice opportunity how the employment of a dental hygienist could be managed financially and could provide needed care to the persons currently receiving other health care within that institution.

3. Invite a recruiter from each of the armed services to describe employment opportunities for civilian dental hygienists or for dental hygienists who wish to join the service for a number of years.

4. Conduct a survey of local dental hygienists to determine what functions they perform in their respective settings and to determine the scope of responsibility and the degree to which they call upon their educational preparation in the daily activities they perform. Use the task analysis provided in ADHA's *Curriculum Essentials* to form a baseline of activities dental hygienists could perform as a result of their educational preparation.

REFERENCES

1. Barnes, Donna P.: Social perspectives on community dental health, Dent. Hyg., **50:**457.
2. Berg, Bettina: Group practice: The role of the dental hygienist in a health care delivery system, Dent. Hyg., **48:**231.
3. Carnegie Council on Policy Studies in Higher Education: Progress and Problems in Medical and Dental Education, San Francisco, 1976, Jossey-Bass, Inc., Publishers.
4. Caveny, Mary: The dental hygienist in hospital practice, Dent. Hyg., **50:**205.
5. Dentistry and Allied Services, 1975-1976, Manpower Analysis Branch, U.S. Dept. of Health, Education, and Welfare, PHS-HRA, Bureau of Health Manpower, Division of Dentistry.
6. Federal Register, November 24, 1976.
7. Hawes, Marie Jo: A dental hygienist's role in an areawide comprehensive health planning agency, Dent. Hyg., **49:**360.
8. Hendler, Barry H. and Alling, Charles C.: Inpatient hospital dentistry, Dent. Clin. North Am., **19:**595.
9. Ingalls, Judith A.: The dental hygienist as home consultant, Dent. Hyg., **47:**38.
10. Iranpour, Bejan and Brown, I. Stephan: Ambulatory hospital care, Dent. Clin. North Am., **19:**587.
11. Klyvert, Marlene: Dental hygienists in community programs. Presented before the Twenty-fourth National Dental Health Conference, Chicago, March, 1973.
12. Jerge, Charles R.: Health care in transition. In Jerge, Charles R., and others, editors: Group practice and the future of dental care, Philadelphia, 1974, Lea & Febiger, pp. 3-28.
13. Lewis, Dorothy Jean: A study of dental hygiene practice in the State of Connecticut: 1971, An Essay presented to the faculty of the Department of Epidemiology and Public Health, Yale University, 1972.
14. Lynch, Malcolm, Cormier Patricia P., and Rose, Louis F.: The dental profession, the community, and the hospital, Dent. Clin. North Am., **19:**575.
15. McCollum, Nancy and Jones, Karen: St. Peter's: A lesson in community involvement, J. Am. Dent. Hyg. Assoc., **45:**172.
16. Schnurr, Barbara J.: State of the Association Address, Delivered at the Fifty-third Annual Session of the American Dental Hygienists Association, November, 1976.
17. Wehse, Virginia A.: The hygienist in dental research, J. Am. Dent. Hyg. Assoc., **45:**383.
18. White, Kay Byers: A preventive dental health education plan for preschoolers, Dent. Hyg., **45:**510.
19. Williams, Carlton H.: Are dental hygiene concepts changing? J. Am. Dent. Hyg. Assoc., **45:**30.
20. Williams, Harrison A.: The challenge of tomorrow in dental care delivery, J. Dent. Educ., **40:**587.
21. Winchell, Sue: Rancho Los Amigos Hospital—a hygiene program, Dent. Hyg., **50:**29.
22. Wyshak, Grace and Hoase, Jeannette V.: Profile of dental hygienists, Dent. Hyg., **50:**497.

CHAPTER 20

Preparing a resume

OBJECTIVES: The reader will be able to:

1. Explain how a resume can affect an employer's decision to offer employment to an individual.
2. Specify the usual components of a resume.
3. Identify which items are, by law, not to be considered by employers in offering employment.
4. Prepare a personal resume for:
   a. Clinical practice employment
   b. Employment within an educational institution
   c. Employment in a public health agency
5. Critique several sample resumes for their structure, completeness, and quality of preparation.

If the health care provider entering the world of work hopes to have a number of employment offers from which to choose, it is important to be able to prepare a resume that will be a clear statement of how well that provider will be able to function within the employment setting.

A resume is a concise statement of a person's qualifications. It serves as a formal written introduction of the potential employee to the interested employer. The employer is able to review the person's educational background, work experience, professional association activities, publications, and other pertinent information in order to assess how compatible the person's qualifications are with the requirements of the available work position. Since the resume is often available to the employer prior to an interview, it creates the "first impression" of the person. It can tell the potential employer a great deal about the applicant, including the person's gift for clarity, completeness, organization, and even the person's basic self-concept.

What are the key components of a well-designed resume? How can it be structured so that vital elements of information are easily identified? What are some general guidelines that should be followed in preparing this statement of qualifications?

The applicant's *name, address, and telephone number* should be conspicuously placed at the top of the resume so that the reader can readily identify whose statement of qualifications it is and so that the person's name is associated immediately with the contents. Its conspicuous location even facilitates accurate filing so that it is not lost on a person's desk while awaiting a careful search for the applicant's name somewhere in the application. This information also ensures that the potential employer will be able to contact the person for an interview or to at least acknowledge receipt of the resume.

Educational experience is usually a most critical element in the resume, particularly in health-related fields where specific credentials are required for a person to be accepted for employment. Usually only postsecondary education is listed in a professional resume unless some aspect of high school preparation is particularly relevant to the person's credentials. For instance, if a registered nurse received nurse's aid preparation in high school or if a special biological sciences honors program was included in high school, then it may be appropriate to include it. Each certificate and degree should be listed, chronologically, along with the institution from which it was received and the year it was earned. The major area of study or the discipline in which each degree is granted should be identified as well. Some resume forms recommend placing the most recently earned degree first on the list, then proceeding backwards chronologically to the first earned educational credential. This may be wise if the list of degrees is lengthy. But for the health care provider just beginning a career, the listing may include no more than one or two entries. In this case, reverse order is not necessary, since the reader should have minimal difficulty identifying the most advanced degree or certificate.

States in which the person is licensed should be listed along with professional certification status as applicable.

Following the basic educational and practice credentials should be a statement of work experience. For persons with several years of professional experience there is little need to list nonprofessional employment experiences. However, if the person is seeking a first professional position, it may be wise to include those employment positions held during high school and college years. Employers look favorably upon a resume that shows that the person has been able to assume the responsibilities associated with employment and hold a position for an extended period of time. The statement of work experience should, again, be in chronological order. The places of employment should be identified, along with a brief statement of the nature of the position held and the dates of employment in each position.

For persons seeking employment in a research or teaching institution or in a public health agency, it is best to subcategorize work experience into clinical practice, laboratory or clinical research, teaching experience, or community projects. For persons applying for an administrative or consultative position, the resume should specifically reference work experience that relates to administrative or consultative roles. These subcategories are usually not even necessary to mention in the resume of a person who is just beginning a career.

If the current employer is listed in the work experience category, it may be helpful to state whether or not it is appropriate for the potential employer to contact him or her as a reference. This can be a sensitive matter if the current employer is unaware of the employee's search for another opportunity. When the call is placed, asking for a reference, it may be met with a shocked response and the employee may be in a most uncomfortable position as a result. However, if the current employer is aware of the employee's intention to change positions and can provide a favorable recommendation, the potential employer should be aware that this is an appropriate reference to call.

Professional activities usually comprise the next category of information in a resume. Membership, committee activities, officerships, and special projects assignments in student organizations and then graduate organizations should be specified chronologically with a brief description of the positions held in each of the organizations. Having assumed a reasonable amount of responsibility within a professional association can be viewed as an indication of commitment beyond the day-to-day work activity of the profession.

It is important to point out that not all employers respond positively at first to obvious extensive involvement in associations. Some employers fear that association business will be conducted over the office telephone and that the political aspects of such a role may conflict with the goals of delivering care. Others view association activity as highly commendable and will offer to support such efforts with secretarial assistance, the use of the office telephone, and a limited number of release days for conducting professional association business. The point is that it is helpful to list memberships and leadership roles in associations and to follow up their entries at the interview with a candid discussion of the degree of commitment and with appropriate assurances that such involvement will not detract from the employment arrangement. If it appears that the level of involvement will affect daily employment activities, then expectations should be carefully described so that neither party encounters unpleasant surprises after the position is offered and accepted.

Clinicians may wish to list continuing education courses attended (and ones they have designed and conducted) and units (CEU's) earned. This may be particularly important if the clinician is in a profession where role changes are occurring and where newly delegated functions have been incorporated.

If the person seeking employment has participated in clinical or pure research resulting in publications, the citations should be listed under that category. This category may be most relevant for persons seeking employment in a research or educational institution or a public health agency. It is a category most often applicable to persons who have had a research component in their master's or doctoral programs or for those who have extensive employment experience with opportunity for research.

Other items of information that may be included are age, marital status, sex, number of dependents, and race. A picture can be attached to the resume, also. However, many people now omit these items because they have been known to be factors that have tended to prejudice employers for or against an applicant regardless of the professional credentials described in the resume.

Some employers may automatically exclude male applicants, persons under 20 or over 45 years of age, black persons, or a married, childless woman. The laws now make it unnecessary for applicants to list age, race,

or sex because of this prejudicial element, which places persons falling in the "wrong" stereotyped group at a great disadvantage. In fact, persons who can prove that they were discriminated against in being hired because of age, race, sex, creed, or national origin may prosecute.

If the applicant wishes to include that information on the resume, he/she may. However, it is difficult to identify how any of those factors should relate directly to the person's ability to perform the job as defined. It might be wisest to limit the resume content to relevant data.

The amount and kinds of information included in a resume can say a great deal about the person's ability to concisely state the essential elements to be considered in assessing suitability for a position. Tremendous detail regarding high school social club activities or church circle responsibilities may not offer the employer the information he/she is seeking and may detract from other, more pertinent items. Scant information regarding previous employment or missing chronological links because of failure to include time frames of school and employment may leave doubts in the reviewer's mind (such as, "I wonder what happened between 1970 and 1975?"). No mention of references, or a limited range of persons cited as references, may prompt the reviewer to wonder what trail of havoc was left behind by the person. And it does not permit the reviewer to quietly follow up references prior to the interview.

The happy medium is to include as much helpful data as possible without cluttering the resume with extraneous commentary.

One certain way an applicant can say a great deal about his or her personality is to include an autobiography. Usually placing a limit of 250 to 300 words on the length of the "life story" forces the applicant to decide what is relevant, what says the most about a person's successes, ambitions, roadblocks, and values, and yet doesn't cause the reader to doze off at "Chapter 3—When I Learned to Roller Skate." An autobiography says a great deal to the observant reviewer about the person's self-concept and helps to prepare for meeting the person in an interview situation. The reviewer gets to know the applicant on a more personal level prior to the session and has something with which to open the discussion.

In writing an autobiography, the applicant should let his/her natural personality show. The writer should use an individual style and mix personal and professional milestones as appropriate. It is important to remember the basic writing skills of coherence, unity, clarity, reasonable paragraph transitions, and grammar. This will facilitate the reader's understanding of what the applicant is attempting to express, and it is an obvious statement of the person's ability to think logically and use written communication skills, which are two qualities the employer may be seeking in an employee. Despite the trend toward devaluing the skills of good grammar and spelling (and their subsequent deemphasis in the content of the secondary school curriculum), potential employers often do focus in on these skills, particularly if the employment role calls for preparing charts and correspondence. People often evaluate intelligence in terms of writing skills, and sometimes in terms of handwriting. Regardless of the applicant's view of the necessity of good writing skills, care and attention should be paid to the preparation of the autobiography in terms of its structure as well as its content. The autobiography should be neat and either typewritten or legibly handwritten. A reasonable mastery of the English language is also often evaluated in terms of the variety of the vocabulary and the appropriateness of word usage. So while it is not necessary to seek out unusual words in the thesaurus, it does help to have some variety in word selection.

The rules of clarity, neatness, coherence, unity, and good grammar apply not only to the autobiography but to the entire resume. It should be an attractive document that reads well. The resume definitely should be typed and proofread. It should make use of headings and appropriate spacing so that the reader's eye can easily focus on relevant categories quickly. It helps to use plain bond paper (rather than the erasable bond) since it is less likely to smudge and leave its imprint on shirt cuffs and other papers on the reader's desk. It may be an obvious copy of an original (photostat or dry stencil product), but it should be readable and of high quality.

It generally is not necessary to use fancy folders or engraved letterhead. Sometimes these extreme approaches to the preparation of a resume speak more of frivolity and compulsiveness than of functionality and neatness. A well-prepared resume with a brief, introductory cover letter is usually what an employer expects or wants.

The cover letter should briefly mention the attached biographical data and should specify the type of position for which the person is applying. If a specific position has been listed as available, it is wise to identify that specific job title and to mention where the position's availability was posted or listed. This assists the reviewer in matching resumes with openings.

The letter should specifically state an interest in obtaining employment; it should identify whether the applicant wishes an interview, and it should suggest how contact may be made. For instance, the closing lines of the letter may say, "Please inform me of the availability of this type of position in your corporation. If you wish to arrange for an employment interview, I will be most pleased to meet with you. Below are listed my address and telephone for your convenience."

The well-prepared cover letter makes the point immediately and courteously asks for follow-up. It permits the reader to rapidly scan the page for the essentials and plan whatever follow-up is needed. It should invite the reader to review the attached resume, not only because it is referenced in the letter but because the cogent style says, "You want to know more about me."

It is a careful balancing act to be assertive without being demanding. Requesting a response and providing a ready means for the response to be made is a reasonable approach. Using phrases such as "I expect you to call me . . . ," or "I will call you for an interview . . . ," or "Have your secretary call me . . . ," are generally construed to be pushy. In contrast, the phrases, "I know you must be very busy, but I would be so elated if you could take a moment to answer me . . . ," and "I hope you will give me a chance . . . ," are too mushy and sound more like "begging" than "requesting" on an adult-to-adult level. Besides, these overqualified, modified, super-humble requests take up a great deal of space in a letter and add words through which the reviewer probably does not wish to wade.

While the resume may be a duplicate, the cover letter should be an original, single copy correspondence. It should, if possible, be addressed to a specific person, and it should contain (as noted previously) references to the particular position available or the work setting. The mass duplication approach with only the reviewer's name and address typed at the top creates in the mind of the reader visions of resumes flooding the land in the hopes that someone will respond. It definitely helps to personalize the cover letter, even if it is only so that the employer feels some sense of potential significance in the applicant's life.

Fig. 20-1* shows a cover letter that is not atypical of those received by potential employers. It is typed (at least) on a postcard and displays many of the no-nos that can cause the initial, albeit written, contact between applicant and reviewer to be less than favorable.

It is addressed to no one in particular. It is not dated. Nor does it have much useful information, despite the fact that it covers the available space. It refers to a curriculum vitae (resume) which is to follow, necessitating that the reviewer hold and match arriving correspondence. Because it is on a

Text continued on p. 219.

---

*No entries in the cover letter and resumes shown in this chapter are to be construed as facts related to any actual person.

```
To whom it may concern:

    I am very interesting in persuing with you the possibility of a job
in your hospital, if you will take the time to call me and arrange for
an appointment sometime soon, at your convenience.  I am sure there
must be many opening for persons such as myself who are interested in
employment.  You could send me a list of what is open or we could
discuss it at the interview.  I have two years of education and have
nursing experience.  My curriculum vitae will be in the mail to you
soon so that you may review it before our interview.  What are the
chances that I will be hired?

                              Yours truly, Gerry Paddington
                                            281-0660
```

Fig. 20-1. An example of how *not* to initiate correspondence with a potential employer. The postcard is undated, contains little useful information, has a misspelled word and grammatical errors, includes only one method for replying, and does not have an accompanying resume.

March 10, 1977

Personnel Director
Rabash Hospital
5758 Main Street
Fordham, OH 55455

Dear Director:

    I am a registered dental hygienist with three years' clinical and supervisory experience in a hospital in Pennsylvania providing routine preventive dental care for extended-care patients and hospital out-patients.

    Your advertisement in <u>Dental Hygiene</u>, the Journal of the American Dental Hygienists' Association, indicates that you have a position open for a dental hygienist which would include similar functions. I am interested in applying for that position and have enclosed my resume for your review.

    Should you find that I possess the appropriate qualifications, I would appreciate the opportunity to meet with you. You may contact me at either of the numbers listed below. My address is also listed for your convenience.

               Yours truly,

               George Herrick

               George Herrick, R.D.H., B.S.
               42 Marble Road
               Bedford, PA 19002

Home: (626) 881-2262
Office: (626) 872-6437

Fig. 20-2. An example of a concise, informative, attractive cover letter for a resume. It refers to the specific position, briefly describes the applicant's qualifications, refers to an enclosed resume, suggests that contact be made for an interview, and provides information for contact to be established. It is assertive but not aggressive.

```
                                     Resume


          George Herrick, R.D.H., B.S.
          42 Marble Road
          Bedford, PA 19002
          Home:  (626) 881-2262
          Office:  (626)  872-6437


          PROFESSIONAL EDUCATION:

            The University of Southern California        1967
                Certificate in dental hygiene

            The University of Pennsylvania               1971
                Bachelor of Science in health care
                management (with high honors)


          CLINICAL EXPERIENCE:

            Dental hygiene practice in                 1967-1969
                periodontics (full-time)
                Dr. Linda F. Homan
                58 Westfield Drive
                Lindwood, CA 99210

            Dental hygiene hospital                    1971-1975
                practice (full-time)
                Bedford General Hospital
                61 Miami Blvd.
                Bedford, PA 19002

            Dental hygiene practice in                 1975-present
                pedodontics (full-time)
                Dr. Elmer Bloomquist
                78241 Randall
                Bedford, PA 19002


          LICENSURE:

            National Board Certificate                   1967
            California licensure (current)               1967
            North East Regional Board Certificate        1970
            Pennsylvania licensure (current)             1970
```

Fig. 20-3. An example of a concise, well-organized resume. It has appropriate categories, reasonable amounts of pertinent information, grants permission to contact references, and is basically unpretentious.

CONTINUING EDUCATION:

"Local Anesthesia"   3.5 CEU's   1974
   The University of Pennsylvania

"Expanded Functions in   3.0 CEU's   1975
   Pedodontics"
   Temple University

"The Effects of Systemic Disorders   1976
   on Oral Tissues"   1.0 CEU's
   Montgomery County Community College

CLINICAL RESEARCH AND PUBLICATION:

The effects of preventive measures on
dental disease as manifested in transplant patients
medicated with corticosteroids, Dental Hygiene,
49:416, 1975.

Note: Current and former employers may be contacted as references.

Fig. 20-3, cont'd. For legend see opposite page.

```
                              Resume


        Education:

           H.S. diploma in Anaheim            1965
           Cert. in dental hygiene            1967
           Penn.-B.S. degree                  1971
           Continuing education               1974 to 1976
             (total of 7.5)

        Work:

           Practiced hygiene for two          1967-1967
             dentists
           Worked in a hospital               1971-75
           Plaque control in hospital.  Got   1975
             published


        Age:  28                              George Herrick
        Married                                 (626) 881-2262
        Two children:  Amy-5
                       James-2                Hobbies:  cooking,
        Wife:  Elissa, age 27                            carpentry
               Unemployed                     Novels read:  Catch 22,
        Weight:  170                          All the President's Men
        Height:  5'10"
```

Fig. 20-4. An example of how a poorly prepared resume can underrate a person's competencies. Information is incomplete and jumbled. Extraneous data are included, but crucial items are missing. It should be contrasted with the resume presented in Fig. 20-3.

Content

1. Are name, address, and telephone number conspicuously spaced at
    the top of the first page?   _____

2. Is education (beginning at the postsecondary level) listed
    chronologically?   _____

3. Are certificates and degrees earned listed with the discipline or
    area of study identified?   _____

4. Are licenses and/or certificates of competence listed, including
    state or region and date achieved?   _____

5. Are places of previous employment listed chronologically with
    addresses and a brief description of the scope of activity or
    responsibility?   _____

6. Are dates provided for each work experience with an indication
    of full- or part-time employment?   _____

7. Are references that may be contacted marked (including whether
    or not the current employer should be contacted)?   _____

8. Is a listing of continuing education courses with credits earned
    included?   _____

9. Are research activities, publications, and consultant roles
    identified as appropriate?   _____

10. Is an autobiographical statement of approximately 250 words attached
    (optional)?   _____

11. Does it contain all (but only) necessary information?   _____

Fig. 20-5. Checklist for evaluating a resume.   *Continued.*

Form and structure

1. Are categories readily identifiable? ⟶

2. Is spacing appropriate to highlight main components? ⟶

3. Is it typed (neatly)? ⟶

4. Are words checked for accurate typing and proper

   spelling? ⟶

5. Is the finished product attractive but unpretentious? ⟶

Fig. 20-5, cont'd. Checklist for evaluating a resume.

postcard, it may well be lost in the paper shuffle on the desk top (if it is not purposely discarded) before the resume arrives. It refers to no specific available employment opening. And it does not offer much clue as to the category of employment for which the person is qualified. Besides that, it contains a misspelled word, errors in grammar, and only one means of contacting the person, without an area code.

What is the likelihood that this "cover letter" creates a positive response in the reader?

Contrast this postcard variety of initial contact with the cover letter in Fig. 20-2. It is neatly prepared, concise, includes a reference to the specific job opening and how the person learned of the opening, and a reference to an enclosed curriculum vitae (see Fig. 20-3). The letter's style is assertive but not aggressive, and it provides information for readily establishing follow-up contact.

A review of the resume shows good categorization of information, chronological order within each category, and a reasonable amount of data accompanying each entry.

Fig. 20-4 shows how the same information could be buried or missing in a poorly prepared resume. It is relatively easy to predict the relative impact these two forms would have on potential employers. The latter version contains jumbled categories, incomplete data (including gaps in time), and extraneous information probably of minimal interest to the potential employer.

The safest way to prepare a resume that will be attractive to the reader is to write it using the guidelines (placed in checklist form in Fig. 20-5) and then ask one or more people, who are involved in making decisions regarding employment, to review it and offer suggestions. With one or two drafts, a highly acceptable document can be prepared that may lead to the next step in finding employment: the interview.

Review questions

1. Why is a well-written resume an important part of seeking employment?
2. List five usual components of a resume:
   a.
   b.
   c.
   d.
   e.
3. Which biographical items are, by law, not to be considerations in selecting job applicants?

ANSWERS

1. A resume is often the first contact between an applicant and a potential employer. If well prepared, it can assist the reviewer in identifying how a person's qualifications match with the available position. It can lead to an interview.
2. a. Name, address, telephone
   b. Educational background
   c. Licensure or certification status
   d. Work experience
   e. Research, publication, continuing education
3. Age, sex, race, creed, or national origin

GROUP ACTIVITIES

1. Invite an employment agency officer to discuss the importance of resumes in obtaining positions and to suggest alternative styles.
2. Prepare a professional resume. Evaluate it in terms of the checklist in Fig. 20-5.
3. Write a cover letter to accompany the resume that could be sent to potential employers currently advertising positions in the professional journals or in the classified sections of the newspapers.
4. Critique each other's letters and resumes, offering suggestions for improvement.
5. Cover various actual resumes that have been received by the personnel office so that the writers are anonymous. Critique the style, content, and structure of each. Make suggestions for improvement.

CHAPTER 21

The interview

OBJECTIVES: The reader will be able to:

1. Explain briefly the purpose and significance of the interview in finding employment.
2. Describe the respective roles of the job applicant and the interviewer in the interview process.
3. Prepare for an interview session by using "preinterview" techniques, including:
   a. Conducting a personal inventory of skills, characteristics, and goals.
   b. Analyzing the probable interests, expectations, and attitudes of the interviewer.
   c. Verbally "adapting" the findings of the personal inventory to these probable interests, expectations and attitudes.
   d. Organizing key points for their greatest effectiveness.
   e. Practicing the interview and establishing a positive attitude toward the encounter.
4. List the four basic phases of the interview.
5. Describe briefly the interviewer's evaluation process.
6. Summarize basic methods for carrying out a successful interview, when:
   a. The interviewer appears to be experienced and the preinventory procedures were accurate with regard to the characteristics of the employer.
   b. The interviewer appears to be satisfied with minimal information.
   c. The interviewer "takes over" the interview.
   d. The interviewer plays a very passive role in the interview.
   e. The interviewer appears to be less than anxious to participate in the interview (appears distracted, preoccupied, or even angry).
7. Outline follow-up procedures that can enhance the effectiveness of the interview and perhaps increase the possibility of receiving an offer of a position.

SIGNIFICANCE OF THE INTERVIEW

The interview is probably the most important part of the placement process to the person seeking employment. An appropriate resume and cover letter can do a great deal to create the expectations the employer may have of the applicant, but the greatest impact that will be made on the employer is the applicant's behavior during the interview encounter. The interview is clearly a time of assessment and evaluation. The reviewer begins the assessment process the moment the applicant arrives (or before that time if the applicant is late). And each successive moment of the interview allows the employer to focus on the applicant in an effort to determine if this is the kind of person he/she wishes to have in the practice setting, firm, corporation, or other establishment. There are some unique features about the kinds of employment interviews that health care providers are likely to encounter, but generally speaking, the interview process is quite similar from one situation to another. It is perhaps *the* big "final exam," with rarely an opportunity for a retake. Based on a few minutes or hours of conversation, the employer will decide whether a position ought to be offered.

The interview also is a time for the applicant to learn as much as possible about the potential position so that he/she can make a reasonable decision about whether an offer from the employer ought to be accepted. It is not possible to use a decision-making grid for selecting an employment situation unless there is considerable information available about the characteristics of each position available. Therefore it is important for the applicant to make use of the interview to learn a great deal about the working environment, the scope of responsibility, and other factors determined to be of importance. As each bit of information is gathered, the applicant is assessing and evaluating the attractiveness of this particular employment situation.

ROLES IN THE INTERVIEW

The interview is a time for mutual evaluation. Both the employer and the potential employee are under scrutiny. The degree of scrutiny each feels will depend upon how sought after the parties in the interview are for their skills (in the case of the interviewee) and in the opportunities they offer (in the case of the interviewer). If many applicants are seeking employment in a nearly ideal practice setting, for instance, each applicant may feel more in the role of the observed than in the role of the observer. When there are few employable, qualified people available for a position and the applicant is being interviewed by a number of potential employers, the employer may be wishing to put his/her best foot forward so that the applicant will look favorably upon the situation being offered.

The "ideal" interview situation for both parties would be when the scrutiny element is about equal, that is, when both parties have a reasonable desire to receive a very good evaluation and when both parties are interested in carefully assessing the other. In most interview situations the ideal is unlikely to occur.

In the realm of health care providers the interview situation was quite out of balance when there were only 9.8 active dental hygienists for every 1000 active dentists.[2] This situation occurred in the early 1960s. A den-

tal hygiene program graduate could expect to choose from a flood of opportunities for practice. With four or more offers certain, the graduate could practically conduct the interview. Many dentists complained that they had little opportunity to interview the applicant because of the applicant's overriding interest in what each setting had to offer. The fact that a hygienist had a pulse often was considered sufficient qualification for that person to be offered a position. The situation was out of balance not only because of the few hygienists available but because many dental practitioners could plan on suffering great losses in time, energy, and money if the practice (which was often dependent upon the presence of a dental hygienist) had to function without the hygienist. Patients expected regular recall appointments, and in practices where a hygienist had practiced full time for several years, that meant a full schedule of recalls to be kept each month. For the dentist to perform those services would mean that little other care could be delivered. So recalls suffered and patients were not called for appointments, which meant some would go elsewhere for care or those who did obtain an appointment, would need more care than if they had been seen on schedule.

In order to avoid this problem, dentists were willing to accept the license to practice as proof enough that the hygienist would be an appropriate addition to the practice setting. This desire to hire also caused salaries to rise for dental hygienists. In an effort to keep the attractiveness of the employment situation high, the dentist would offer a slightly higher amount of money, which over a period of 5 years caused daily salaries to rise from an average of $18 to $20 per day to $50 to $60 per day. One dentist in the upper peninsula of Michigan advertised for several years that he would offer the services of his private airplane to bring a hygienist to his town to practice. Another advertised a mink coat, a Cadillac, and 4 weeks vacation each year to a hygienist who would practice in his particularly remote location.

But the balance has shifted from being weighted in favor of the hygienist, to being equal, and now to being in favor of the dentist. The salary levels are no longer rising. A graduating hygienist, in some locations in the United States, is relieved to have even one interview. And accordingly, the hygienist is the one feeling scrutinized. The potential employer can now look beyond the license and the pulse to the specified qualities and qualifications of the applicant.

The evaluation skills the hygienist uses to assess a potential employment site are by necessity a bit more complex today than they were 15 years ago, also. With employment opportunities that go beyond the private solo practice dental office, the hygienist has a greater number of factors to evaluate in terms of how the practice setting meets his/her needs. One hygienist may have only three interviews, but one may be in a hospital setting, another in a penal institution, and only the third in a general dental office. With perhaps ten or more hygienists also interviewing for each of those positions, the hygienist has to be well prepared to succeed in the interview in making him/herself the most logical selection for the position. The hygienist also has to have well-developed skills in ferreting out the needed information about the setting so that if more than one offer is made, he/she is in a position to make an informed decision.

Therefore, the applicant and the interviewer serve a dual, simultaneous role— that of scrutinizer and the one being scrutinized. Fortunately, being an active, tactful inquirer (a characteristic necessary for a person to gain the needed information) is often a trait the other person is hoping to see. As a result, the dual roles are usually quite compatible or even complementary.

It is not the role of the applicant to sit back and "be interviewed" with the full responsibility of the discussion falling upon the shoulders of the interviewer. It should be a mutual exchange of information, inquiry, and discussion, with the applicant having equal input with the interviewer.

PREPARATION FOR THE INTERVIEW

Being the expert applicant for a position requires some preparation. The best way to develop interview skills is to participate in a preinterview process, which includes careful analysis of what factors should surface during the discussion, which are likely to, and how to address each one.[1] How can the applicant's attributes best be presented? And how can those attributes be related to the functions and responsibilities the employer expects the applicant to assume?

The first step in the preinterview preparation is to assess carefully and honestly one's capabilities and qualifications with regard to the position available. The obvious, and perhaps easiest, qualifications to examine are the educational and work experience factors that are related to the position applied for.

A medical technologist with a special concentration of study and experience in blood analysis may find her credentials ideal for the position open at the newly established blood bank. But a nurse requesting employment as an administrator in a research center may need to more carefully analyze his credentials for the sources of expertise that cause him to believe he is qualified for the job. It is a helpful exercise to return to the written resume and jot down how each of the entries has helped prepare the person for the available position. Then the notes should be set aside, and the applicant should describe aloud, convincingly, how each component of education and experience relates to the job applied for. This can be done alone while the applicant is looking in the mirror so that mannerisms and other aspects of the delivery can be seen from the point of view of the other person.

Once the more professional aspects have been analyzed, the applicant should practice some introspection and analyze his/her personal characteristics. To focus on the positive, the applicant can begin by listing and describing aloud personal successes. Listing one or two successes each, of early childhood (ages 1 to 8 years), adolescence, college years, the most current year, and the last week and describing aloud in the mirror why each of those is viewed as a "success" can be quite an experience. However, it is essential that the successes be explained *aloud*. Even though it is highly unlikely that such an autobiographical survey will unfold during the interview, certain elements of the success chain may be quite appropriate to reveal during the interview, and having already verbalized the vignettes may make it much easier to describe the events and the feelings the person has about them.

A step further is to analyze personal failings in terms of how they enhanced growth. Even what appears to be a major setback can have a positive effect, depending upon how the person reacts. These so-called failures should be explained aloud in the mirror, also. This may be the most difficult portion of the process. It is usually difficult to rationalize away personal errors while looking in the mirror. It forces a person to see how easily self-deception can be perceived by "the other." Human nature often causes people readily to claim credit for their achievements and to place blame elsewhere when they perform below expectations. Explaining into the mirror that the reason for the failing grade in chemistry is that the teacher was "out to get me" can stimulate some second thoughts about self-honesty. It is better to view one's own self-deceptions and analyze them before parading them in front of a prospective employer.[1]

An appropriate way to discuss weaknesses or failings is to admit them openly and then to cite how they have caused growth and how their "owner" is coping with their planned modification.[1] No employer expects an employee to be perfect and he/she probably has little interest in hiring a person who has deluded him/herself.

Once the successes/weaknesses identification and analysis are complete, the applicant is prepared to follow a more conventional approach to preparing for the interview by:

1. Describing, in general, what kind of person he/she is.

2. Stating whether his/her grades reflect real potential and explaining why.
3. Explaining what he/she considers to be the most meaningful part of formal education.
4. Listing and explaining his/her most important short range goal related to personal and professional life.
5. Listing and explaining his/her most important long range goals related to personal and professional life.
6. Identifying school, community, and volunteer activities in which he/she has been involved which reveal important personal characteristics, qualities, skills, abilities, or maturity.[1]

This more conventional series of problems should still be answered aloud and in the mirror.

The applicant should then move on to analyze what the interviewer may be interested in knowing.[1] What are the probable interests, expectations, and attitudes of the interviewer? This is not always easy to predict, especially if the interviewer is not a skilled conductor of employment interviews. The dentist an hour behind schedule may feel less than resourceful at the time of an interview and may ask questions related strictly to clinical skills and experience. With a little more time available, that same dentist may choose to initiate a discussion of how auxiliaries ought to be integrated into the practice of dentistry, along with a philosophical discussion of the political and legal considerations involved in such changes.

The verbal skills and tact required of the applicant are quite different in the two situations. In the direct-and-to-the-point interview, the applicant will need to offer considerable, positive input in a short amount of time. Every word spoken will count doubly, since the decision to employ will be based upon a restricted amount of contact. The applicant will have to be certain that the crucial positive elements surface and that the information needed to assess the practice is obtained without having to fire a series of questions while being ushered to the door. In the latter encounter, more information than planned may surface. Also, the applicant will have to decide what game the employer is playing: Is he/she simply taking this opportunity to voice convictions with little expected response from the potential employee? Is he/she attempting to determine whether philosophies are compatible? Or is the employer attempting to measure the applicant's ability to think, articulate responses, and behave in an assertive yet nonaggressive manner in a face-to-face discussion? In addition to deciding the "game," the applicant will need to ensure that the crucial exchange of basic information occurs and that it is not subordinated to the philosophical discussion, regardless of how interesting it is.

It is relatively safe to assume that potential employers expect: (1) evidence of competence (education, experience, and licensure), (2) a pleasant disposition, (3) an energetic approach to the potential position, (4) honesty tempered with diplomacy and a positive attitude, and (5) in instances where the position includes contact with people, an ability to communicate easily both verbally and nonverbally. Experienced interviewers also expect that the applicant will have researched the background of the firm or practice and will be familiar with the goals, objectives, and accomplishments of the organization.[1] A frequently asked question based on this expectation is: "How do you feel you will be able to contribute to the goals and objectives of our organization?" It should be obvious that such a question requires not only forethought but some homework on the part of the applicant prior to the interview.

The self-analysis process described previously should help prepare the applicant to meet the expectations related to items 1, 4, and 5. If the applicant learned to smile, sit up, established good eye contact and acquire a reasonably relaxed manner as a result of the conversations with the mirror, items 2 and 3 may have at least partial preparation.

The employer probably does not particularly desire to offer a position to someone who is "ho-hum" about the idea of functioning in the described role. He/she is more likely to hire the excited, energetic person who sees the position as an opportunity to accomplish great things. Some people need a great deal of practice in being excited. For those who have difficulty revealing their positive feelings, it is probably best to return to the mirror.

Sitting forward with eyes sparkling compared with slouching with lids at halfmast should provide at least one example of how nonverbal behavior can portray interest. In beginning a discussion of the actual available position, it helps to include statements such as: "I've always wanted to work in this kind of practice environment," "I'd love to try out some of the approaches to patient care you hope to introduce," "That would be an ideal way for me to put to use the skills I learned that I enjoy most," or "The position you describe is really exciting. It would be a fantastic opportunity." Coupled with the nonverbal energy signals, these phrases can help the employer determine the applicant's interest in the position.

Employers have varying expectations of employees in terms of responsibility, management participation, and professional growth. Some view their employees as basically subservient, support staff with strictly defined task-oriented roles. Others invite critical input, decision-making, and signs of a need for increased responsibility. It probably is not wise to anticipate the expectations of the employer and slip into a role that is unnatural to the applicant. First of all, the attempt may backfire. Second, the attempt may be seen as an act. And third, if the applicant is hired as a "nice girl who knows her place" and then emerges in a few weeks as a real thinking human being, the applicant may be back at the mirror preparing for more interviews. In this category of concern, it is probably wisest to assess the expectations as they emerge in the interview and then decide how compatible or tolerable they are in terms of the goals and needs of the applicant.

The "research" element of the preinterview procedure includes acquiring some advance information regarding the employer's expectations of employees. This can sometimes be accomplished by means of a conversation with former employees. The gathering of background information may include an identification of the employer's goals and objectives. In an innovative group practice, an educational or research institution, or in a public health agency it may be fascinating to discover what the goals and objectives are, particularly if it is possible to compare them with measured results.

With a reasonably accurate idea of the employer's mission, the potential employee should begin identifying, first in writing and then aloud, how his/her interests and qualifications can match or contribute toward it. Interviewers are generally impressed by a person's desire to "join the effort" and to become a contributor toward attaining the mission.

Regardless of the ill-defined or simplistic nature of the goals, few employers will be excited about hiring a person whose range of interests is limited to hours to be worked, duties to be fulfilled, and money to be earned. The role of the applicant is to provide as much information and conviction as is reasonable and possible to help the interviewer see the merits of hiring the person. This can be done without affectation and yet with a great deal of polish by means of the self-analysis, the analysis of the likely needs of the employer, and the matching of needs and expectations prior to the interview.

PHASES OF THE INTERVIEW

The presentation, however, needs some organization and timing for it to be effective. The matter of organization of the interview can be addressed in terms of its basic phases. There are four basic phases regardless of its length or sophistication. The first is the *introduction*, which includes the critical initial contact, the exchange of the basic amenities, and the establishment of rapport. The second phase is the discussion of the *candidate's background* when the interviewer asks questions and the applicant makes use of a great deal of the preinterview mirror talk. The third phase is the *matching of the candidate with the position* when the discussion of goals commences and the position itself is described. The last phase is the conclusion or *closure* when it will be apparent how successful the interview has been. Plans for follow-up will be discussed, or there will be a definite farewell.[1]

With these phases in mind it is possible to plan the organization of presenting key items of information, asking key questions, and using nonverbal cues to best advantage.

During the introductory phase the applicant should do his/her best to establish positive, open communication. The tone of voice should be friendly yet gentle and respectful. The eye contact should be positive without being a stare and accompanied by a smile and an energetic approach during the walk toward the person and the handshake. There is no need to mazurka into the room or turn the handshake into an arm wrestle, but a hesitant-free walk forward with a genuine, firm handshake can do a great deal to assist the initial encounter. There is nothing quite so disgusting as a "dead fish" handshake nor anything so initially negative as a hesitant approach with a slippery slump to the most distant chair. The approach should not make the interviewer suspect that the applicant's mother forced the person to appear. And the handshake should assure the interviewer that the applicant is alive and possessing some nerve endings in the hands, which are sensitive to other human beings.

A bit of excitement at the initial encounter is usually expected. It is softened by a "safe" discussion of the weather, the trip to the interview, or other recent events generally considered of mutual interest. It cannot be emphasized too greatly that the first 4 minutes are indeed critical.[3] This is the time during which most people decide whether or not they wish to continue the relationship, based on nonverbal as well as verbal expression. It is difficult to undo these first impressions, especially if the less than favorable ones relate to honesty (really security) and encounters with obstacles (desire to succeed).

The person who trips over the rug and knocks over an umbrella stand and squeaks out, "Oh, I'm so glad I'm not nervous," may be met by a sympathetic, knowing smile or with a glance heavenward. The person who missed a train and was taxied ten blocks out of the way by a foreign-speaking cabbie and who can find amusement in the incident rather than rage may score points.[3]

Trust is the key element that needs to be established. It may, almost magically, exist between two people from the first eye contact. Or it may take some time for it to be established. Sometimes it never happens.

Hopefully it will happen before the second phase. It is less than a comfortable position to be describing one's attributes while still attempting to establish trust. It is in this instance that the honesty of the mirrorside self-talks may be very handy. The start of the second phase is often marked by a question. The "small talk" shifts to a more interrogatory mode. And the applicant finds him/herself describing the educational aspects, work experience, and interests that were carefully analyzed during the preinterview process. Questions such as, "Why did you leave that position?" "What did you like best about your clinical experience?" and "Why did you decide to enter this field?" are likely. The responses should build on the trust established and avoid "cute" remarks or a degeneration into apathy. Information should be offered. And each question should be used as a springboard to provide the precious kernels of knowledge that were all explained in careful terms to the mirror.

When the attention shifts to career goals (short and long range), the third phase has begun.[1] The employer is beginning the matching process of candidate and position. Well thought out personal objectives and careful research of the employer's needs become invaluable. The interviewer will probably describe the available position. Or the applicant may ask about it—in a cautious,

yet assertive, gesture of interest. If the match-up is apparent, the applicant should inject a measure of energy and excitement into the conversation, indicating interest, challenge, and commitment. This may be the key moment in securing the position if the overall interview has been positive.[1]

If the interviewer begins to "sell" the position by elaborating on its merits or by agreeing that it matches well with the applicant's credentials, it is usually an indication that the interviewer recognized the match, also.

The fourth phase begins with a discussion of follow-up procedures.[1] The employer may offer a simple, "We'll call you," or may suggest a second meeting and a discussion more related to specific benefits and discussion of roles. In any case, it is essential that both persons agree to whatever the follow-up plans are. As the interview draws to a close, the applicant should reiterate or summarize those plans and seek the interviewer's nod of agreement. This can be accomplished during the final handshake, by pausing at the end of the summary and giving one last shake when the nod is given.[1] If ushered to the door, eye contact at the parting should not be broken until the nod is obtained. It should be relatively easy to obtain the nod as long as what is being summarized is an accurate feedback of what the interviewer said. This is no time to put words in the mouth of the interviewer. If the interview points out that personal characteristics and the position do not match, it is better to part with an honest good-bye and to maintain trust than to attempt a futile follow-up procedure.

SUCCESS WITH THE INTERVIEWER

The evaluator/interviewer is basically assessing the applicant from the first to the last contact, eliminating negative elements rather than building positive ones.[1] If the applicant is on time, the interviewer crosses off the negative element of discourtesy or tardiness. If the person smiles and is generally pleasant to talk to, the interviewer eliminates grouchiness and dullness. If the applicant is interested, eager, and qualified, the traits of apathy and incompetence are erased. The key to success is to not fit the negative aspects that are anticipated and to have enough uniqueness and attractiveness that the interviewer remembers the person and the interview. A job offer may follow.

If the interviewer is a professional and the preinventory procedures appear to be working well, the secret is to relax and make the most of the success. Attentiveness to what is said and what is asked is important. If an item of information in the resume is misstated by the interviewer, tactfully provide the accurate information. To ignore the error may be a mistake if the interviewer made the "error" as a means of evaluating listening and diplomacy skills.[1] If a question is asked that is unclear to the applicant, he/she should ask to have it repeated by saying something similar to, "I'm not certain I understand your meaning. Could you rephrase it for me, please?" It is unwise to say, "You didn't say that very well. What are you asking?" If the meaning is still unclear, a simple feedback strategy may correct the situation. The applicant should say, "What I understand you are asking is . . ." If the applicant's interpretation is correct, the interviewer will agree and the answer can be supplied. If the interpretation is inaccurate, the interviewer can ascertain where the misunderstanding lies and can then correct it.[1]

Timing for the inclusion of key elements of information is important. It is best to plan to include key elements according to the typical topics of the four phases. As each phase unfolds, the applicant can feed into the discussion the preplanned selling points and questions.

This is particularly important in instances when the interviewer doesn't request or offer much information. And in cases where the applicant feels rushed as the fidgeting interviewer continues to glance at his/her watch, the tendency may be to blurt out a series of statements and questions at such speed that the impact of each is more negative than positive. In an obviously disastrously brief interview situation, it might be best for the applicant to suggest a second appointment. The interview requires the development of trust, and this is not possible when the introduction is limited to a "hello" and the subsequent components fly by like Keystone Cops.

It also may be a feat to provide and gather the needed information in instances where the interviewer seems to "take over" the session, conducting each phase in a directive manner. The interviewer asks the questions, moves the session from phase to phase, and may allow little opportunity for the applicant to initiate topics or ask questions.[1]

The polar opposite is the nondirective interviewer who sits back and responds to how the applicant develops the flow of the interview. This is a technique that often is used to assess a person's ability to function in a structure-free situation.[1] Some interviewers will begin in a directive manner and then adopt a nondirective style.[1] The preinterview planning related to each of the four phases will help the applicant facilitate the development and the progress of the session. It will be possible to provide the needed personal background data, inquire about the position, match characteristics, and achieve closure with relative ease if it has been preplanned.

There may be times when the applicant finds a weary, distracted, or even angry interviewer. It is rarely the case that an interviewer approaches the visit with the same air of excitement and interest that the applicant has.[1] So the applicant should prepare for at best a moderately interested person and at worst one who wishes to be somewhere else. When confronted by a harried interviewer, the most appropriate behavior is to be as positive as possible, with a continuous warm smile. The objective becomes to be the highlight of the person's day. It may not be very difficult to compete with his/her earlier experiences if the mood is obviously a dour one, and to fall into a grumpy state rather than to remain positive may result in the interviewer subconsciously heaping the blame for the day's catastrophes on the applicant. In any case, few job offers are given to grumpy people on an already bleak day.

FOLLOW-UP OF THE INTERVIEW

Regardless of the outcome, it is appropriate to send a letter of appreciation to the interviewer thanking him/her for the time and the opportunity to share.[1] The letter should contain whatever additional information the interviewer has requested. Even if the closing of the interview was not filled with hope, such a gesture may result in a second interview particularly if other applicants did not perform much better.

The note of appreciation also provides an opportunity to add omitted or new information. The letter should, once again, be impeccably neat with a concise, coherent message. It should provide the interviewer with a pleasant reminder of the encounter.

The interview experience can be a rewarding one that leads to offers of employment if it is prepared for and conducted with a measure of self-assurance and honesty. To do otherwise may result in extended efforts at obtaining employment and plenty of opportunity for practice.

Review questions

1. What is the purpose and significance of an employment interview?
2. List four ways in which the applicant can prepare for the interview:
    a.
    b.
    c.
    d.
3. What are the four basic phases of the interview?
    a.
    b.
    c.
    d.

True or false:

4. The interviewer often assesses the applicant by eliminating negative elements rather than by building positive ones. _____
5. If an interviewer misstates some item of information about the applicant, it is best to ignore it. _____
6. An interviewer who seems satisfied with little information should be allowed to leave the encounter with whatever he or she chose to learn. _____
7. An interviewer who uses a nondirective approach is probably inexperienced in evaluating people. _____
8. The angry interviewer is a lost cause. The applicant should just get through the encounter and hope for the best. _____
9. A follow-up letter should contain no more than a thank you. _____

ANSWERS

1. The interview provides a potential employer and an applicant an opportunity to meet and evaluate each other in order to determine whether the characteristics of the available person match the requirements of the available position.
2. a. By self-assessing job qualifications such as education and work experience.
   b. By self-assessing personal strength and weaknesses and describing how weaknesses can be overcome.
   c. By anticipating the interests, expectations, and attitudes of the interviewer and adapting the identified qualifications to those interests, expectations, and attitudes.
   d. By organizing key points and practicing (especially with a mirror).
3. a. Introduction
   b. Candidate's background
   c. Matching of the candidate with the position
   d. Closure
4. True
5. False. It should be tactfully corrected.
6. False. It is important that the applicant offer any key items of information for the interviewer even though the interviewer has not asked.
7. False. The interviewer may be assessing the applicant's response to an unstructured encounter.
8. False. It should be the applicant's role to become the highlight of the interviewer's day.
9. False. It may contain additional information and even another expression of interest in the position.

GROUP ACTIVITIES

1. Role play several interviews between employer and applicant including:
   a. The directive interviewer
   b. The nondirective interviewer
   c. The angry interviewer
   d. The rushed interviewer
2. Prepare a series of trigger tapes showing selected discussion prompting responses to each of the kinds of interview situations practiced in the role play.
3. Discuss the probable effects the various applicant responses may have on obtaining the desired position.

REFERENCES

1. Amsden, Forrest M. and White, Noel P.: How to be successful in the employment interview: A step-by-step approach for the candidate, Cheney, WA, 1974, Interviewing Dynamics.
2. Dentistry and Allied Services, 1975-76, Manpower Analysis Branch, U.S. Dept. of Health, Education and Welfare, PHS-HRA, Bureau of Health Manpower, Division of Dentistry.
3. Zunin, Leonard and Zunin, Natalie: Contact: The first four minutes, New York, 1972, Ballantine Books, Inc.

CHAPTER 22

Establishing priorities in selecting a practice setting

OBJECTIVES: The reader will be able to:

1. Identify at least ten factors that health care providers often express as important considerations in selecting a practice setting.
2. Select categories of concern that are important to him or her in selecting a practice setting.
3. Identify any additional categories of concern that should be considered in assessing how a practice setting meets his/her priorities.
4. Establish a decision-making grid in determining what practice setting is most appropriate.
5. Explain how a formal decision-making process applied to selecting an employment setting can clarify the strengths and weaknesses of each possible decision.
6. Describe goal orientation as a tool for planning change.

Very often a new graduate of a health care program has unclear or idealistic expectations of what the practice of his/her profession will be. The educational environment focuses on the ideal, in many instances, and may not necessarily provide the person with an externship program that familiarizes the student with the economic and logistical realities of practice. The delivery of health care is rarely idealistic. Each practice setting may measure up to some of the student's expectations and fall short in others. Each practice setting will be different in what it offers and in what it expects of the practitioner who is employed.

FACTORS IN SELECTING
A PRACTICE SETTING

In a profession where the scope of practice is changing and where role delineation in practice is either not keeping pace with or is ahead of the educational preparation of the graduate, there are multiple factors that need consideration in seeking and accepting employment. These factors are both person-

al and professional. They are economic, emotional, logistical, and peculiar to each individual making the decisions and choices.

What kinds of factors do new graduates often consider in seeking employment? Basically, they fall into two main categories: personal need and desire to serve. Often, for persons who have spent a large amount of time and money in obtaining their education, the personal need factor is the primary consideration. The new graduate is anxious to earn some money for a change and to have a reasonably comfortable and secure position in employment. For others, the primary motivator is the desire to provide the care where it is needed. These persons are willing to make sacrifices in the areas of personal need in order to fulfill a more altruistic desire to serve those segments of the population that do not usually have access to health care. Ideally, a recent graduate would be able to fulfill both categories of expectations for practice, earning a reasonably comfortable living in a reasonably comfortable, secure position while serving segments of the population who have a definite need for care. Since this panacea of practice is unlikely to exist for many providers, it can be helpful to examine each category of expectation and to establish those personal priorities that will affect a graduate's decision to accept employment and the likelihood that the provider will be happy in that employment situation.

Salary and fringe benefits

Under the personal need category, there are many considerations that practitioners cite as important. The amount of the *salary* is a prime consideration. Is the salary offered commensurate with the amount the provider hoped to earn? Is it reasonable for the locale, for the degree of education required of the provider, and in relation to the economic income that will be generated for the practice setting? Closely related to salary is the amount of *fringe benefits* available to the provider. Many times a low level salary will be counter-balanced by a sizeable fringe benefit package, including vacation time, sick pay, insurance programs, inservice training and opportunities for continued formal education, free personal and family health care, parking, professional dues payment, and other various benefits. In order to assess the relative merits of the benefits package, the prospective employee should total up the dollar worth of the benefits and add it to the salary before comparing it to a position that has a high salary but limited benefits. Insurance and any of the other items listed can be costly if paid out of the salary. Many benefits are not subject to income taxation, which makes them even more economically attractive. Therefore, it is important to consider more than just the weekly take-home pay before making a decision regarding the economic benefits of employment.

Location

One consideration closely related to economic benefits but that also has other factors related to it is the *location* of the employment setting. The farther away the practice setting, the more time and money it will cost

to travel to and from work each day. If public transportation is available, how much will it cost each day? If the travel requires a car, how much will it cost in terms of gasoline and other mileage expenses? And how much is parking, if it is even available? Is there some likelihood that the car will be damaged while parked? If so, will insurance rates for the car rise?

Location can have other importance for prospective employees, too. If the position available is in a rural area, in the heart of a big city, or nestled in the suburbs, the location may have a different priority ranking for the people considering the position. The country lovers may be miserable in the city, whereas the city lovers may be stir-crazy in the mountains. Those providers who prefer the flavor of the suburbs may place little positive value on the other two locations. Isolation, crowding, atmosphere, availability of entertainment and services, and opportunity for rest and relaxation are all important considerations associated with the location of a practice setting. How far will the provider have to move in order to accept the position? Will the cost of living and availability of housing pose special problems? Whenever the opportunity requires a substantial change in location for the provider, these elements are important.

Security

Security is a reasonably important factor for health care providers, too. What is the likelihood that the person will be able to retain the position? Is it a grant-funded (soft-money) position that may disappear from the face of the earth if the grant is not renewed or when the contract is complete? Does the employer have a high turnover rate among employees? Is there a union to protect employee's rights in an instance of unfair severance of employment?

Perhaps the most important consideration is whether security is a very important consideration to the potential employee. Usually, security becomes an increasingly important factor as the provider assumes new responsibilities, such as raising a family, or as the provider ages. The loss of income and the inability to find another place to work can be frightening prospects when there is a family of three to clothe, feed, and shelter or when a provider is nearing retirement. It is true that some people seem minimally troubled by this employment factor when they accept employment, but they may wish to consider that the relative importance of security may change during employment. With time, security may be an increasingly significant factor for the provider, but the benefit of security may not necessarily increase in the employment setting with longevity.

Opportunity for advancement

Opportunity for advancement and upward mobility are important factors for many health care providers, particularly if they view their profession as a lifetime career. Providers may wish to see possible opportunity to assume supervisory roles or to acquire education or skills that will enable them to move up the structure of the practice setting or prepare them for more responsible roles in other employment settings. Persons who are "upward oriented" may place a great deal of importance on how the offered employment will enhance their experience and improve their chances to succeed. It has been the plague of some health care professions that advancement opportunities were extremely limited, because of either the law or the structure of the practice setting or the employer's view of the "appropriate" role of the employee.

In many ways, women struggle with this problem more than men because of the stereotyped approach to the ability or desire of women to stay in practice for longer periods of time and to function well as managers of people. Women have for decades generally viewed professional life as a stopover between high school and marriage and as a source of security if the husband should turn out to be a poor financial provider. Women averaged few years of economic productivity and were willing to wear the label of short-term, low-commitment workers in a male-dominated professional world. These two factors are changing as women less and less fit the mold and do look forward to lifetime careers and opportunity for advancement.

Role and responsibility

The *role* or position offered to the health care provider at the time of initial employment is even more often a primary consideration than opportunity for advancement. Will the provider have responsibility in decision making? Will there be an opportunity to exercise the judgment skills developed in school? Is there an opportunity to be creative and innovative? How well is the role defined, and what is the relationship between that role and the roles assigned to co-workers? Providing specific, predictable, often repeated services each day is ideal for some employees who view the predictability as "security." For others, it is intellectual death. It may be wise to assess just how mentally stimulating and challenging a position may be for the individual provider in comparison to the stimulation and challenge the person was confronted with each day while in the educational program. There is some chance that the daily routine of practice, if barren of responsibility and creativity, may be quite a letdown from the daily activities of succeeding in school.

Variety of services

Related to role is the amount of learning the provider will be able to draw upon in practice. Will a relatively low percentage of skills be drawn upon, or will the provider be able to provide a full range and *variety of services?*

Therefore it might be wise to carefully assess what abilities the practice setting will draw upon in employing the health care provider. This can tie in with potential for advancement and upward mobility in that it can be worthwhile to accept a position initially that is not completely drawing upon the ability of the person but that can lead to a position that is more demanding and based upon success in the performance of the practical, albeit banal, experiences of the lower level position.

Interpersonal relations

While assessing the challenge of the position, it is also wise to assess the people with whom the health care provider will be working. Observing the cheerfulness and thoughtfulness of the personnel in the practice can provide some indication of how pleasant the *interpersonal relations* may be among the workers and how generally satisfied they are with their respective roles and responsibilities. In the majority of private practice settings, the number of employees is relatively small and relations among the workers must be good if there is to be some harmony. Generally there isn't room for avoidance of conflict and there is a great deal of opportunity for confrontation. Paying close attention to the communication frequency and the tone of the communication can provide a fairly accurate assessment of the "group" development among the team. It certainly can point out whether there is a team or merely a number of individuals who happen to be employed in the same setting and who perhaps are not even very happy about it.

Working environment

In addition to the personnel in the office, there is the *physical working environment* itself. Is the equipment to be utilized in providing care adequate and operative? Is there adequate emergency equipment to handle medical/dental emergencies that may occur? Is the setting clean and relatively neat? Are proper sterilization procedures observed, and is the space adequate to provide care?

It is amazing how the physical limitations of an area can have such an effect on the attitudes of the personnel and sometimes on the quality of care delivered. For some people, physical setting can be a primary consideration in selecting a practice setting, whereas for others it may be a factor that can be outweighed by other positive elements.

Needs of people

One instance in which physical setting is often offset by another plus factor is the health care delivery setting located in a less than plush area, where care is being provided for people who usually would have little or no access to health care. Many government-assisted programs or programs carried out largely by charity donations and volunteer efforts are not located in high priced quarters with the very latest in equipment. However, for those persons who choose to provide care where it is really needed, the luxury of the setting is not the most important factor and it may be sacrificed in return for the genuineness of the caring of the personnel and for the satisfaction derived from *providing care where it is needed most*.

What other factors can be defined that will be looked for or expected in a practice setting? Others may be added to the preceding list of ten primary factors, preparing an individual to begin analyzing which are the most important, which are less than crucial, and which matter little if at all.

DECISION-MAKING

Once the factors are identified, they can be weighted on a scale of one to ten. Those factors that are absolutely essential or very desirable are weighted with a high number, whereas "nice to have" factors are weighted with a lower number. Once each factor has been reviewed for its relative importance, the potential employee is ready to compare the available opportunities in relation to those factors and make a decision regarding what practice setting is the most likely to satisfy the person. The perfect position probably exists nowhere, or at least it is unlikely that it will be found immediately upon graduation from a health care program. Unless it is possible to be among the ranks of the unemployed for some time, the health care provider may find him/herself in a position of accepting employment that does not satisfy all needs but that satisfies at least a reasonable percentage of the stated needs.

Refer to Table 6 for a quantitative analy-

Table 6. Decision-making grid for selecting a practice opportunity

	Personal weighting		Opportunity 1	Opportunity 2	Opportunity 3
Salary	5	×	3 = 15	1 = 5	3 = 15
Fringe benefits	5	×	3 = 15	2 = 10	3 = 15
Location	6	×	2 = 12	1 = 6	2 = 12
Security	2	×	3 = 6	1 = 2	3 = 6
Opportunity for advancement	8	×	0 = 0	3 = 24	0 = 0
Role/responsibility	9	×	1 = 9	3 = 27	1 = 9
Personnel relationships	9	×	3 = 27	3 = 27	1 = 9
Working environment	5	×	3 = 15	1 = 5	3 = 15
Need of people	10	×	1 = 10	3 = 30	2 = 20
Variety of services that can be provided	10	×	1 = 10	3 = 30	2 = 20
	Preference points:		119	166	121

sis of a number of practice settings available to a health care provider. The potential employee has been interviewed by three potential employers and is awaiting their offers. Before the offers are made, the applicant decides to assess his/her own "druthers" weighting each preference on a numerical scale of one to ten. Salary, fringe benefits, and working environment are weighted equally at five. A relatively low value is placed on security, whereas opportunity for advancement, scope of responsibility and role, personnel relationships, need of the people, and variety of services that can be provided are rated high. Location is only slightly more important than the salary/fringe benefit category.

With each factor weighted, the three practice settings are weighted from one to three according to the degree to which each lives up to the hopes of the applicant as assessed during the interview. Opportunities 1 and 3 are in private practitioners' offices. One of them is a solo practice; the other is a group practice. The opportunity labeled 2 is a government funded health clinic operating on a grant due to be renewed in 1 year. It should be apparent from the weightings that the two private practitioners' offices provide the best salary, fringe benefits, and security as well as scoring well in the areas of personnel re-

lationships (in one of the two offices) and working environment. They do not offer much in the category of opportunity for advancement nor in variety of services that can be provided by the interviewing provider. The role and responsibility that could be assumed by the provider also appear to be less than ideal in the private practices.

The government clinic offers the lowest salary, some fringe benefits, location in a less than ideal area, minimal security, and a relatively poor physical working environment. Its plus factors include the opportunity for advancement, the role and responsibility the health care provider will be able to assume, personnel relationships, the need of the people, and the variety of services that the health care provider may actually perform. Because of the weighting of factors, the government clinic earns more points than the two private practice settings. If opportunity 2 is offered, and if the health care provider was honest with himself or herself in weighting the factors, the answer should be "yes." The quantitative assessment of the wants and needs of the provider match best with what the government clinic has to offer, and the health care provider will therefore probably be happiest in that position.

If opportunity 2 is not offered, but either opportunity 1 or 3 *is* offered to the person,

Table 7. Decision-making grid for selecting a practice opportunity

	Personal weighting		Opportunity 1	Opportunity 2	Opportunity 3
Salary	8	×	3 = 24	1 = 8	3 = 24
Fringe benefits	8	×	3 = 24	2 = 16	3 = 24
Location	10	×	2 = 20	1 = 10	2 = 20
Security	8	×	3 = 24	1 = 8	3 = 24
Opportunity for advancement	4	×	0 = 0	3 = 12	0 = 0
Role/responsibility	5	×	1 = 5	3 = 15	1 = 5
Personnel relationships	8	×	3 = 24	3 = 24	3 = 24
Working environment	8	×	3 = 24	1 = 8	3 = 24
Need of the people	3	×	1 = 3	3 = 9	2 = 6
Variety of services that can be provided	4	×	1 = 4	3 = 12	2 = 8
	Preference points:		152	122	159

the health care provider had best decide whether to look further for an opening more compatible with his/her personal wants or needs or to accept the job with the idea that he/she may be able to adapt to the position despite its drawbacks or find a better opportunity later. This choice is often a difficult one to make since the need for income may be the prompting factor to take the position and since a person's performance level may not be at its best in an employment situation incompatible with the person's goals. A lowered performance level seldom leads to advancements and hardly ever leads to good recommendations.

It is important to realize that given the same numerical assessment of the same three job opportunities on a scale of one to three, a different person may arrive at quite a different conclusion regarding which setting is the most appropriate one to accept. For instance, a classmate of the first applicant for a position may also interview at opportunities 1, 2, and 3 and could even arrive at the same judgments regarding their relative offerings in the same ten categories. Given a different personal weighting of the ten factors, in terms of their importance to the applicant, the numerical values ultimately tallied for each opportunity will be quite different.

See Table 7. The only significant difference between this ranking of opportunities and that described in Table 6, is the personal weighting. Notice that salary, fringe benefits, location, security, and working environment assume a much greater importance for this person than they did for the first person described. Opportunity for advancement, degree of role or responsibility, need of the people, and variety of services that can be provided are ranked lower on the scale of one to ten. As a result, opportunity 3 appears to be the best opportunity for the potential employee. Opportunity 1 is almost equal, but opportunity 2 is less appropriate for this person. An offer from either opportunity 1 or 3 should be readily accepted, but an offer from 2 should be assessed in terms of how satisfied the health care provider will be. It is possible that advancement and challenge could make up for the shortcomings the facility and location have, but there is a large possibility that the person will continually be watching for a practice setting that better meets her wants and needs.

Not all people are alike in their respective wants and needs in employment, which is why it is important for each individual to carefully assess just what is important to him/her. Once this has been decided, it is relatively easy to assess how closely a potential employment site meets those wants and needs.

Honesty is, however, a crucial element in this decision-making process. Many persons would like to believe that they are altruistic and that a pleasant office with a fat salary is unimportant. If they rank their personal weightings based on how they wish they were rather than on how they really are, they will end up accepting a job that they really are uncomfortable with, or they will abandon the decision-making system and simply accept the position they "really want" without realizing why. If a person's internal reaction is contrary to what turns up numerically on the decision-making chart, then the tallies ought to be recalculated with an eye to greater self-honesty.

PLANNING CHANGE

Another important factor to remember is that a person's wants and needs do change with time. A person may have a more mature approach to the need for money after the first few years have seen the emphasis on material possessions lessen. It may be wise to reassess the individual's wants and needs periodically, particularly if the employment situation seems to be less than satisfying. One sign that a person is not pleased with the current role or position in a practice setting is if he/she has little if any inclination to start work each day. Lying in bed wishing it were Saturday may be a sign of fatigue, but it may also be a sign that the challenge or the attractiveness of the person's employment situation needs a careful review. Sometimes a person can inject his/her own excitement into the job by developing some new approach to the daily routine or by generating some clinical study that intrigues the provider while working in the same practice setting. The addition of a new employee who seems to be compatible with the health care provider can also spark new interest in a position.

However, the genuine reluctance to go to work each day is often the first sign that one ought to begin looking for a change in employment. The bored or frustrated employee is seldom viewed with a positive eye by the employer or by the patient, despite the provider's abilities to perform. It is better to seek new employment on one's own than to be asked by the employer. This kind of self-imposed termination is difficult for most people, particularly if security is of high value. Employers often then do it *for* the person.

People often read termination (which is a nice way of saying "fired") as a failure, which is not always an appropriate interpretation. Being terminated from a position can often be the best thing that can happen to a person who has become fixed in a rut and finds little excitement in the current employment situation. Termination can actually rejuvenate a person into a new approach to life and success and can prompt a person to seek and find a position that is far more rewarding.

Some personnel advisors say that a person should change positions or working environment every 5 years in order to retain a dynamic, healthy approach to living. Others are content with changing some facet of their lives every 5 years, but not necessarily jobs. It is probably true that a person who is happy with his/her success and who is invigorated by the challenge of what he/she is doing will have opportunity for advancement far more often than every 5 years, so the person's need to single-handedly initiate a change in role or function may not be necessary. Perhaps the most critical point in all of this is that change is not necessarily bad—even when it is forced change. Change is often a very good thing. Planned change can be even better.

Planning for change is often termed "goal orientation." What is the person's goal for change? Are today's activities contributing toward the achievement of that goal?

For instance, it is quite possible that while a certain health care provider is very excited about clinical practice and the current practice setting in which she is employed, she may have tucked away in her brain the idea that she would like to be a consultant for the efficient operation of health care facilities. While being employed in the facility, she may be observing how the practice is efficiently or inefficiently operating and she may have registered for one or two advanced education courses related to management and economics. The practice experience will help establish credibility for the person for having been "in the salt mines" for a period of time, actually participating in the day-to-day delivery of care. The course work may provide a broader base of knowledge and lead toward a credential that will further establish credibility.

Attending appropriate professional meetings and establishing professional relationships with persons who are currently active as efficiency experts may establish some inroads to the profession and actually start the woman on her new career. The truly goal-oriented person assesses a large part of the activities on the current day in terms of how they build toward the future. Every request to assume a responsibility that can lead toward the goal is responded to with a positive answer. New challenges are exciting because they provide a broader range of understanding and because they can lead to even more exciting endeavors. With each new challenge the risk of failure is inherent, but the risk becomes less and less apparent with each new success. Perhaps the key is to assume those challenges for which the person is prepared, with a small edge of the unknown or the untested left to peak the brain power and logic of the person so that one continually adds to abilities with each new challenge rather than simply calling upon old abilities again and again.

The goal-oriented person is growing—intellectually and emotionally as each new experience adds to the person's ability and self-concept.

The antithesis of goal orientation is security orientation. The desire to remain in one secure position with minimal change and minimal challenge (minimal risk) results in a basically stagnant approach to life that can

be devastating if the source of the security is taken away. A person who remains in one job position for 20 years performing the same tasks and learning very few new things can be overwhelmed if that job is taken away by the death of the employer or by a physical disability that makes continued performance impossible. Women who remained housewives for years and then were confronted with either the death of the husband or divorce have had to undergo tremendous change for which they often were not prepared because of the "security" of their unchanging worlds.

Generally the best preparation for such change is to build constant change into one's life so that the psyche is accustomed to the risk element and so that the prospect of risk is not so great as to impair the person's ability to respond to change and grow with it. Coping with change is a mental process that relies upon a person's ability to see the growth that can come from it, how the change will improve the person's world, and how there is some element in change that is positive regardless of the short-term tragedy that may accompany it. Loss of a loved one is a change that deserves grief and a time of adjustment, but it also can be a spark that causes a person to find new sources of strength and ability to succeed.

The goal orientation concept may be the best protection against the current tumultuous changes in technology, life style, the family, acceptable behavior patterns, and the resultant demands upon a person's ability to cope with each change. However, it needs to be tempered by a certain serendipity—or ability to see the natural flow of events and to accept the external forces that cause changes to occur, which may not be a part of the person's master plan for the future. Human beings have some control over the future, but not total control. So in order to avoid inevitable frustration and disappointment, the serendipity element is a crucial aspect of coping with change.

Life planning has been minimally emphasized in educational programs; the stuffing of knowledge into students has been more in vogue. However, the ability to call upon and use all that knowledge relies upon some skill in applying it to one's life. A person's com-mitment and quality of performance rely in large part upon a person's world view toward growth. This aspect of learning may well be the most important.

Review questions

1. List ten factors that are often important considerations for health care providers seeking employment:
   a.
   b.
   c.
   d.
   e.
   f.
   g.
   h.
   i.
   j.
2. List the factors that are important to *you* and weight each on a scale of one to ten.
3. Design a form that will permit classifying each of several job opportunities according how well each meets the weighted preference factors.
4. What could be the possible difficulty if the total preference points in a decision-making grid point to an opportunity as the best selection contrary to the person's internal reaction?

ANSWERS

1. a. Salary
   b. Fringe benefits
   c. Location
   d. Security
   e. Opportunity for advancement
   f. Role/responsibility
   g. Variety of services that can be provided
   h. Personnel relationships
   i. Working environment
   j. Need of the people
2. The answer is yours to design.
3. A form similar to that shown in Tables 6 and 7 will probably meet your needs.
4. Either the calculator needs new batteries or the health care provider ought to be more honest with him/herself regarding the weighting of factors.

GROUP ACTIVITIES

1. Discuss how individuals in the class weighted the ten critical factors in evaluating a practice setting. Explain why the factors were weighted as they were.
2. Describe what the "ideal" practice setting would be for each person, according to the factors.
3. Share long range goals for employment, outlining how each person hopes to achieve his/her personal goals.
4. Debate the statements: "Change is always good," "To build toward a better employment position is a self-centered approach to daily work," and "Women have a relatively short-term commitment to employment."

CHAPTER 23

Employment contracts; the role
of collective bargaining in health care
delivery

OBJECTIVES: The reader will be able to:

1. Define an employment contract.
2. Construct a sample employment contract that could be utilized in an employment agreement in a health care delivery setting.
3. Explain the reason for preparing an employment contract.
4. Identify the likely responses such a request may generate in the employer.
5. Define collective bargaining.
6. Cite examples of professional associations that include collective bargaining as one of their functions.
7. Explain how collective bargaining for dental health care providers is different from that which is used for health care providers in group settings, such as hospitals.
8. Predict the effect collective bargaining could have upon dental auxiliaries in health care delivery.

The arrangement that an employer and an employee agree to with regard to the terms of the employment is a contractual agreement. It obligates both parties in the contract to some specific duties, and it is voluntary in nature. In many employment situations, there is a written statement of those terms, which both persons (employee and employer) sign and agree to uphold. However in the vast majority of employment arrangements, particularly where no union is involved, the agreement is oral. In some situations it is even implied.

The typical employment arrangement between the dental auxiliary employed in a practice and the employing dentist has been the verbal, express contract. The dentist offers a certain amount of salary or commission and specifies the numbers of days and hours to be worked. He/she may request that certain attire be worn and indicate

whether there is any allowance for vacation or travel to professional meetings.

The applicant for the position either agrees to the terms or requests some other arrangement. He/she may request additional benefits or indicate that certain ones offered are not of use.

Once the two parties have reached an agreement, the contract is complete. One would then assume that the needs of both persons are well defined and all that is left is a pleasant working relationship with predictable paychecks and predictable services in return for the remuneration.

Frequently, however, the employment agreement has been so lacking in specificity that the expectations of the two parties are not matched by the performance of their counterparts. The employee may expect that sometime during the first 6 months a raise will be provided. When no raise occurs,

248

the expectation is unmet and the employee feels frustration. On the other hand, the employer may expect that the employee will be willing to assist with other duties in the facility, such as radiographic processing, records maintenance, and the sterilization of instruments and supplies whenever a patient is not available for treatment because of a cancellation or the completion of a treatment in less time than was provided for in the schedule. When, instead, the employee moves to the laboratory for a cup of coffee and chooses to read a journal for that 15-minute period, the employer may be feeling a high level of frustration.

THE EMPLOYMENT CONTRACT

A large source for misunderstanding and malcontent in a practice environment is the unexpressed, unmet expectations of the persons involved. One way to prevent that frustration is to have a written, preplanned employment contract that directs the two parties' attention to many of the typical concerns that can cause difficulty but that rarely surface in the employment interview. To use such a form may at first seem less than trusting—particularly if the presentation of the employment contract is done in a fairly chilling manner. Many employers confronted with such a document for the first time in their professional careers of hiring auxiliaries may be quite taken aback. An employer less than pleased with the new assertiveness shown by auxiliaries in recent years may decide to change his/her mind about the employment agreement. However, if it is used with some finesse and its advantages are pointed out to both participants in the agreement, it can be a valuable mechanism.

An employment contract generally has several categories to be addressed in discussing the terms of the working agreement. The categories are:

1. Title of the position and a listing of basic functions to be performed.
2. Hours to be worked and, if appropriate, days of the week to be worked.
3. Amount of remuneration to be paid for

the completion of the employment activities, as well as:
a. Pay period schedule
b. Benefits to be deducted from the paycheck according to government schedules
c. Manner in which remuneration is to be calculated (including the precise formula if commission, or salary plus commission, is to be used as the means of calculating the payment)
d. Identification of who calculates the paycheck amount and whether calculations are available for evaluation by the employee
4. Schedule of review for raises (particularly if the raises are to be based on merit) and continued employment (probationary period).
5. Method of evaluation upon which the raise reviews will be based. (What outcomes are expected? What criteria will be used? Who will evaluate? What will be the form of the evaluation?)
6. Fringe benefits available:
a. Paid days for illness or bereavement
b. Paid days for participation in professional activities, including continuing education
c. Funding of travel or tuition for continuing education
d. Participation in insurance programs (What type? What benefits are included?)
e. Participation in profit sharing (How often? How are shares calculated? Does seniority affect amount accrued?)
f. Participation in retirement program (Are funds transferable to another program if the employment agreement is severed?)
g. Availability of cost-free health care (In the facility? Or at the physician/dentist of the employee's choice?)
h. Paid holidays (Which ones?)
i. Paid vacation (How many days?)
j. Uniform or lab coat allowance
k. Parking allotment

1. Days paid when the employer is not present in the facility (if the law stipulates the health care provider may not work without the direct supervision of the employer)
7. Opportunities for professional advancement (if any) that exist within the setting for which the employee may at some time qualify.
8. Method by which the employment contract may be severed (appropriate notice, reason for severance, etc.)
9. Specific expectations with regard to the employment situation as perceived by the parties of the contract, which are not covered above.

If all nine components of the employment contract or agreement are discussed in the course of the employment interview and both persons agree to these specified terms, it is a relatively easy matter to complete the contract form and share it with the employer as a confirmation of the discussion. The form doesn't have to be whipped out for use during the interview, although it is helpful to have notes regarding the key items to be discussed in hand so that each area is covered and some agreement reached. It is far more tactful to make brief notes and then prepare the contract after the interview is complete. Each category can be completed with the data agreed to and typed for review. If there are categories not yet agreed to, this can serve as a springboard for further discussion of those points and hopefully their resolution. Reading the document together can be quite a symbolic act in establishing the employer-employee relationship on an even, professional ground.

It will serve to remind the employer of the agreed upon elements, and it will provide the employer with the knowledge that the employee is aware of the expectations that were discussed and that they are indeed in writing (a written contract). It may not even be necessary to require the signing of the document for it to be useful. If it appears that the employer is quite willing to do so, then it can be requested (and probably should be if the employee hopes to make any parts of it hold up in court). Otherwise simply handing a typed copy to the employer while folding his/her own copy for safekeeping may assure the employee of a binding arrangement.

Many readers may feel that this procedure is laughably unworkable, that there is little reason to go to such lengths in order to record the verbal agreement, and that to attempt such an approach to the employment agreement would end in early dismissal from the job. However, health care providers have indicated that once there is a sufficient number of qualified persons available for any given practice position, the employer can become unscrupulous in the hiring and firing process and maintain an employment relationship with a health care provider only until another comes along for the position, who is willing to work for less. A survey of hygienists in the State of Michigan has indicated that at least 20% of active hygienists fear that they may lose their positions because another hygienist might work for less— particularly those just graduating from programs in dental hygiene.[2] Also, when there are large numbers of hygienists available to practice, the employer acquires a much shorter memory about raises, agreed upon benefits, and opportunity for advancement, since he/she may have little desire to ensure that the person stays in the position for an extensive period.

Job security and an awareness of professional rights in the employment situation are relatively new in the field of dentistry— largely because of the nature of the practice of dentistry. Dentistry is housed largely in solo practice settings with little or no relationship with each other. Each practice setting is an entity unto itself, and each employs a limited number of persons or auxiliaries. For this reason, the employing dentist has been able to operate with little external control in paying employees and in upholding verbal agreements.

Other health care providers are often housed in large practice settings, such as hospitals, and are a part of a system that may use contracts routinely in specifying salary amounts, benefits, and conditions of terminating the employment agreement. This procedure simply may be practiced for administrative record keeping of employee data and job descriptions. Other times it is because the employees within that large facility have unionized and through a collective bargaining process have been able to help formulate policy that governs the amounts of salary each category of employee is eligible for and that delineates the fringe benefits and working conditions for each category of employee.

COLLECTIVE BARGAINING

Collective bargaining refers to the process representatives of the union and the employer utilize to formulate and agree upon policy and procedure with regard to the employment of union personnel. The federal law provides employees with the right to vote to unionize and to be recognized by the employer as a force that represents the interests of the employees. Unionization allows many small voices to be banded together to form one strong voice. If the employer does not wish to accommodate the demands of the union, the employees can take a strong action, such as striking, or take other actions such as work cutbacks or refusal to perform certain procedures until the employer decides to bargain more "equitably." The employer, when confronted with outrageous demands, can simply let the employees strike, which of course closes down operations but also places the employees in a salaryless position until a settlement is reached. It can become a long-term standoff as has happened many times in industry.

Industry was the birthplace of unionization, prompted by the abuses workers suffered during the Industrial Revolution when outrageous working conditions and very low salaries characterized the plight of the factory worker.[3] Strong unions developed, which

drove up salaries and benefits and caused working conditions to improve significantly.[3] They also caused prices to rise since the corporations had to pay for the increased salaries and the better conditions. Money for higher wages was rarely extracted from corporate profits; rather it was taken from the consumer in the form of higher prices. So in many ways, the persons working in the factories who achieved the new benefits paid for those same benefits when they purchased the goods and services made with their own efforts. Some economists blame the inflationary spiral in this country on the increased costs to business caused by the demands of the unions. Others blame the corporations for not permitting a more equitable distribution of the wealth by absorbing some of the cost of certain employment benefits.

With industrial workers and later various service persons earning higher and higher wages, the professional people, including teachers and nurses, began to examine collective bargaining as a way of increasing the benefits they were receiving. It was incredible to them that unskilled workers often were earning more than they, when nurses and teachers were required to have professional training and college degrees. The National Education Association and the American Nurses Association examined the role of collective bargaining in professional groups and opted to support such efforts. Special units affiliated with the state constituents of those associations provide union opportunities for groups of professionals who vote to be represented in collective bargaining.

It is possible to belong to the professional association without being represented in a collective bargaining setting. The association's separate union unit provides and promotes this opportunity for its interested and desiring members.

When a group of employees decides to unionize, they must file a formal petition and the state labor relations board will conduct an election, at which time the employees cast their ballots in favor of either unionization or remaining nonunionized. Sometimes the election will provide employees with an option regarding which group will represent them. The American Federation of Teachers, for instance, is a union of teachers competing with the National Education Association's constituents. Those voting to unionize may cast their ballots for affiliation with one or the other group.

Usually the employer will vigorously oppose the unionization movement, citing how such a move will reduce the quality of employer/employee relations and increase the cost to the employee because of union dues. The employer attempts to demonstrate how well the employees have been taken care of in the past and to show that unionization will not improve the quality of their benefits or their working conditions. Those persons striving for unionization counter those statements with statistics showing how salary levels have not achieved the levels they should and how certain persons have not been fairly dealt with in the evaluation process or in the termination of the employment agreement.

If the employees vote in favor of a union, they elect officers and, for purposes of employment contracts, become an adversary of the employer. It is infrequent that the collective bargaining sessions have been warm, sharing, pleasant encounters. Usually they take on all the characteristics of an outright fight. The union pushes for everything it can win, and the employer fights to retain every cent and every right he could offer the employee. It becomes a game in many instances but may degenerate into all-night sessions, strikes, professional people resorting to emotional name-calling, and a general breakdown in trust.

It *can* result in higher salaries, better fringe benefits and working conditions, more clearly defined evaluation mechanisms, and a grievance procedure to protect the rights of workers in unfair severance of employment.

UNIONIZATION AND DENTISTRY

The newspapers are filled with the tales of collective bargaining breakdowns each Fall as teachers prepare to return to classes—but only with a contract negotiated by the union. Occasionally there will be reports of nurses or other allied health personnel who have cut back services at a hospital over the lack of a contract or because of the unwillingness of the employer-hospital to bargain in "good faith." Unions have been voted in for police, firefighters, and practically every other category of worker.

But unionization has not affected dentistry—largely because it is such a fragmented cottage industry. The only way it could be introduced would be to unionize in *affiliation with* but technically separate from the constituent structure of the American Dental Hygienists Association and the American Dental Assistants Association. By law professional associations may not themselves carry on union activities.[2] Collective bargaining would have to become a statewide or at least component activity, with personnel appearing for work only if bargaining continues in good faith and if ultimately a contract is prepared, which is mutually agreeable to both parties. It would demand full participation—a problem since not all employed hygienists and assistants are members of the professional association and may choose to abandon the idea of collective bargaining.

Another difficulty lies in the fact that these two professions are comprised largely of women, many of whom work part-time and may feel little inclination to survive the perils of collective bargaining. Despite the fact that they may wish to earn a reasonable wage, they may still feel that their salary is secondary in the family income. This, of course, may change as women begin to have a different perception of their roles in the family as financially responsible members who should be adequately paid for the work they perform. Another interesting quirk in the profession of dental hygiene that could affect the success of collective bargaining is that many women who are dental hygienists are married to dentists and work in their offices for no salary! The persons conducting an employment survey in Michigan found this situation to be surprisingly frequent.[2]

There has been periodic discussion among association leaders of the need to unionize in order for auxiliaries to earn respectable incomes for the vital work they perform in the provision of dental care. Efforts to work directly with dentists have not proved fruitful.

What might happen if unionization could be realized for dental auxiliaries? First of all, the labor relations board would be quite busy conducting hearings of reported instances of unfair labor practices involving the firing of persons active in the labor movement. That is prohibited by the law, but the widely distributed settings and the subsequent unlikelihood that each case could be investigated and resolved would tempt some employers to react harshly, putting many auxiliaries out of work immediately. Some might do this because they are unfamiliar with the law governing such acts.

Secondly, the adversary relationship that would be established between dentistry and the dental auxiliaries would quickly negate many of the efforts to establish interdependent programs of mutual interest and concern. Auxiliaries have been attempting to demonstrate a new assertiveness in planning their own futures and in refusing to rely upon what they see as the fatherly leadership of dentistry. This new assertiveness has in itself been met with quick, authoritarian-style rebuttals.[4] Any headway that has been made to demonstrate cooperation and a desire to work toward common goals on a common ground could be overshadowed.

Thirdly, the success of any collective bargaining activities would certainly drive up the cost of health care. There is little reason to suspect that the dentists would be willing to absorb the increased benefits' cost from their own profit. The cost will be passed on to the consumer, as it has been in most other industries.

Dental auxiliary professional associations will probably be faced with the decision to unionize—regardless of whether it is a local union or a national movement. The costs and the benefits will have to be measured carefully before such a decision could be made.

The costs of unionization will be high, if collective bargaining is to be successful. Dues assessed each participating member must be sufficient to cover the cost of employing collective bargaining agents—ones who fully understand the needs of the client and who are successful at winning important benefits. When collective bargaining requires 10 hours each week for 2 months, the hourly cost of such an agent (often $50 or more) can amount to a great deal.

Dental auxiliaries may acquire a great deal of practice in decision-making if this issue surfaces soon. It may well be a key issue in the decade ahead.

Recently unionization has been a topic of interest among professionals such as dentists and physicians. However, the reasons are not poor working conditions or low salary. The "cause" of this trend toward unionization is related to dentists' (in particular) opposition to third-party payment trends, which they believe are disrupting and even destroying the dentist-patient relationship. The unions have been formed to provide a mechanism for "negotiating with the organizations that provide dental insurance to the public, discussing items such as fee schedules, uniform claim forms, and rules concerning practice procedures and the dentist-patient relationship."[1]

Physicians' unions are interested in hospital control issues as well as third-party payment policies.[1]

With this new breed of union developing, the provisions of the 1935 National Labor Relations Act are difficult to apply. Most dentists are self-employed and have little claim to the purpose and regulations included in NLRA regulation of employee-employer relationships. It is possible that the strength of the "union" despite its not being covered by the NLRA may make it a viable force in "collective bargaining" for professional rights—even for dentistry's cottage industry. The court decisions regarding the right of these unions to be recognized may well decide the growth of the organizations.[1]

Collective bargaining may be a force to be reckoned with in the years ahead.

Review questions

1. What is an employment contract?
2. Why is it wise to prepare a written employment contract when agreeing to an employment situation?
3. Identify five key components in an employment contract:

   a.

   b.

   c.

   d.

   e.

4. What is collective bargaining?
5. Identify two professional associations that sponsor union activities, including collective bargaining:

   a.

   b.

6. What primary difference exists between dental care delivery and other forms of health care delivery?
7. What are three costs that dental auxiliaries may suffer if they elect to implement collective bargaining?

   a.

   b.

   c.

ANSWERS

1. An employment contract is the set of terms to which the employer and employee agree with regard to role, working conditions, salary, fringe benefits, and other relevant factors. It can be verbal or written. Sometimes it is even implied.

2. A written employment contract specifies the terms agreed to and creates a more permanent record so that the terms do not change at the whim of either party and so that it is more likely the terms will be followed.

3. a. Title and basic functions to be performed
   b. Hours to be worked; days to be worked
   c. Amount of remuneration and its method of calculation
   d. Schedule or review for raises
   e. Method of review (evaluation) for raises and continued employment.

   (Others include: fringe benefits, opportunities for professional advancement, methods by which the employment contract may be severed, and specific expectations with regard to the employment situation that are not covered above.)

4. Collective bargaining is the process representatives of the union and the employer utilize to formulate and agree upon policy and procedure with regard to the employment of union personnel.

5. a. Teachers—American Federation of Teachers, National Education Association
   b. Nurses—American Nurses Association (its constituent bargaining units)

6. Dental care delivery is primarily a cottage industry with individual dentists providing care at scattered sites with few numbers of auxiliaries at each site.

7. a. Initial loss of employment
   b. Adversary relationship with dentistry
   c. High dollar cost of collective bargaining

GROUP ACTIVITIES

1. Invite a representative of a local professional union to discuss the procedures involved in collective bargaining. Request information regarding how unionization has affected salaries, fringe benefits, working conditions, and the cost of professional membership.
2. Request information of the national professional associations regarding their recommendations for employment contracts. Determine whether the association has addressed the issue and if they recommend any particular format for practitioners seeking employment.
3. Outline the procedures that are followed (in detail) in organizing a union and in beginning contract formulation through collective bargaining.
4. Analyze the power sources in the collective bargaining processes of negotiations at the table, the strike, the lock-out, and the work cutback, and other tactics. How does each power act affect the economic well-being of the employer and the employee involved in the struggle?

5. Introduce the idea of collective bargaining at a local component meeting of the dental hygiene or dental assisting professional association. Record the responses of the group with regard to the interests they see will be enhanced or undermined by such a move.
6. Simulate the formation of a union with the group, agreeing upon minimum salaries that will be accepted (upon graduation), minimum fringe benefits, and other specific employment characteristics. Analyze what could be gained by such a group agreement. Describe aloud any reasons for being reluctant to form such a group.

REFERENCES

1. Barnett, Peter: Professional unions, Insights, **9**:3.
2. Judge, Susan P. and Malvitz, Dolores M.: The survey of dental hygiene in Michigan, Dent. Hyg., **50**:463.
3. Pelling, Henry: American labor, Chicago, 1960, The University of Chicago Press.
4. Schnurr, Barbara J.: State of the Association address, Delivered at the Fifty-third Annual Session of the American Dental Hygienists Association, November, 1976.

CHAPTER 24

Insurance

OBJECTIVES: The reader will be able to:

1. Identify the basic reason for purchasing insurance coverage.
2. Explain briefly how insurance is financed.
3. Describe the reasons for and the benefits of:
   a. Malpractice insurance
   b. Health insurance
   c. Disability insurance
   d. Life insurance
   e. Retirement programs
   f. Personal liability insurance
   g. Household and other personal property insurance
4. Describe some key variables in coverage that should be assessed in the written policy when purchasing insurance.

Upon entering the world of work, career-oriented people take on a number of risks that perhaps have never existed for them before—or at least were not as obvious or as great.

The risks can include damage to other persons or their property, the loss of their own livelihood through illness or death, or the loss of personal property through natural disaster or theft. Generally the ultimate loss associated with the risks is money. The purpose of insurance is to have some assurance that money will be available to cover the costs of the "risks-come-true."

The insurance company reviews the relative likelihood of the disaster actually striking the person requesting insurance (based on actuarial data that provide "probabilities") and decides whether or not to insure. If the risk is too great, the insurer may decide to refuse insurance. If the probability is relatively high that the carrier may need to pay out against a claim but remote enough (according to their calculations) to insure, the

company (or *carrier*) may grant insurance but charge a high premium.

A *premium* is the amount of money a person pays to purchase insurance. It may be paid monthly, quarterly, yearly, or at some other interval depending upon the arrangement made with the carrier. The premium paid varies with the amount of coverage purchased and with the degree of likelihood the carrier will have to pay a claim.

For instance, in the case of malpractice insurance, if a dental hygienist requests $100,000 coverage (the maximum amount the carrier would need to pay if he/she were to lose a malpractice suit with damages of $100,000 or more to be paid the plaintiff), the premium payment will be higher than for $50,000 coverage. The insurance company may charge a higher premium of a dental hygienist working in an area where malpractice suits are frequently filed against such health care providers, since the risk may be higher. The carrier may refuse to insure a provider who has already been sued, or worse yet, who has lost a suit, because the risk is considered too great.

Explained in simplest terms, the carrier and person to be insured are, in a sense, making a bet with each other.[6] The carrier has predicted statistically that disaster will not strike and that the company will be able to collect premiums for an extended period of time without paying out to the insured person. The insured concludes that the risk is significant enough that he/she ought to be protected from having to pay large amounts of money if disaster strikes. Insurance companies advertise their services on the basis of "needed protection" and hope to attract large numbers of premium payers who will not need to file claims. To be successful they must collect enough premiums to more than offset payouts on claims.[6] Insurance companies also build buffers against the cost of payout against claims by investing a portion of collected premiums so that the dollars earn money for the company.

MALPRACTICE INSURANCE

As mentioned previously, one type of insurance that should be considered by professionals is malpractice insurance. Purchase of malpractice insurance protects the person against financial loss from a successful negligence or technical assault suit or, with certain limitations, against a charge of breach of contract. Costs that may be covered are damages paid to the plaintiff, court costs, and attorney fees. The policy offered by the insurance company should be evaluated in terms of actions covered and maximum benefits in each cost category. Some policies maintained by physicians or dentists will also cover persons acting as their agents (assistants, hygienists, nurses, or other personnel), if both the employer and the agent are sued. However, it may not cover the agent who is sued separately. Or the maximum benefit allotted to the agent may be relatively low. Therefore, it is a wise precaution for allied health personnel to carry their own malpractice insurance. Usually the cost is low enough to be unprohibitive and

the charge is a deductible business expense for income tax purposes.

HEALTH INSURANCE

A second kind of insurance frequently purchased by health care providers is health insurance.[3] Health insurance protects the person against the costs of illness, usually physician's costs, hospital fees, and, sometimes, medications. The policies vary with regard to their coverage of office calls to the physician, the length of hospitalization and the daily rate that will be paid, the kinds of illness or surgical treatment, and the amount allocated to cover various procedures.[3]

A policy may have a "deductible amount," a threshold amount, which the patient pays before the insurance company begins covering costs.[3] It is an amount deductible from claims paid to the insured. For example, the policy may specify a $50 deductible amount for all physician costs. If the insurance person incurred $150 in covered expenses, the company, subtracting the deductible amount, would pay only $100. Depending upon the policy, the deductible amount might apply only once in a specified period of time (the more common arrangement) or it might be required with each new treatment. In other policies there may be a provision where a flat percentage of the cost is paid. If the policy specifies that it covers 50% of hospital costs, the patient will need to pay for the other half. The type of shared-cost arrangement is known as "co-insurance."

Another variation among policies is the kind of services for which the insured is covered. It is important to determine which health care services are covered and which are not. Some policies cover dental care and corrective eye lenses. But the premiums are high because so many people have a need for these services, which means the carrier is going to be paying out a great deal in claims. Most policies do not cover preventive services such as physical examinations or nutritional counseling.

It is wise to carefully assess the policy to

see what is being purchased with the premium cost. Policies do vary greatly.[3] The worst time to find that out is when the hospital bills are astronomical and the benefit payments are minimal.

DISABILITY INSURANCE

Closely related to health insurance is disability insurance. When a person is ill, financial burdens of getting well are compounded when the income of the person drops or stops. There may be a certain allowance by the person's employer for sick days when the usual salary continues, but it may be financially impossible for the employer to pay full salary for 2 weeks or more. So how does a hygienist with a broken wrist earn income for the 8 weeks it takes to heal? Or what if a skiing accident strains the back muscles of a nurse so that he/she must spend 4 months in traction? What if the person is disabled for life by arthritis, a brain tumor, or an accident?

Insurance carriers do offer insurance against disability. After a certain period of documented disability, the carrier begins paying regular dollar amounts to the insured. The amount for which the person is insured should be at least equal to the regular income of the person so that financial hardship is minimized. If the health insurance purchased does not cover medications or the cost of a home nurse, it might be wise to purchase a level of disability insurance that would cover these costs as well as providing the usual income level.

LIFE INSURANCE

The career person who has a family dependent upon his or her income ought to purchase life insurance. Even if no other person is specifically dependent upon the income, a person may consider purchasing insurance sufficient in amount to cover funeral costs. Such a topic is often unpleasant to consider since purchasing life insurance is an admission that the person will die. Most persons prefer to forget that fact. Young persons, in particular, readily scoff at the idea of life insurance, which is financially unfortunate. The annual life insurance premium of a 40 year old is a great deal higher than that of the 20 year old. By purchasing coverage at an early age, a person may secure the lower rate, which will remain constant throughout the entire term of the policy. Furthermore, life insurance may become less available for a particular individual as his/her age increases.

There was a time when women were rarely encouraged to purchase much insurance. Typically, a family was supported financially by a man. A woman with children and no career was lost financially if her husband died leaving no insurance or only a small amount. It was presumed that the man, already the financial provider, could carry on after the death or disability of his wife.

With women acquiring greater financial responsibility in the family, two changes should occur. The more obvious change is that the woman will begin purchasing larger amounts of insurance. The second trend is that the amounts purchased by each will be more modest, since the death of either person will not drive the family into poverty. When both earn a reasonable salary, the continued income from the remaining partner can feed and clothe the family even if one partner dies. The risks remains, however, that both partners could die, leaving children with bare essentials and little aid for educational costs if little or no insurance is provided. The orphaned toddler will require a great deal of money to survive before reaching adulthood, and the charity level of the extended family should not be relied upon to provide it. The wisest route is to assess the financial needs of the greatest disaster that could strike and plan reasonable insurance coverage on that basis.

There are several types of life insurance that can be purchased. Some plans permit money to return to the insured at retirement. Others simply pay benefits at the time of death.[3] The type the person purchases should be based on the individual's financial plans and his/her short- and long-term needs. If the person plans to invest in stocks and bonds and to build a strong retirement program other than in life insurance, the minimal costs and benefits of *term insurance* may be appropriate.[3] But for a person who does not wish to invest, it may be wiser to let the insurance company make the investments and pay into a *whole life* policy or one of its limited payment period variants. Term insurance provides financial protection in the case of death. It is not a savings plan. Term insurance premiums increase with the insured's age. In the early years, premiums are lower than those incurred with whole life (also called "straight life") policies. Whole life policies provide savings (cash value) as well as protection. Premiums are usually the same from year to year, and while term insurance usually cannot be renewed beyond age 65 or 70, whole life insurance continues to provide protection regardless of age.[3]

RETIREMENT PROGRAMS

Life insurance can provide for retirement. But there are other retirement programs designed specifically to provide regular income after leaving full-time employment.[3] Pension plans can be available through the employer. Professional associations may sponsor such opportunities. While retirement may seem terribly remote to a beginning professional, its financial realities are best considered early. Social Security may provide basic retirement income, but for most people this government pension will not be sufficient to allow them to maintain a life style close to that which they enjoyed before retirement. The cost of living will likely be higher in years to come, and income should be sufficient to meet that inflation. In order for a savings plan to be minimally draining on current income and yet sufficient to pay for retirement living, the habit of allocating some income to retirement should be practiced as soon as employment begins. Long range planning is essential, especially when retirement programs are not provided or encouraged by the employer.

Many employers do provide such programs. However, accruing sufficient sums may depend upon longevity and continuity of employment. Some plans pay back lump sums of retirement savings to the employee when changing places of employment, causing considerable temptation to spend the money rather than to reinvest it. In some pension plans the employer matches some portion of the employee's investment in retirement. That portion of the savings may be lost when employment is severed for reasons other than retirement.

Some teachers have a system whereby retirement funds are basically unaffected by a change in employment positions. TIAA-CREF (Teachers Insurance and Annuity Association–College Retirement Equities Fund) is a program accepted by numerous schools and colleges. This permits continuity of the savings program when a person changes from one participating institution to another.[5] Hospitals and certain other institutional employers in the health care field have a similar program available to them, known as the National Health and Welfare Plan.

Prior to the 1960s, physicians were not able to incorporate their practices and gain for themselves—and their employees—the favorable pension benefits that business corporations can make available to their employees. In 1962, the "Self Employed Individuals Tax Retirement Act" (the Keogh Act) was passed by Congress, allowing all self-employed persons to establish a tax shelter for a limited portion of their incomes and thus to build up retirement trust funds somewhat like the corporate pension plans. The individual retirement plans authorized by the Keogh Act—often referred to by its prepassage bill number, H.R.10—were not nearly as favorable as the corporate plans, but they were a first step toward equality of treatment for physicians and their employees. To obtain the benefits of a Keogh plan, the physician is required to make contributions into the plan on behalf of all employees as well.

During the 1960s, most states amended their laws to allow physicians and other professionals to form "professional corporations," which, although not like business corporations in all respects, did allow more favorable tax treatment of pension plan contributions. Many physicians responded by incorporating their practices and setting up pension plans, thus avoiding the tight limitations of the Keogh plans.

In 1974, a new federal law, the "Employee Retirement Income Security Act" (ERISA), substantially liberalized the rules controlling H.R. 10 plans and thus made them a much more attractive vehicle for funding retirement benefits for physicians and their employees. The new rules allow the physician to make tax-deductible contributions of up to 15% of annual income to a retirement fund, with a maximum of $7500 per year. Moreover, these maximums can be exceeded if the individual is older when the retirement account is begun, in recognition of the fact that savings will have to be made at a faster rate to build the reserves to provide an adequate pension base. This fast-accumulation approach is available through what is called a "defined benefits" plan.

A physician or other individual who sets up a Keogh plan must also provide for all employees with 3 or more years of service— including auxiliaries, receptionists, and others—by contributing annually to the fund the same percentage of income which is set aside for himself. Thus, a physician earning $40,000 who sets aside 15% of his income, or $6,000, for his own retirement must also contribute an equivalent percentage of each employee's income. If the sole employee was an auxiliary paid $10,000 annually, the physician would have to contribute $1500 per year toward the auxilliary's retirement fund. The equal percentage requirement applies, however, only to the first $50,000 of the physician's taxable income; above that amount the physician may use a formula to reduce the contributions for employees below that

which a straight equivalency would require.*

Another recent change in the law allows persons not covered by a pension plan through their employers to set up their own Individual Retirement Account (IRA) and to contribute up to 15% of annual earned income, with an annual maximum of $1500. Amounts so set aside in any year are tax deductible to the individual for that year, and all interest earnings on the fund are nontaxable until the individual retires and begins to receive the retirement income. An individual may have an IRA regardless of whether his/her spouse has one or is covered by an employer's pension plan. This legislation is important for auxiliaries, since they may find themselves working in positions where no other retirement-fund mechanism is available. This would be the case, for example, where an auxiliary changes jobs frequently enough that employers are not bound to make Keogh plan contributions on her account (assuming that the employers even have Keogh plans, of course).

PERSONAL LIABILITY AND PERSONAL PROPERTY INSURANCE

There are other kinds of insurance that persons may wish to purchase regardless of their employment status. One kind is personal liability insurance; the other is household and personal property insurance. Often the two will be included in one policy. Personal liability covers a person against damages for having harmed another person or property through negligence—outside of professional activities[3] or the use of a motor vehicle. The person who falls on the snowy path left unshoveled or the person who falls in an unmarked trench in the front yard may incur harm for which the property owner must pay.

---

*For example, if the physician's income was $60,000 and he set aside 4% of that figure for his own retirement, he would have to set aside an amount equal to only 3.33% of his nurse's salary for her fund. The formula is as follows: $\frac{\$50,000}{\$60,000} \times 4\% = 3.33\%$.

Such policies may also pay for damage to the insured's house caused by fire, wind, flood, or other natural disaster. Coverage can be purchased for loss by theft. Usually a comprehensive householder's policy covers all these needs related to the home. Also, many people just entering a career do not realize how much it will cost to replace personal property if an apartment burns. A renter does not need to have insurance on the dwelling itself but will need coverage on contents. Coverage can include burglary and vandalism, but it can be very expensive in city areas where such incidents are frequent. Automobile insurance packages also may cover liability, theft, and damage related to the auto.[3] Savings can sometimes be realized by purchasing all personal liability and property insurance in one package. Once again it is important to read what is covered and under what special circumstances, what dollar limits are imposed, and whether there is a deductible or percentage of coverage clause.

PURCHASING INSURANCE

Virtually anything can be insured if the purchaser is willing to pay the premiums. The important point is to decide what risks the health care provider should or should not be willing to take in terms of potential financial loss. In the areas where a risk-come-true is devastating, it is probably wise to purchase coverage.

Some forms of insurance (malpractice, health, disability, life, and retirement) are often available through professional associations at lower premiums than would be available through individual plans. When a large group of people is purchasing insurance, the carrier can usually offer the coverage at a lower cost, because marketing costs are lower than if the company were to sell to numerous individuals. A large source of potential insured persons may lead to a large number of premiums. Professional associations take advantage of this fact and advertise package group insurance as a benefit of association membership.[1]

Insurance coverage is frequently a negotiable item for fringe benefits. It may be wise to accept insurance as a fringe benefit in place of some monetary compensation. A hardy side benefit is that tax laws may exempt the dollars spent on insurance benefits by the employer from taxation as income to the employee. Tax laws are constantly changing and should be consulted for the current applicable provisions. There may be some tax advantage for the employer. It may be wise to investigate whether such provisions could be funded and discuss them with the employer for possible implementation.

Regardless of what procedures and special packages are available, it is in the interest of a career person to establish financial security. Insurance is one way of accomplishing that.

Review questions

1. What is the basic reason for purchasing insurance?
2. How can an insurance company afford to pay the insured amount when a claim is filed?
3. List seven kinds of insurance coverage that may be purchased:
   a.
   b.
   c.
   d.
   e.
   f.
   g.
4. Describe why each of the above kinds of coverage might be a reasonable purchase for a health care provider:
   a.
   b.
   c.
   d.
   e.
   f.
   g.
5. Identify three key variables that should be kept in mind in assessing policies when purchasing insurance.
   a.
   b.
   c.

ANSWERS

1. A person entering employment assumes a variety of new or greater risks that can be financially disastrous unless there is some source of money to pay for the unexpected costs.

2. An insurance company assesses the likelihood that the need for benefit payment will occur and covers only those persons where there is a probability that a claim will not be filed or where there will be a considerable delay before a benefit will be collected. The idea is to collect more premiums than there are claims paid out. Also, the premiums collected are invested so that the dollars earn money.

3. a. Malpractice
   b. Health
   c. Disability
   d. Life
   e. Retirement
   f. Personal liability
   g. Household/personal property

4. a. A patient may win a case charging a tort or breach of contract.
   b. Hospital, physician's costs, and medications may be high if illness strikes.
   c. If the ill person cannot work, some income will be needed.
   d. The person may be leaving dependent persons without an income and with cost of the funeral.
   e. To continue living, there will have to be some income after retirement.
   f. A person harmed by the insured's negligence will need damages covered.
   g. An apartment or house and its contents may be destroyed and need replacement.

5. a. Amount of coverage
   b. Special exempting clauses
   c. Deductible or percentage clauses

GROUP ACTIVITIES

1. Invite an insurance representative to discuss various insurance programs, including the options available in policies, how claims are paid and how premiums are determined.
2. Define personal needs for insurance and compare several policies that could provide coverage. Select the policy that best meets the stated needs.
3. Compare regular individual commercial coverage and rates for insurance with comparable coverage and rates available through a professional organization package.

REFERENCES

1. American Dental Hygienists Association: Publicity releases concerning available insurance programs for members, 1976.
2. Concise Explanation of Pension Reform Law, Employment Retirement Income Security Act of 1974 (ERISA), Englewood Cliffs, N.J., 1974, Prentice-Hall, Inc.
3. Denenberg, Herbert S.: Getting your money's worth: Guidelines about insurance policies, health protection, pensions and professional services, Washington, D.C., 1974, Public Affairs Press.
4. Kalish, Arthur and Lewis, Patricia G.: Professional corporations revisited (after the Employee Retirement Income Security Act of 1974), Tax Lawyer, **28:**471.
5. Kramer, Henry T.: What about pensions?, Nurs. Clin. North Am., **9:**513.
6. Sarner, Harvey: The proper use of insurance, Pennsylvania Dent. J., **44:**28.

PART VII

PLANNING FOR GREATER RESPONSIBILITY FOR DIRECT PATIENT CARE DENTAL AUXILIARIES

There is no single solution to the problems of improving health care. The answer or at least the point of change, will probably result from a confluence of solutions. As incremental changes fit together, perhaps the larger picture of a logical system of care that measurably improves the health of the people will form.

The forces that have been identified in the early portions of this text encompass the primary sources of influence on change. The educational system, credentialing agencies, the state and federal governments, professional organizations, and groups of associations, such as the American Society of Allied Health Professions, will all help shape whatever stasis or change health care delivery realizes in the years ahead.

Primary to those forces is the concept of professional responsibility, which, in its various interpretations, defines what each professional holds onto and works toward when grappling with the problems of providing better care to more people in a more patient-centered system. Professional responsibility has been cited as the reason for not fully utilizing available auxiliaries. It has been identified as the reason for spending a year or more providing care in a remote rural area despite the attractions of the metropolitan areas, so that people who usually have no access to care may have the services available to them. Likewise it has been cited as the stimulus for improved patterns of individual practice and as the reason for closing down experimental programs.

Whatever value system underlies a person's "professional responsibility," it probably is the single greatest source of influence in the move toward or against change.

CHAPTER 25

Leadership development

OBJECTIVES: The reader will be able to:

1. Describe the key characteristics of leadership.
2. Identify how the socialization process and life experiences mold leadership skills and how this process may have affected leadership development in dental auxiliaries.
3. Describe each of the six stages of problem solving.
4. List the five steps involved in problem formulation.
5. Describe and give examples of decision-making that occurs by means of:
   a. Lack of response
   b. Authority rule
   c. Minority rule
   d. Majority rule
   e. Consensus
   f. Unanimous consent
6. Reconstruct the continuum of leadership behavior.
7. Contrast leadership with authoritarian directiveness.
8. Discuss the impact leadership and authoritarion directiveness have on the development of leadership skills within followers.
9. Identify the sources of leadership that have typically been acknowledged as the guidance system of the dental auxiliary professions.
10. Use ten measures of group maturity to assess professional organizations' state of development and growth.
11. Develop inquiry and decision-making skills in analyzing key issues confronting the profession with regard to health care delivery patterns.

LEADERSHIP CHARACTERISTICS

The research related to leadership traits and patterns continues to show that personal characteristics are very closely related to a person's ability to function as an effective leader.* Leaders seem to emerge rather than to have learned the skills in any predictable or definable manner. Leadership behaviors are probably learned (or extinguished) throughout life, based on a reward pattern and society's expectations. Persons who have been expected to have little leadership behavior may have been able to stifle any such natural tendencies.

Leaders are often characterized as intelligent, enthusiastic, dominant (especially in establishing a position of leadership), self-confident, socially participatory and egalitarian.[5] These lifelong or early developed traits breed the leaders that emerge in primary childrens' groups, in high school social groups, in college and business world groups, in the family, and in other groups of people. A person who is able to develop those traits early in life and then to use them continues to be the leader. The person who possesses many of those traits but who is punished for displaying those talents may find leadership less of a ready position in later life.

*See references 1, 3, 5, 8, 23, 27.

The research, not reflective of recent changes in women's assertiveness, shows that women are generally *responsive* in groups rather than *initiative* of activity. This is particularly true in mixed groups of men and women. *Men direct* the activity; *women respond* to others' ideas and play a largely social-emotional role.[21,22,24] Once again, the fact that most dental auxiliaries are women may be a significant factor in the current and future status of the group. While some people may still believe that women naturally are not good leaders, there is reason to believe that the dearth of leadership or managerial skills among women in years past was the result of the effectiveness with which society taught young women to hide their leadership capabilities and to play a more reticent role in groups.[17] Intelligent, articulate women held back their contributions or were viewed as masculine by the other group members. The threat of being a masculine woman was often sufficiently awful (especially in an era when women's primary role was seen by many as attracting men and competing with other women in that sphere) that the source of most leadership in important decision making was men.[17]

More recent literature seems to substantiate that most peoples' expectations are that women will contribute to groups in this reticent manner. Women who have managed to develop leadership skills and who attempt to initiate change or activity in groups of men have great difficulty being accepted as leaders. Ideas they represent are rarely acted upon in a positive manner until miraculously one of the male members presents this "new" idea. The amazed women often find that the other males in the group do not even recognize the topic or suggestion as having been raised earlier.[22]

If the professional woman who is an educational and functional peer of the men with whom she interacts in groups has difficulty establishing equality of input and leadership, imagine what the element of the very title "auxiliary" must have in discrediting the input of women in allied dental health roles in attempting to shape change and participate in groups of dentists (usually males). Because auxiliaries play supportive, "helping" roles in the employment aspect of the dentist-auxiliary relationship, it is difficult to adopt a more equal ground in peer relationships such as exist between two professional organizations (one representing dentists and the other representing a dental auxiliary group) or between two faculty members (one who is a dentist and the other a dental auxiliary) of equal rank.[5a,6,10,20]

For women who have served in leadership positions in the American Dental Hygienists Association and in the American Dental Assistants Association, the rejection or discounting process has been felt more than once in encounters with dental organizations.

It is an instance of role confusion and role discrimination in which an auxiliary's ideas and abilities to project the future and suggest change are judged less than worthy because of the person's professional preparation (auxiliary level) and usual role function (helper), regardless of the person's advanced degrees or administrative responsibilities and experiences beyond the worker, auxiliary level. The male dentist is responding to a *woman* (expected to be responding and facilitating) who is an *auxiliary* (created and trained to follow directions and to help).[5a]

Perhaps for these reasons, a good many auxiliaries' attempts to work with dentists on state boards of dentistry and through dental associations have been minimally productive. Group process research does seem to substantiate that thesis.

The problem is even more severe for the auxiliaries, however, when it is recognized that large numbers of auxiliaries do not see themselves as leaders or initiators of change. Many individual dental hygienists and assistants may see themselves as properly in the role of responder and in the role of facilitating social-emotional relationships.

Once again the literature shows that

women have been socialized to respond largely in the "child" state and in the "parent" state (in the terminology of transactional analysis) in nurturing and succoring tendencies. The woman has learned to react with love, anger, jealousy, and fear very well—generally expressive of emotions and responding to others' similar emotions. Likewise she has learned to care for the needs of others. With these attributes typically belonging to the "properly socialized" woman, there is little doubt that a role calling for those kinds of responses will seem natural—particularly if the role of "adult" has been minimally developed or even repressed by the social expectations of men and other women.

The male dentist who wishes to be surrounded by short-skirted "pretty" auxiliaries to whom he refers as "his girls" may be just what the eager-to-please female ordered. Those women's libbers who challenge the appropriateness of the pat on the head (or elsewhere) attitude are often highly resented *by the auxiliaries* as threatening their source of strokes and security. An organization of "girls" with such needs and with such limitations will hardly muster sufficient leadership to be able to work with dentistry on a local, state, or national level. When the organization is fortunate enough to have intelligent, articulate, "adult" women move to the top, the response of the dentists in peer roles in their own organization is understandable. They are baffled by what they see. The assertive role does not fit their expectations.

The assertiveness of the woman may be labeled "aggressiveness" and "impertinence." Challenges may be viewed as lack of cooperation. Confrontation may be so uncomfortable as to be avoided; meetings may be cancelled or structured so as to minimize meaningful interaction. Auxiliary persistence to have points of disagreement addressed may be labeled as useless haggling.

It is unfortunate in terms of the goals of providing meaningful, well-designed systems of health care delivery and of developing a team approach to care delivery that the roles

in which society has cast many women and the roles dentistry created for its co-workers are so antithetical to the development of a cooperative, egalitarian group.

PROBLEM SOLVING

Involvement of many points of view and perspectives can have a significant positive impact on the ultimate decisions and actions a group generates, as it is involved in the problem-solving process.[5,8,12] Problem solving that involves a functioning, task-oriented group is more likely to be accurate in its data gathering, its problem formulation, and the appropriateness of its plans for action and their ultimate evaluation. Health care providers' mutual problem is the confrontation with present and imminent change and with the massive changes that may occur in the decades ahead. How it deals with the challenge of change can be a very revealing vignette of the maturity of their professional groups in decision making and in leadership.

Problem solving can be described in terms of two phases of activity with a total of six stages.[18] The first phase is characterized by problem formulation (defining the nature of the difficulty), the generating of solutions that could be applied to the resolution of the problem, and the "forecasting of the consequence of solutions proposed."[18] The second phase is marked by planning for appropriate activity, carrying out the activity, and evaluating the outcomes of the activity, often with a reinitiation of the problem-solving cycle.[18] (See Fig. 25-1.)

A large measure of failure on the part of groups to effectively solve problems lies in the groups' failure to adequately define what the problems are. They may be initiating an action program aimed at a nonexistent problem or at the symptom of a problem rather than the problem itself. A case in point is a professional organization's refusal to work with consumer groups to design an improved system for access to health care. The consumer group and its activism may be viewed as "the problem" when indeed the poor access to health care is the real problem. The

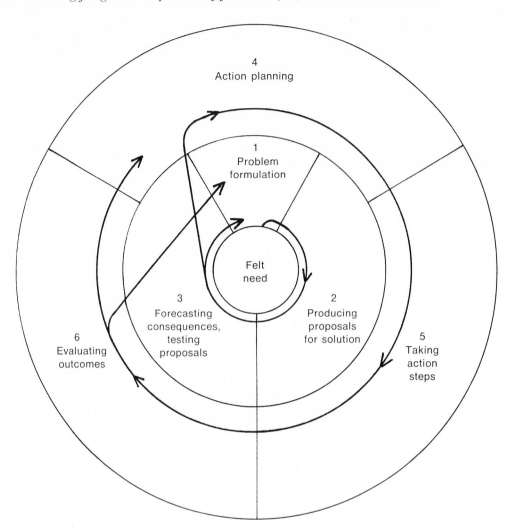

Fig. 25-1. The problem-solving cycle. (Schein, Edgar H.: Process consultation; its role in organization development, Reading, Mass., 1969, Addison-Wesley Publishing Co., Inc.)

organization may better rid itself of the consumer thorn under the belt by solving the actual problem than by denying its obligation to cooperate with interested laypersons.

What steps are involved in problem formulation that can better ensure that the "real" difficulty is identified? One suggested process is shown in Fig. 25-2. The first step is to clearly describe the feelings and frustration and tension that seem to identify that some problems exist. The next step is to identify and describe specific incidents or occurrences that have stimulated those feelings of

uneasiness, anger, fear or whatever were described. "By carefully going over these incidents in detail and trying to identify what was going on which actually triggered the frustration, it is often possible to define the real problem. The essential step is to examine the concrete incidents and to generalize the problem from these."[18]

Basic styles of group decision making

When the problem has been adequately defined in terms of the frustrations it has generated and the incidents that have caused

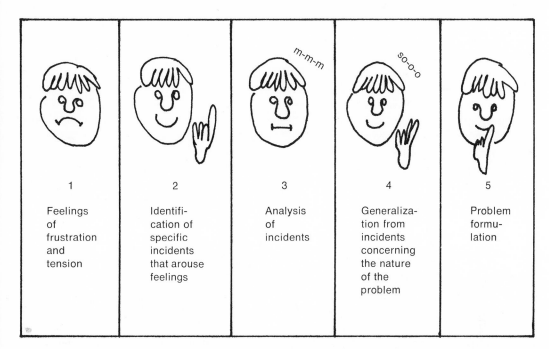

1	2	3	4	5
Feelings of frustration and tension	Identification of specific incidents that arouse feelings	Analysis of incidents	Generalization from incidents concerning the nature of the problem	Problem formulation

Fig. 25-2. Problem formulation process. (Schein, Edgar H.: Process consultation; its role in organization development, Reading, Mass., 1969, Addison-Wesley Publishing Co., Inc.)

frustration to emerge, it is possible to move toward the proposal of solutions. The crucial factor is that adequate data must be gathered and careful analysis must be used to attempt to make sense of the available data and to determine whether more is needed in order to clearly define the problem.

The maximum amount of data can be gathered if all group members are involved in its identification and in bringing it to the group's attention. Likewise the analysis and the formulation of the problem, along with the formulation of possible consequences of solutions and the initiation and assessment of activity, benefit most from total group input.

It is at this point that the degree of group involvement deserves careful analysis as it relates to leadership style and group development. The six basic styles of group decision making are highly descriptive of the leadership style and the group maturity.[18] The first is the "plop" style or the decision by *lack of response*. In this method, members may pre-

sent various ideas or solutions that are not discussed. They are passed over by the group as new ideas are introduced, or they are met with total silence, eventually broken by a member whose comments do not relate to the "plopped" idea. The group in this case is making a decision without discussing the idea introduced. The second method is decision making by *authority rule*. The leader introduces the problem, the solution, and the action for the group to discuss, but it is clear that the leader will make the final decision after having heard discussion (and not necessarily in keeping with the direction of the discussion that has taken place). It is a highly efficient, time-saving, method for decision making, but it often lacks the commitment or the full understanding of the group for the implementation of the decisions, which makes the process highly inefficient in its action phases.[18]

The third approach to decision making is *decision by minority*, when a small sub-group of the "decision-making" group has decided ahead of time how the plan should be formulated and effected. The rest of the group may feel that their input is merely a polite allowance for the sharing of opinions and that the ultimate decisions are railroaded through. The leader of the group may ask for input, and if there is no immediate response, he/she moves on to the next point with a comment that summarizes the group's "obvious" support for the concept. The difficulties of implementation are as common to minority rule decision making as they are to authority rule decision making.[18]

Majority rule, the fourth style, should generate additional support for implementation, but it often does little better than previously described styles. Despite the fact that a larger portion of the group supports the plan than that part which does not, decisions made by the vote, especially a split vote, may not earn the full support of the group because the minority group is concentrating more on how to "win" the next vote (battle). The voting process divides the group into camps. The competitive nature of the losers may rise to the fore, especially if that group feels their input was insufficient to really impact the decision-making process and if their general feeling is that they were misunderstood and discounted in the discussion process (shades of the dental team?). So while the major health care provider organizations use a highly efficient majority-rule parliamentary process for decision making, the position statements and programs that result from such a style may not receive full implementation or support.[18]

Citing evidence of the inefficiencies of the majority rule and other styles of leadership in terms of implementation and ultimate success of programs, the backers of the *consensus-seeking* decision-making process offer their approach. The group members are able to openly and completely describe their concerns, to question the components of a problem or of the plan, and to have sufficient input that outcomes of the session reflect the efforts of the groups' members. If the discussion and feedback process is sufficiently open and honest, the group members may feel that the ultimate decisions (while not completely in keeping with their own preferences) do reflect group input and at least are understood by all members of the group. The frustration level of the group members is low, and the resultant implementation of the group plan is good. The time span in discussion may be a small price to pay for the effectiveness with which plans are carried out.[18]

A step further down the road involves *unanimous* group decisions. The issues are hammered out until all members of the group agree upon the plan. The degree of support and success of implementation may be the highest with this method (if the members care to even think about the issues for one moment longer), but the costs of time in discussion and in generating frustration in the agreement process are great. The actual implementation of plans may be delayed for long periods of time (even past the time when action is meaningful), and the ultimate plan may be little better than the one that was fully understood months earlier but about which a few members still had reservations.[18]

Styles of leadership

The art of leadership is to guide the group through the decision-making process so that all members are able to participate openly, so that as decisions or points of agreement develop within the group they are identified and summarized, and so that the group can move ahead with its discussion through the phases of problem formulation and solution identification and implementation. The good leader is a facilitator, a manager of the decision-making process.[5,18] Fig. 25-3 shows the continuum of managerial styles ranging from the authoritarian to subordinate-centered leadership.[25]

It is important to recognize that leadership and authoritarianism are not synonymous. Authoritarian leaders are seen as self-oriented, being "rather hostile persons with a driving need to be in the center of the

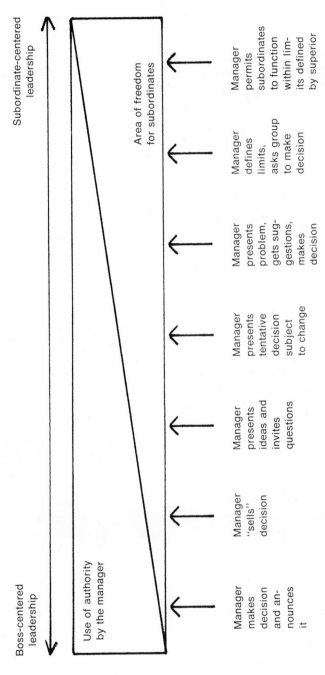

Fig. 25-3. A continuum of leadership behavior. (Tannenbaum, R., and Schmidt, W. H.: How to choose a leadership pattern, Harv. Bus. Rev. **36:**95, 1958.)

group's activities,"[5] whereas the egalitarian is viewed as group-oriented, being "able to reduce tension in a group, work toward a group goal, and take a follower role when it is appropriate."[5] An appropriate exercise in understanding this contrast is to apply these definitions to the director of an educational program, to the leader of the dental team, and then to the teacher in the classroom. They can also be applied to the health care provider in relation to the patient seeking care. Who makes the decisions? Is it the director, the dentist in the team, the teacher, or the health care provider in planning care for the patient? Applying the descriptions of the relative costs of time and ultimate implementation of plans, how could authoritarian leadership in any of these positions affect the ultimate outcome?

LEADERSHIP THROUGH EDUCATION

The next question is, "What kind of educational program would generate egalitarian leadership patterns in the students?" Is it possible that the authoritarian role model creates authoritarian health care providers who view patients as objects *to* whom they provide care, rather than as persons *for* whom they provide care? Turning again to communications research, it is possible to identify the two groups that would be most likely to be compatible with authoritarian leadership, which perhaps also defines those persons most likely to be "successful" in the program directed by an authoritarian. The submissive person, who requires little controlling behavior toward others and likewise submits readily to strong control from others, is one type of person who is able to work in spite of authoritarian leaders. The other type of person is the authoritarian who readily submits to strong external control and who likewise assumes a controlling position when in a position defined as powerful. The democratic person who has a balance of controlling behaviors (able to assume leadership when it is needed) and submitting behaviors (able to recede into the group as other contribute

their strengths) and the anarchic person (who neither controls nor is controlled) do not develop well under the authoritarian leader. It is difficult for the democratic or the anarchic personality to tolerate submitting to the authoritarian who dictates what will be learned, how well it will be learned, how each hour of the day will be spent, and who enforces the mandates with fear arousal.[5,8] Is it possible that there are numerous program dropouts who had these leadership styles and who left the program because of the incompatibility of needs and expectations?

The students who sit quietly in their seats taking copious notes during hour after hour of lecture learn to hear what is said, write it down, and then rewrite it on tests. Such students have little opportunity to engage in knock-down-drag-out inquiry regarding the validity of time-honored beliefs, the appropriateness of certain conclusions, or the importance of certain facts. They have little time to create anything. They have little, if any, reward for original thought in the form of challenge and search and discovery learning. Students who watch faculty monitored by an authoritarian, or dominating, director may have little opportunity to discover any other form of managerial style.

Such training in school prepares the person for more external direction after graduation, perhaps handily supplied by the employer. It would be interesting to note how many national and state leaders in professional auxiliary associations were labeled troublemakers in the schools where they learned the didactic and technical aspects but showed little aptitude for the authoritarian mode. Perhaps some gained strength from having survived the system, where to disagree or challenge openly on an adult-to-adult level may have been considered impertinent or at least annoying behavior. Perhaps others who had the strength to disagree, but insufficient political skills to protect their survival, are now in other fields because they did not have the opportunity or the fortitude to exist within the system.

Are there schools of dental hygiene and

individual faculty members whose leadership modes were sufficiently democratic and open that others were able to develop their own style of cooperative leadership and go on to association leadership? Each reader should be able to plot a point on the axes in Fig. 25-4 that represents the control behavior of the faculty person who has most influenced him or her in developing a leadership style.

Some readers may have a classic authoritarian with the point plotted in the upper right quadrant, but most likely there is some mixture of behavior that could cause the axes to be decorated with the control patterns of the faculty who have taught in dental hygiene programs. Hopefully, many fall near the intersection, at the democratic point.

The key points to be made are that students learn leadership styles from their role models and that various leadership styles attract or dissuade students to or from continuation in the program. What students learn in educational programs and the leadership/follower styles that are likely to survive in the educational system define what resources the profession will have in organizational leadership.

EVALUATING GROUP MATURITY

The source of leadership for dental auxiliaries was long considered to be in dentistry, largely by transferring the dentist-auxiliary practice relationship of the work environment to other relationships, such as those affecting the educational, credentialing, and economic realities of auxiliary practice. For years, dentists were believed to be the most qualified to direct auxiliary programs, evaluate clinical competence, and assess the economic impact of auxiliaries on practice productivity. This attitude is easily generalized to the process of defining the future. Who should be involved? Should dentistry lead the way, with auxiliaries following or "helping"?

Is it reasonable to expect that dentistry would be able and inclined to protect the interests of the auxiliaries to a greater extent than the organized auxiliaries themselves?[19] At what point is the "protection" element destructive rather than supportive? Perhaps that point is best identified when dentists move to open the law to permit the performance of numerous direct patient services by any person the individual dentist determines to be competent, or when they hope to revise the law to no longer require educa-

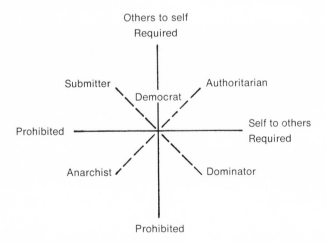

Fig. 25-4. A paradigm for role analysis in the control area. (Hare, A. Paul: Handbook of small group research, New York, 1962, The Free Press.)

1. Adequate mechanisms for getting feedback:

Poor feedback   1   2   3   4   5   Excellent feedback
  mechanisms   mechanisms

2. Adequate decision-making procedure:

Poor decision-   1   2   3   4   5   Very adequate
  making   decision-making
  procedure   procedure

3. Optimal cohesion:

Low   1   2   3   4   5   Optimal cohesion
  cohesion

4. Flexible organization and procedures:

Very   1   2   3   4   5   Very flexible
  inflexible

5. Maximum use of member resources:

Poor use   1   2   3   4   5   Excellent use
  of resources   of resources

6. Clear communications:

Poor   1   2   3   4   5   Excellent
  communications   communications

7. Clear goals accepted by members:

Unclear goals--   1   2   3   4   5   Very clear goals--
  not accepted   accepted

8. Feelings of interdependence with authority persons:

No interde-   1   2   3   4   5   High interdependence   pendence

9. Shared participation in leadership functions:

No shared   1   2   3   4   5   High shared
  participation   participation

10. Acceptance of minority views and persons:

No acceptance   1   2   3   4   5   High acceptance

Fig. 25-5. Criteria of group maturity. (Schein, Edgar H.: Process consultation; its role in organization development, Reading, Mass., 1969, Addison-Wesley Publishing Co., Inc.)

tional preparation or a standardized credentialing process. Perhaps it occurs when an entirely new breed of auxiliary is introduced to provide care, despite the already available, educationed personnel who possess the needed skills or could be easily upgraded to perform advanced skills.[10]

The literature of the late sixties and seventies is particularly revealing of the desire of some dentists to see dental hygiene, in particular, decide to set its own course and to become more assertive in assuming the role of the direct patient care auxiliary in expanded roles.[4,7,26] And certainly there has been considerable stimulus at least recently from within the auxiliary professions to become assertive. The editorials in the journals and the president's messages, as well as the series of leadership workshops sponsored by the ADHA Boards of Trustees in the mid-seventies, point out how the leaders of the national and state organizations have promoted self-direction and leadership development among the ranks.* Workshops on managerial skills, decision making, and defining roles and goals have been sponsored to improve the skill of the leaders and members.

However, until the individual auxiliary educators and practitioners have fully developed skills in these areas, the progress toward a true team integration in dentistry will be slow, if existent. The auxiliaries need to acquire these skills. And dentistry's leaders need to see auxiliaries continuously not

---

*See references 2, 9, 11, 13-16, 19, 26.

fitting the mold that dentistry's (males') prejudices have created. The group development of auxiliary members should continue to progress toward a maturity that will enable well analyzed, appropriate decisions and plans to be carried through according to the defined needs of the group.

Schein suggests a series of criteria for measuring group maturity.[18] (See Fig. 25-5.) The questionnaire is based upon criteria that can be applied to individual development/maturity. They are:

1. Does the group have the capacity to deal realistically with its environment to an optimal degree?
2. Is there a basic agreement within the group about ultimate goals and values?
3. Is there in the group a capacity for self-knowledge? Does the group understand why it does what it does?
4. Is there an optimal use of the resources available to the group?
5. Does the group have the capacity to learn from its experiences? Can it assimilate new information and respond flexibly to it?
6. Is there an integration of the group's internal processes—communication, decision making, distribution of authority and influence, and norms?[18]

Development of these attributes is not usually enhanced by "professional" meetings that feature fashion shows and sewing circle activities. They can be developed through sessions that focus on current issues impacting health care delivery and, as a result, the profession.

Review questions

1. Describe briefly why it is possible that decision-making skills and leadership development are hampered in auxiliary groups because the large percentage of the membership is women.
2. Explain the likely frustration a woman with leadership skills may feel when in a meeting with men who have a typical perceptive set of the woman's input to the meeting.
3. How are leadership and authoritarian directiveness different?
4. How does authoritarian directiveness affect leadership skill development in followers?

ANSWERS

1. Communications research has shown that the roles women play in group process are largely those of responding to others' ideas and of facilitating social-emotional communication. This may be the result of the socialization process women have endured, which rewards their behavior when it follows this expected pattern and punishes behavior that is "masculine" in nature, such as initiating ideas, prompting decision making, and initiating activity. Auxiliaries are usually women. Their group process may therefore be hampered by this socializing process, if few leaders are available as a result of the socialization.

2. Men have been shown to expect responding behaviors and social-emotional behaviors rather than valuable input from women. Women who do offer input often find that their contributions are ignored until some other member amazingly raises the idea. The group often does not even recall that the woman introduced the idea earlier in the group meeting.

3. Leadership implies facilitating group effectiveness, with feedback of consensus as it develops and allowing group resources to be used maximally to develop group decisions. Authoritarian directiveness connotes one person making the decisions with the group discussing the issues and decisions more as a rubber-stamp exercise than as a procedure that will have any predictable impact on the ultimate decisions and their implementation. The former method is group-centered; the latter method is leader-centered.

4. Authoritarian directiveness is most compatible with submissive followers and with mutually authoritarian followers, both of whom demonstrate a need to be led when not in a power position. The authoritarian follower is able to assume a strong directive, controlling position when in power. The submissive is unable to perform in such a position. In either case, the follower learns the style of directiveness and learns to obey it and to replicate it as the need arises (at least in the case of the authoritarian personality). Democratic persons may have less opportunity to develop leadership skills in this environment.

GROUP ACTIVITIES

1. Practice problem formulation, solution identification, projection of likely outcomes, and methods of implementing action for each of the following key issues that may confront (or have confronted) organized health care providers:

   a. A new auxiliary has been proposed by the federal government, which is defined as providing nearly the same skills as one of the currently existing auxiliaries.

   b. The law is to be changed to permit a less formally educated person to perform certain services that currently are performed only by licensed personnel with high levels of educational preparation.

   c. Two auxiliary associations are considering amalgamating into one for purposes of legislative strength, consolidation of resources in management and communications, and in an effort to jointly solve the manpower muddle of "which auxiliary will perform what services."

   d. The law in one licensing jurisdiction is being changed to eliminate formal educational requirements from the preparation of certain personnel for licensure as direct patient care providers.

   e. The local dental society agrees to pay no more than $30 per day to the licensed auxiliaries in the office and begins lowering salaries of the health care providers so that all practice settings are in conformance.

2. Observe an executive board meeting in which there are many men and one woman member. Tally the number of contributions the woman makes, the number that initiate an idea or activity, the number that are in response to an idea or an activity, and the number that "plop."

3. Review the presidents' messages in the American Dental Hygienists Association and the American Dental Assistants Association official publications for the indicators of the stages of professional maturity within the organizations over the last 10 years.

4. Videotape a class or meeting to assess the level of maturity in decision making that the group exhibits. Apply the scale of group maturity identified in Fig. 25-5.

5. Evaluate a class or meeting to determine the leadership style used by the elected officers in achieving group agreement.

6. Design a script that depicts each of the six styles of group decision making. Role play each of the scripts for the entire class. (The class can be divided into six equal parts to develop and dramatize each of the six scripts.) Discuss what each type "costs" in terms of time spent in the decision-making process and ultimate implementation of decisions.

7. Discuss how the "dominator" in Fig. 25-4 could cope with a democratic leader, an authoritarian leader, or a submissive leader.

REFERENCES

1. Cattell, R. B. and Stice, G. F.: Four formulae for selecting leaders on the basis of personality, Hum. Relat., **7**:493.
2. Cavicchio, Patricia Monahan: Building a future into dental auxiliary careers: An attempt to meet population needs, Presented at the Third International Symposium on Dental Hygiene, 1972.
3. Chevaleva-Ianovskaia, E. and Sylla, D.: A study of leaders among children, J. Psychol., **26**:604.
4. Dummett, Clifton: The role of the dental hygienist in community dentistry, Dent. Hyg., **50**:24.
5. Hare, A. Paul: Handbook of small group research, New York, 1962, The Free Press.
5a. Ehrenreich, Barbara: The status of women as health care providers in the United States. In Proceedings of the International Conference on Women in Health, Washington, D.C., June 16-18, 1975.
6. Hein, John W.: Dental hygiene USA—New duties and responsibilities, unpublished paper.
7. Hillenbrand, Harold: Prospect for tomorrow: dental hygiene, J. Am. Dent. Hyg. Assoc., **45**:12.
8. Luft, Joseph: Group processes: An introduction to group dynamics, ed. 2, Palo Alto, California, 1970. Mayfield Publishing Co.
9. Luke, Donna J.: Letter to the editor, J. Am. Dent. Hyg. Assoc., **45**:14.
10. Luke, Donna J.: President's message: Reach out beyond the operatory! Dent. Hyg., **50**:490.
11. Luke, Donna J.: Someday, somebody, Dent. Hyg. Newsbriefs, October, 1976.
12. McCain, Diane F.: Toward proliferation in the allied oral health professions, J. Am. Dent. Hyg. Assoc., **45**:349.
13. Motley, Wilma: Generation gap, J. Am. Dent. Hyg. Assoc., **44**:16.
14. Motley, Wilma: Misoneism, Dent. Hyg., **47**:10.
15. Nantz, Irene: Dental hygiene's changing self-concept, J. Am. Dent. Hyg. Assoc., **45**:373.
16. Reynolds, Barbara: Development and continuity, Bull. Mich. Dent. Hyg. Assoc., **6**:3.
17. Sargent, Alice G.: Fourth world issues and beyond, Supervisor Nurse, **4**:16.
18. Schein, Edgar: Process consultation; Its role in organization development, Reading, Mass., 1969, Addison-Wesley Publishing Co., Inc.

19. Schnurr, Barbara J.: State of the association address. Delivered at the Fifty-third Annual Session of the American Dental Hygienists Association, November 13, 1976.

20. Schwerin, Ursula: The maturation crisis of a profession, Dent. Hyg., 48:145.

21. South, E. B.: Some psychological aspects of committee work, J. Appl. Psychol., 11:348.

22. Steege, Michele McGann: Women in medicine and dentistry, Health Affairs, 2, Spring/Summer 1976.

23. Stogdill, R. M.: Personal factors associated with leadership: a survey of the literature, J. Psychol., 25:35.

24. Strodtbeck, F. L. and Mann, R. D.: Sex role differentiation in jury deliberations, Sociometry, 29:3.

25. Tannenbaum, R. and Schmidt, W. H.: How to choose a leadership pattern, Harv. Bus. Rev., 36:95.

26. Woodall, Irene: Dental hygiene tomorrow too . . . If we take the opportunity, Dent. Hyg., 47:94.

27. Zeleny, L. D.: Characteristics of group leaders, Sociology Soc. Res., 24:140.

CHAPTER 26

Projections for assuming greater responsibility in health care delivery

OBJECTIVES: The reader will be able to:

1. Identify the key issues confronting health care providers and the public in developing a health care system that meets the needs of the public and draws upon the available resources.
2. Summarize how these key issues affect the auxiliary health care providers' role in the health care delivery system.
3. List the ways in which the individual health care provider can contribute to the development and success of the health care system.
4. Identify those projects that organizations of health care providers can undertake to enhance the development and success of the health care system.
5. Project what the nature of the future health care delivery system may be.

The discussions included in the previous chapters of this text have provided explanations of many of the problems, trends, and issues related to the provision of care. The discussions have addressed the development and direction of contemporary systems; the roadblocks of stereotyped roles and limited self-concept; the limitations imposed by state laws and "customary" approaches to health care services; the roles of professional associations, the consumer, the government; ethical, legal, and practice management implications in providing care; and the role auxiliary health care providers can have in expanding their scope of practice, creating a more favorable practice environment, and assuming a more creative and progressive approach to their careers and the care they provide. From all of these discussions there arise four key issues of which all the other topics are subsets.

KEY ISSUES FOR HEALTH CARE PROVIDERS

Those four key issues are the *cost* of health care, *access* to health care, *quality* of health care, and the manner in which *manpower* is used to meet the need/demand of the people.

There should be little need to further discuss the actual *cost* of health care. Someone must pay for the costs of rent, supplies, utilities, equipment, salaries, and other ever-present financial realities. Health care is never free. The primary issue is *who* is to pay for care and *what mechanism* should be employed in its payment.[4] Should dental health care (in particular) remain on a fee-for-service plan, or should it continue its trend toward third-party payment systems where insurance groups, the government, or other agencies administer the financing of health care, as in the case in most medical care? How can costs be reduced? And will a concerted plan to reduce health care costs point toward an equalization of income among health care providers?

If care is funded, will it be *accessible* to the people who need it most?[4] Will care be available in the inner city and on the farm as well as in the suburbs? Will people needing care be able to obtain an appointment with relative ease and minimal red tape? Will the hours during which care is provided be compatible with the hours the people can visit the facility? Will there be programs for homebound patients and for persons needing transportation? Access to health care must be assessed in terms of the resources and special problems each community has rather than in terms of how an outsider perceives the community's special situation. Even with the logistical roadblocks to care removed, there will remain the sociological problems that will continue to cause care to be denied to certain elements of the community because of the provider's prejudices. Resolving this problem may require the greatest effort of all.

Quality is the third major issue.[4] If care is paid for and accessible, it is still of little use unless it is of high quality. A system for ensuring quality care, which is reasonable to implement in a practice environment and which answers to the consumer as well as to peers, must be operable before quality can be assured. A system for prescribing and providing continuing education for providers who need to improve their skills will have to exist in order to make the evaluation system meaningful.[2]

The fourth issue, which arose as a focal point for debate in the early 1960s, is the *manpower* issue. The statistics showing that insufficient numbers of dentists and physicians existed to meet the rising demand for services have been cited again and again,[9] ignored by many and frequently challenged by the skeptics as misleading. The government and private foundations funded numerous programs and projects to evaluate what functions could be performed by auxiliaries and to teach auxiliaries to perform those services.[3,6,7] For the most part those educated auxiliaries have been confronted by unchanging legal constraints, by employers unwilling to utilize such auxiliaries, and by the trend to utilize on-the-job trained auxiliaries for expanded roles rather than the formally educated, credentialed person.[6] Educational institu-

tions have been enjoined to stop teaching controversial expanded functions. The research data demonstrating the effectiveness with which auxiliaries can provide care and the costs that can be saved have been greatly ignored.

Out of all these issues emerge the conflicts between provider and consumer, provider and government, consumer and government, and among the various health care providers. They should provide the brewing kettle for a new system, which hopefully will evolve from the debates of the day.

The forces of the consumer, dissatisfied with high cost, inaccessibility, and poor quality of care, will demand a new system.[6,12] And if government responds to those dissatisfactions, legislation supporting new systems may prompt their development. Professional organizations, can contribute to those revisions through systems of practice management, credentialing, peer review,[8] and continuing education designed to increase productivity and improve quality.

How these issues of alternative delivery systems are eventually resolved will, of course, greatly affect the people needing care. The resolutions can also have a staggering effect upon the individual health care provider. Defenders of the current process by which people receive care are careful to point out that projections for manpower requirements are often based on people's *need* for care rather than on the number of persons who actively *seek* care. The "low dental IQ" of the masses of people who have dental problems that are not being prevented or treated is cited as the reason "need' is unlikely to become "demand." They argue that even with accessible, fully funded care, the masses will resist care out of ignorance. With this basic premise established, they conclude that the manpower shortage scare is unfounded.

One fact that they fail to recognize is that even among patients who actively seek and receive dental care, health levels are not enviable. Persons who visit their dentist regularly often require a periodontist to attempt to rectify the years of supervised neglect that has resulted in extensive periodontal damage. Regular seekers of care often still lose their teeth.

Missing entirely from most discussions of need versus demand is the premise that health care providers have an obligation to create demand for care by stimulating people to recognize their need to have oral health and the care that can help the patient achieve it. Missing, also, is the ultimate goal that might be appropriate guide all discussions of health manpower: The efforts of health manpower should indeed have a strong impact on the health levels of people who *are not* seeking care.

Complacency with the amount and levels of care provided could result in fewer programs to teach physicians and dentists to function effectively with allied health personnel and subsequently in fewer allied health programs as employment levels of support personnel drop, federal financial support diminishes, and applications from potential students dwindle.

Despite the fact that many dentists and physicians who have realized the cost benefit of direct patient care allied health personnel will probably continue to employ and efficiently utilize such persons, the trend of the early 1970s could reverse, with the late 1980s resembling the late 1950s in terms of manpower, and subsequently cost and access.

However, if the public and selected groups of health care providers continue to believe that an obligation is owed to provide care to all people in order to raise national health levels to the optimum, funding will continue to rise to promote auxiliary utilization programs, to educate auxiliary personnel, and to provide readily available, quality care. The role of the auxiliary will be more vital, more appreciated, and more gratifying.

It should be apparent that the level of social consciousness of the public, the government, and regulating agencies will be a determining factor in the growth and development of auxiliary personnel and that the role of the auxiliary will be a major contribution toward achieving optimal health for the people of the nation.[3,12]

CONTRIBUTIONS OF AUXILIARIES TO HEALTH CARE SYSTEMS

There are many ways in which the individual health care provider can impact the effectiveness of the health care delivery system. A primary way is through adopting a professional view of his/her career. If it is viewed as a lifetime career, it is likely that many of the complaints regarding the longevity of auxiliaries in practice will no longer be applicable. If the goal of employment and practice is seen as raising health levels and if care is evaluated in those terms, then greater respect should be accorded to auxiliaries. It is important to shed the stigma of being procedure-oriented, time-conscious, dollar-directed "workers" with little stake in the overall productivity, achievements, and philosophy of the practice setting. It is important for the auxiliary to "join" the team and become a full member.[1]

An auxiliary can contribute a great deal by genuinely caring about the ultimate outcomes of the practice and by actively participating in its definition, implementation, and evaluation. To accomplish this, the auxiliary will need an extra ounce of drive, commitment, and maturity to participate in decision making and problem solving. Once the auxiliary is viewed as a person with a genuine interest in the practice, he/she may be able to contribute special expertise in prevention programming, patient relations, and the management of time and motion to the overall development of the practice setting. The contributions may be more readily accepted once the vested interest is more apparent.

A second contribution is to adopt an attitude toward the delivery of care, which focuses on the well-being of the patient and on the prevention of disease and the maintenance of health. While this may sound a bit platitudinous, it is relatively easy, particularly in certain sectors of health care, to be distracted by the monetary return the delivery of services can provide. When a practice structure is centered around the comfort and well-being of the provider rather than the comfort and well-being of the patient, the delivery of care (the actual delivery of services) does less to minimize the problems of cost, access, and quality assurance the people seeking care face.

Perhaps a less obvious role that can be taken by the individual health care provider lies in the person's self-concept development. Among auxiliary personnel who typically work under the direction of a physician or dentist, the idea of role delineation and esteem-building needs to be more fully addressed. Can the auxiliary be a part of the decision-making process with valid input? Should women providers begin to shed the title "girl" and accept a full scope of professional responsibility as women? Can the individual health care provider *facilitate* the formation of the team?

CONTRIBUTIONS OF ORGANIZATIONS TO HEALTH CARE SYSTEMS

Another way in which an auxiliary can contribute to the health care delivery system is by supporting an organization of providers whose goals and objectives *and programs* reflect a strong interest in improving health care rather than in merely perpetuating the profession.[9] A carefull assessment of the organization's position statements and ongoing programs should indicate the organization's priorities. This can usually be accomplished by reviewing the organization's publications and by attending their annual meetings. A delegate's manual will provide a handy summary of its current activity and direction.

An organization that has reasonable goals, objectives, and programs can provide an excellent forum for the identification and resolution of problems, for the mustering of strength for influencing other organizations and the government, and for self-improvement.[10] An individual may simply contribute dues and participate in local meetings or may elect to participate more actively in the organization through committee work or by holding office. Such activity can take place at the local, state, or national level, and involvement can be relatively minor or nearly a full-time commitment. Such a role should assist the group in remaining goal-oriented and in striving for greater self-reliance and greater impact on the health care delivery system.[9]

What kinds of projects should a professional association of health care providers undertake if they are to be considered active participants in the resolution of the issues of cost, access, quality assurance, and manpower?

The organization may be actively participating in assessing and improving the efficiency with which education is provided for people entering the field. If the educational process is so drawn-out and tortuous that persons are unduly delayed in their attempts to enter practice, the cost of education rises, placing a substantial burden on the public funding of those programs and on the private resources of the students. The public must wait longer for the provider to be available for practice. The organization may be actively recruiting persons into the field who are likely to remain in practice for a lifetime, thus reducing the high cost of personnel turnover and the cost of educating the replacement workforce. Its members may be actively involved in improving the efficiency of practice through improved clinical procedures, materials, staffing patterns, and through the better management of time and motion.

The organization may be actively pursuing credentialing procedures that enable providers to obtain licensure with minimal delay when moving from one jurisdiction to another. Or they may be seeking legislative change to permit practice patterns with less restrictive supervision requirements so that access to care is improved.[9]

Systems of peer review, self-assessment, continuing education and evaluation for competence may be under development or in operation. And there may be great activity in promoting a resolution to the problem of who should perform what services in providing care. Experimental models in developing health care systems may be ongoing projects of the organization. Or the members may be engaged in a consumer awareness programs to improve the public's concern for available preventive care[8] and to promote new positions for health care providers in the community.

In an organization that uses sound decision-making processes, the personal aspirations and individual goals or "agenda items" of members are tempered by the collective wisdom of the group. Each person contributes ideas, attitudes, and effort. And by means of the group process that occurs among participating members, each person is able to grow in self-awareness and in his or her world view. The professional association provides a source of camaraderie for its members, and it can be a source of intellectual and emotional stimulation.

If the provider's investigations of the nature of the association do not prove that it is a group with the best of goals and principles, it is always possible for the member to join and work for change in the association leadership.

THE FUTURE HEALTH CARE DELIVERY SYSTEM

Toward what is the organization working? For what is it preparing its membership? What "future" is it anticipating? Projections for what the future will hold vary from flat statements that dental health care delivery will be very much the same as it has been, to detailed outlines of the provision of care in a sophisticated group practice setting or in a neighborhood health center that focuses on prevention as much as on treatment.[4] The speculations are numerous and varied, but with the exception of those of the stoic traditionalists, projections do point toward groups of providers working together with auxiliary personnel well-utilized in the day-to-day operations. Some project that the groups will consist of a few general practitioners with each of the primary specialities represented.

Others say the age of the specialist will decline and that the group will consist almost entirely of generalists who are oral physicians and auxiliaries who perform routine clinical procedures and conduct the preventive program.

Some have labeled this the era of "hygienistry,"[11] since broadly educated, direct patient care auxiliaries will be able to assume most of the clinical care currently provided by most practicing dentists (amalgam and tooth colored restorations, oral prophylaxis, oral examination and chartings, radiographic survey preparation and interpretation, application of caries preventive agents, root planning, soft tissue curettage, preventive orthodontics, pain control, and disease control programs involving patient education, as well as others). The future dentist is often described as a diagnostician, a master of advanced periodontal, orthodontic, prosthetic, and endodontic procedures and as a primary link to the medical component in ensuring complete health care for each patient.

Health care is envisioned as being a fully integrated, team approach with each health care provider having a vested interest in the success of treatment and prevention. The careful role definitions of "doctor" and "auxiliary" are softened by the shared responsibility, and the sex role stereotypes have been obviated by the influx of women into dentistry and men into auxiliary roles. Salary levels have been altered to provide a share of the profits to the auxiliaries without increasing costs to the patient; auxiliaries are no longer subjected to subsistence income levels.[3a,5a]

Practice settings are located in neighborhood health centers, hospitals, penal institutions, health maintenance organizations, and in a few individual practice sites. Auxiliaries educated in providing direct patient care staff these practice sites as well as other community sites such as public and private schools, geriatric centers, centers for the mentally and physically handicapped. The auxiliaries conduct preventive programs and refer patients with complex needs to community dentists for care.

Several "clinics on wheels" carry teams of auxiliaries to remote geographical locations to provide advance screening and preventive care while in contact with the dentist by television. Patients needing advanced care are either transported to the dentist or are scheduled for a subsequent visit by the dentist "on wheels."

Care is available both on a distant mountain top and in an inner city neighborhood. Costs are in careful control by means of continuing cost-benefit analysis and management of resources. An internal and external audit mechanism in addition to a peer review system of clinical procedures ensures quality of care.[5] Consumers, third-party payors, and health care providers work together to ensure that protocols are established and followed.

The laws covering auxiliaries have been revised to permit *educated* auxiliaries to assume a more active, logistically sound role in patient care. Credentialing procedures are competency-based rather than norm-referenced, and evaluation techniques are standardized and reliable.

The educational programs for providers are related to the ultimate functions and decision-making processes the providers will need. The environment is conducive to search and discovery and is egalitarian in its treatment of students.

A system of continuing education exists where learning is measured and where continued competence and learning are related to certification or license renewal.[2]

The entire system functions without strong governmental control or support. And best of all, the health of the public improves measurably each year.

Each element of this panacea has been debated and promoted in the literature, but the United States health care system is a far cry from it. Change will come slowly if the prompts for change are scattered and incompatible. It may come more quickly if the effort is unified and if the quiet force is great enough.

Review questions

1. List the four key issues involved in health care delivery:
   a.
   b.
   c.
   d.
2. How might the resolution of these issues affect the individual health care provider (auxiliary)?
3. Identify three ways in which an individual health care provider can have impact on the health care delivery system:
   a.
   b.
   c.
4. List six key features the "ideal" health care delivery system of the future would have:
   a.
   b.
   c.
   d.
   e.
   f.

ANSWERS

1. a. Cost
   b. Access
   c. Quality assurance
   d. Manpower

2. If the nation becomes less interested in providing care where it is needed and is satisfied with providing care for those demanding it, the auxiliary utilization issue will probably fade away as fewer dentists use auxiliaries, funds supporting such programs diminish, and fewer persons find those role attractive because of low employment. If the nation's interest increases, auxiliaries should be in great demand as one solution to the need for providers of care.

3. a. By viewing auxiliary practice as a lifetime career.
   b. By developing a vested interest in health care outcomes and success of practice
   c. By reassessing his/her self-concept in decision-making
   Others: by joining a professional organization and working for goals that will improve health care delivery

4. a. Generalists, who are oral physicians, are responsible for diagnosis and complex treatment and coordination with medical care.
   b. Teams of *educated* auxiliaries to provide routine care and a full preventive program.
   c. Practice settings where the people are: neighborhood health centers, hospitals, remote locations, inner city areas.
   d. Credentialing that is criterion-referenced.
   c. Educational system that is more relevant
   f. A system of audits, peer review, and continuing education to ensure quality.
   NOTE: Add your own.

GROUP ACTIVITIES

1. Read Waldman and Schoen's article, "Hygien-istry,"[11] and Lobene's, "The role of dental auxiliaries in the future dental health care delivery system,"[6] and identify and discuss the controversial elements in both.
2. Debate the statements: "Direct patient care auxiliaries must be formally educated" and "All auxiliaries must work under the direct supervision of a dentist."
3. Review and discuss the salary survey results published in *The Dental Assistant* in July 1975.

REFERENCES

1. Adelson, Richard, Bass, Robert, and Seremetis, Stephanie: The dental hygienist—a member of the team? Dent. Hyg. Assoc., **50:**25.
2. Cosaboom, Mary E.: This greater need for continuing education, J. Am. Dent. Hyg. Assoc., **46:**267.
3. Diefenbach, Viron: The 1970's—A new era for dental auxiliaries, J. Am. Dent. Hyg. Assoc., **45:**50.
3a. Helgeson, Bee: A depressing situation, Dental Assistant, **44:**15, July.
4. Jerge, Charles R., and others: Group practice and the future of dental care, Philadelphia, 1974, Lea & Febiger.
5. Jerge, Charles R.: Summary of the medical audit procedures utilized at the Promis Clinic, Hampden Highlands, Maine, unpublished paper.
5a. Leibowitz, Teri and Cupkie, Patricia: Salary survey results, Dental Assistant, **44:**29, July.
6. Lobene, Ralph R.: The role of dental auxiliaries in the future dental health care delivery system, Dent. Hyg., **59:**359.
7. Lucaccini, Luigi F., editor: Research in the use of expanded function auxiliaries, Bethesda, Md., 1974, U.S. Department of Health, Education, and Welfare, PHS-HRA, Bureau of Health Resources Development, Division of Dentistry.
8. Motley, Wilma: Friend or foe? Dent. Hyg., **48:**194.
9. Nantz, Irene R.: Dental hygiene's changing self-concept, J. Am. Dent. Hyg. Assoc., **45:**373.
10. Schnurr, Barbara J.: President's message: Keys to progress, Dent. Hyg., **49:**494.
11. Waldman, H. Barry and Schoen, Max H.: Hygienistry, J. Am. Soc. Prev. Dent., **4:**6, 27.
12. Williams, Harrison A.: The challenge of tomorrow in dental care delivery, J. Dent. Educ., **40:**587.

CHAPTER 27

Role delineation for health care providers: present and future

OBJECTIVES: The reader will be able to:

1. Analyze the symbols traditionally associated with health care providers in various roles in terms of how they create sterotypical mind sets or expectations in the observer.
2. Assess traditional symbols regarding their impact on the flexibility and growth of the health care profession associated with those symbols.
3. Develop "objective observation skills" that enable the observer to look past traditional *symbols* to those *signs* that are justifiable in terms of what is observable.

This chapter is composed primarily of photographs of health care providers and their patients. Each shows a dental hygienist, a dental assistant, a dentist, or a student who is preparing for one of those three roles, functioning in some capacity within the scope of his/her practice. Typically, a person viewing these photographs arrives at snap conclusions about what role the provider is playing. A picture of a white-uniformed woman wearing a white cap with a lavender stripe signals "dental hygienist" to those who are familiar with the profession. Those who are not may conclude that she is a nurse. If she is in a dental office, the person may place her in the category of a dental assistant. A man providing dental care is most often labeled "dentist." A person in a lab coat, regardless of the person's sex, is often viewed to be in a position directive of or superior to the uniformed person. A care provider in street clothes may be mistaken for a patient.

The labeling is related primarily to attire (uniform, lab coat, street clothes) and secondarily to sex (males as dentists and females as support personnel). People feel less secure about labeling when the symbols are mixed, such as when a woman wears a lab coat or when a provider of care wears no symbols to distinguish him/herself as a provider of care.

Before sex role stereotypes can be broken down, they must be analyzed for their sources and for the impact they have on a profession if they continue to be used. As stated in previous chapters, most auxiliaries in dentistry are women. Most dentists are men. Because people see this so consistently, they begin to *assume* that a woman health care provider is an auxiliary and a man is the primary deliverer of care. Male nurses and hygienists and female dentists and physicians can no doubt recount numerous episodes of role confusion on the part of people encountering them for the first time. There are no doubt instances of patients reluctant to receive care from a provider who does not match their preconceived notion of what that person should be.

This includes preconceived notions regarding age, race, or other individual characteristics. A student 50 years of age in a class of dental hygienists may be mistaken for a faculty member. A faculty member 25 years of age may be mistaken for a student. Regardless of the *actual* role and skill of the person providing care, the patient may sometimes feel more comfortable in receiving care from someone whom he/she would *expect* to have the role and skill.

These expectations become more serious when a potential employer has them and when a fully qualified person is denied employment on the basis of his/her not matching those expectations. Admission to educational programs may be denied for these same reasons. Federal law has attempted to halt this kind of discrimination both in employment and admissions practices.

However, it is not possible to "legislate away" a person's prejudices and assumptions. Modification usually comes about as a result of continued bombardment by encounters with persons who do not fit the mold prejudice has created. Continued references in education to male hygienists and female dentists is one way. Employment practices that favor members of "minorities" is another way. However, this may be difficult to accomplish if the educators designing materials and the employers themselves have prejudicial approaches to role delineation. Where should or can change begin?

Perhaps the best place to begin is with whomever is willing to learn to strip away traditional symbols and focus on objective observation. This exercise involves evaluating each "encounter" with minimal reliance on preconceived notions. Instead of concluding what a person's role or function is on the basis of symbols, the person assumes as little as possible and rather investigates what the reality of the situation is. It is merely a scientific approach to role delineation. While it is obvious that any preconceived notions people have had may be reinforced by what they learn (since men and women, for the most part, do still often fall into traditional role patterns), at least the mind can begin to practice separating out fact or objective observation from assumption.

If this skill of objective observation is not developed, there is little way in which people can begin to break down their prejudices. There is little way of knowing how many decisions regarding role delineation or expansion of function have been based upon the usual sex, age, or race of the group or person rather than upon the education or skill of the person. What seems important is to separate those issues. They have clear implications regarding manpower utilization if they are left intermingled in the minds of educators, employers, providers of care, and patients.

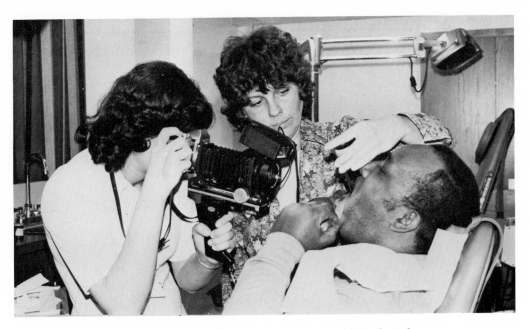

Fig. 27-1. Intraoral photography to document clinical research? Students learning to expose clinical slides? On the basis of what is observable in the photograph, what conclusions can be reached about the activity taking place and the persons involved in the activity?

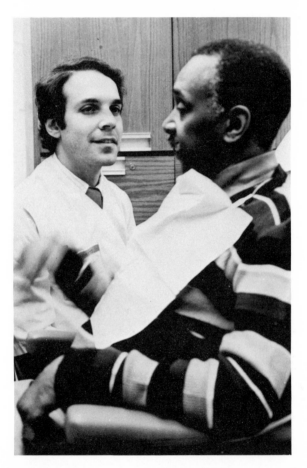

Fig. 27-2. Dental student counseling a patient? A dental hygienist recording a medical history? What symbols trigger "assumptions" or "expectations" about the person providing care?

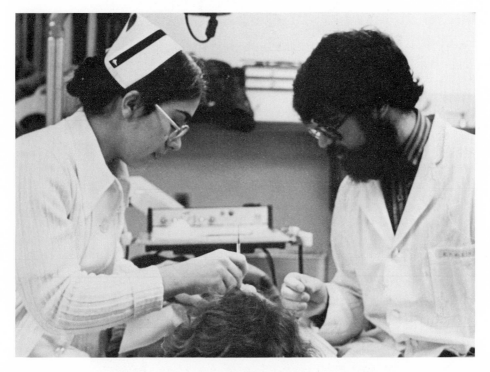

Fig. 27-3. Dentist teaching hygienist? Dental hygienist teaching dentist? Dental hygienists learning from each other? What symbols associated with the two providers of care lead one to conclude the role each is playing in the provision of care?

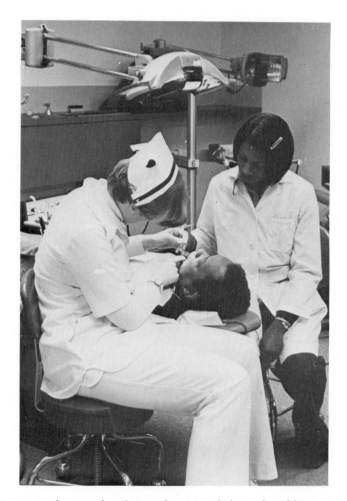

Fig. 27-4. Dentist teaching auxiliary? Dental assistant helping dental hygienist with the delivery of care? What role models do we have that cause us to "assume" the role the person is playing? How does the presence or absence of certain key symbols make differentiation difficult?

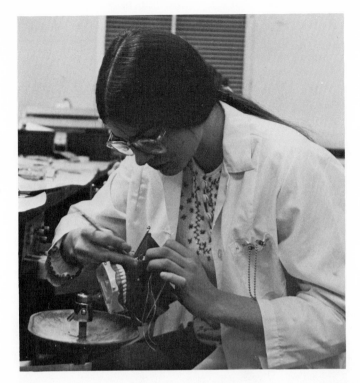

Fig. 27-5. Dental student learning restorative skills? Dental hygiene student learning restorative skills? What signs are present that confuse or clarify what the role of the person is? How does a past encounter with a typical dental student or typical dental hygiene student influence judgments regarding which people "fit" into which roles?

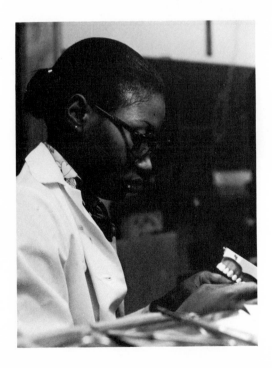

Fig. 27-6. Dental hygiene student? Dental assisting student? Dental student? Or is she a dental faculty member giving a demonstration? On the basis of objective observation of data presented in the photograph, what can be concluded about the person?

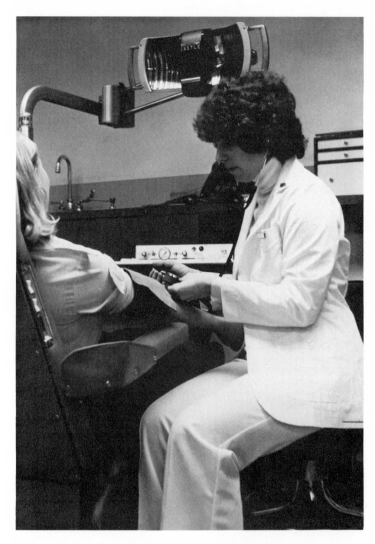

Fig. 27-7. Physician? Nurse? Dentist? Dental auxiliary? What symbols (present or absent) influence judgments regarding who this person is?

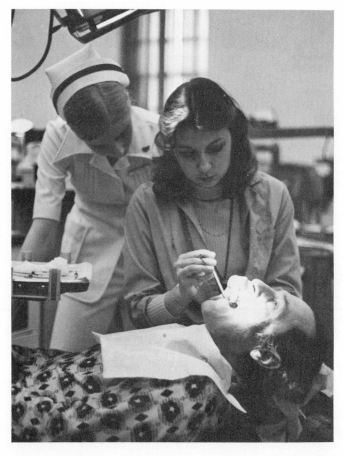

Fig. 27-8. Dental faculty member? Dental hygiene faculty member? Dental assisting student? What can be observed in the photograph to justify the conclusions drawn?

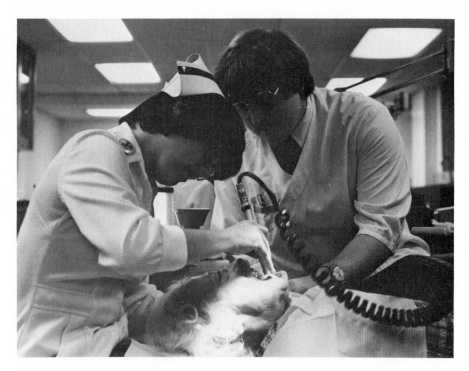

Fig. 27-9. Dental hygiene student teaching dental student? Dental hygiene student teaching dental hygienist? Auxiliary assisting dental hygienist? What assumptions are automatic in viewing this photograph? What is justifiable in terms of objective observation of data?

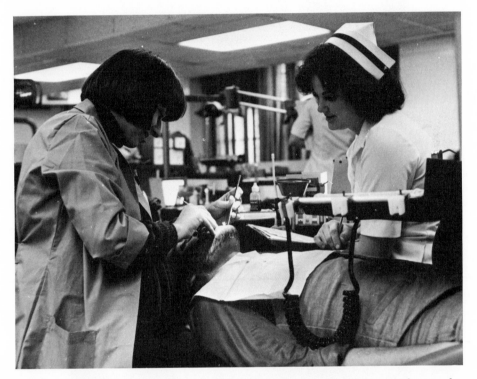

Fig. 27-10. Dental assistant observing dental hygienist? Dental faculty member teaching auxiliary student? What can be observed from the photograph that is a sign of the function of the persons shown?

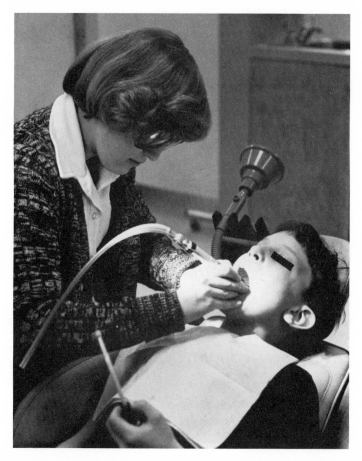

Fig. 27-11. Dental auxiliary preparing a tooth for an amalgam restoration? Dental hygienist polishing coronal surfaces of the teeth? Dentist providing pedodontic care? What observable signs cause us to form judgments regarding the function and role of the person pictured?

GROUP ACTIVITIES

1. Discuss responses to questions posed regarding each of the photos in this chapter.
2. Debate the statement, "Before dental hygienists or assistants are fully recognized as providers of care and not just support personnel for dentists, they will have to abandon their traditional symbols that are associated with subserviance."
3. Return to Chapter 1 and repeat the values clarification exercise. Discuss any changes in perceptions that are apparent in the group.

INDEX

Legislatures, state
 "denturism," 27
 state boards of dentistry, 31-32
Licensure; *see also* Certification; Credentialing
 base for expanded functions, 16
 continuing education, 56
 of dental hygiene, 13
 effects on dental care and on dental hygiene's
  growth, 13
 enforcement difficulties, 41
 institutional, defined, 42
Life insurance, 260
Light, effect of environment on practice, 152
Location, geographical, and relocation as factors in
 selecting employment, 237
Longevity of patients in practice and economy, 182
Louisville, Kentucky, 14, 30

M

Maintenance of facilities, cost of practice, 186-187
Malpractice insurance; *see* Insurance, malpractice
Management, efficient
 effect on income, 182
 styles, authoritarian and democratic contrasted, 131
 use of time and facilities, 131-137
Maryland, University of, 44
Medicare
 American Medical Association opposition, 28
 views of Joseph Califano, 53
Medicine contrasted with dentistry
 confrontation with current issues, 28
 viewed, 26
Men, leadership characteristics, 272
Midwifery, credentialing in nursing, 46
Motions, types, analyzed in time and motion study,
 143
Multi-handed dentistry, 29
Murchison, Irene, on expanded nursing practice and
 legal responsibility, 67

N

Nader, Ralph
 assault on unsafe automobile, investigations, 52-53
 investigation of x-radiation, 52
National Commission on Accrediting, completion of
 study proposed by W. K. Selden, 40-41
National Commission for Health Credentialing Agencies, Steering Committee of, certification
 recommendations, 44
National Education Association, example of collective
 bargaining, 251
National health insurance
 dental coverage possibilities, 185
 description, 184
National Health Service, Great Britain, use of hygienist and restorative therapist, 29
National Labor Relations Act of 1935, provisions, application to new breed of union, 253; *see also*
 Unionization

National League for Nursing
 accrediting role, 40
 "Patient's Bill of Rights," 117
Negligence; *see also* Law, malpractice; Law, negligence
 related to standards of competence, 83
 summarized, 90
New Cross Dental Auxiliary, 15, 29
Newman, Irene, first dental hygienist, 12
"No show" fee and patient appointment scheduling,
 138
Nonverbal behavior and expression in employment
 interview, 228, 229
North Carolina, University of, 14
Nursing; *see also* National League for Nursing
 competency assurance and expanded functions, 46
 regulation as model for dental hygiene, 46-47
Nutrition beyond prevention, 159

O

Ohio College of Dental Surgery, first educational program in dental hygiene, 13
"Open" practice acts
 advantages, 106
 and criminal offenses, 106
 effects on state boards of dentistry, 31-32
Operation motion, analyzed in time and motion study,
 143
Oral prophylaxis related to goals of dentistry, 25

P

Pacific, University of, 14
Paramedical and paraprofessional personnel, 43
Patient cooperation, legal element and effectiveness of
 care, 91-92
Patient education
 ethics, 123-124
 part of prophylaxis, 157
Patient record in fee collection, 98
Patient scheduling, contrast between physician and
 dentist, 137
"Patient's Bill of Rights," National League for Nursing,
 117
Peer review and quality of care, 26-27, 55
Penal institutions as alternative practice, 201
Pennsylvania, University of, dental hygiene periodontal
 experiments at, 16
Personal characteristics in preinterview process, 226-
 227
Personal conduct and ethical codes, 125
Placement, operator
 changes during procedures, 172-174
 relative to patient, 169-172
Planning change in employment, 239-244
Plato, contributions to ethics, 113
Policy shifts in organized dentistry, 28-29
Population growth as stimulus for change in dentistry,
 29
Posture, effect on fatigue, 169
Practice, alternative, types, 201-203